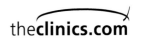

PSYCHIATRIC CLINICS OF NORTH AMERICA

Suicidal Behavior: A Developmental Perspective

GUEST EDITORS
Maria A. Oquendo, MD
J. John Mann, MD

June 2008 • Volume 31 • Number 2

SAUNDERS

An Imprint of Elsevier, Inc.
PHILADELPHIA   LONDON   TORONTO   MONTREAL   SYDNEY   TOKYO

W.B. SAUNDERS COMPANY
A Division of Elsevier Inc.

1600 John F. Kennedy Boulevard · Suite 1800 · Philadelphia, PA 19103-2899

http://www.theclinics.com

PSYCHIATRIC CLINICS OF NORTH AMERICA	**Volume 31, Number 2**
June 2008	**ISSN 0193-953X**
Editor: Sarah E. Barth	**ISBN-13: 978-1-4160-5870-0**
	ISBN-10: 1-4160-5870-2

Reprints. For copies of 100 or more, of articles in this publication, please contact the Commercial Reprints Department, Elsevier Inc., 360 Park Avenue South, New York, New York 10010-1710. Tel.: (212) 633-3813, Fax: (212) 462-1935, E-mail: reprints@elsevier.com.

The ideas and opinions expressed in *Psychiatric Clinics of North America* do not necessarily reflect those of the Publisher. The Publisher does not assume any responsibility for any injury and/or damage to persons or property arising out of or related to any use of the material contained in this periodical. The reader is advised to check the appropriate medical literature and the product information currently provided by the manufacturer of each drug to be administered, to verify the dosage, the method and duration of administration, or contraindications. It is the responsibility of the treating physician or other health care professional, relying on independent experience and knowledge of the patient, to determine drug dosages and the best treatment for the patient. Mention of any product in this issue should not be construed as endorsement by the contributors, editors, or the Publisher of the product or manufacturers' claims.

Psychiatric Clinics of North America (ISSN 0193-953X) is published quarterly by Elsevier Inc., 360 Park Avenue South, New York, NY 10010-1710. Months of issue are March, June, September, and December. Business and Editorial Offices: 1600 John F. Kennedy Blvd., Suite 1800, Philadelphia, PA 19103-2899. Customer Service Office: 6277 Sea Harbor Drive, Orlando, FL 32887-4800 Periodicals postage paid at New York, NY and additional mailing offices. Subscription prices are $213.00 per year (US individuals), $362.00 per year (US institutions), $107.00 per year (US students/residents), $255.00 per year (Canadian individuals), $440.00 per year (Canadian Institutions), $297.00 per year (foreign individuals), $440.00 per year (foreign institutions), and $149.00 per year (international & Canadian students/residents). Foreign air speed delivery is included in all *Clinics'* subscription prices. All prices are subject to change without notice. **POSTMASTER:** Send address changes to *Psychiatric Clinics of North America*, Elsevier Periodicals Customer Service, 6277 Sea Harbor Drive, Orlando, FL 32887-4800. Customer Service: 1-800-654-2452 (US). From outside of the US, call 1-407-563-6020. Fax: 1-407-363-9661. E-mail: Journals CustomerService-usa@elsevier.com.

Psychiatric Clinics of North America is covered in *MEDLINE/PubMed (Index Medicus), Current Contents/ Social and Behavioral Sciences, Social Science Citation Index, Embase/Excerpta Medica,* and PsycINFO.

Printed in the United States of America.

ELSEVIER
SAUNDERS

PSYCHIATRIC CLINICS
OF NORTH AMERICA

Suicidal Behavior: A Developmental Perspective

GUEST EDITORS

MARIA A. OQUENDO, MD, Professor of Clinical Psychiatry, Division of Molecular
Imaging and Neuropathology, New York State Psychiatric Institute and Columbia
University; Vice Chair for Education, Department of Psychiatry, Columbia
University; and Director, Clinical Evaluation Core, Silvio O. Conte Center
for the Neurobiology of Mental Disorders, Division of Molecular Imaging
and Neuropathology, New York State Psychiatric Institute, New York, New York

J. JOHN MANN, MD, The Paul Janssen Professor of Translational Neuroscience
in Psychiatry and Radiology; Vice Chair for Research; Scientific Director,
Kreitchman PET Center, Columbia University; and Chief, Division of Molecular
Imaging and Neuropathology, New York State Psychiatric Institute, New York,
New York

CONTRIBUTORS

ENRIQUE BACA-GARCIA, MD, Adjunct Assistant Professor of Psychiatry, Columbia
University, New York, New York; and Profesor Asociado, Universidad
Autonoma de Madrid; and Department of Psychiatry, Fundacion Jimenez Diaz
University Hospital, Madrid, Spain

DAVID A. BRENT, MD, Academic Chief, Child and Adolescent Psychiatry;
and Professor of Psychiatry, Pediatrics, and Epidemiology, Western Psychiatric
Institute and Clinic, University of Pittsburgh Medical Center, Pittsburgh,
Pennsylvania

JELENA BREZO, PhD, Department of Psychiatry, McGill Group for Suicide Studies,
Montreal, Québec, Canada

BETH S. BRODSKY, PhD, Assistant Clinical Professor of Medical Psychology,
Department of Psychiatry, College of Physicians & Surgeons, Columbia
University, New York, New York

THOMAS BRONISCH, MD, Professor, Max-Planck-Institute of Psychiatry, Munich,
Germany

YEATES CONWELL, MD, Professor of Psychiatry, University of Rochester School
of Medicine; and Co-Director, University of Rochester Center for the Study
and Prevention of Suicide (CSPS), Rochester, New York

DIANNE CURRIER, PhD, Staff Associate, Division of Molecular Imaging and Neuropathology, Department of Psychiatry, Columbia University, New York, New York

KANITA DERVIC, MD, Associate Professor of Child and Adolescent Psychiatry; and Consultant Child and Adolescent Neuropsychiatrist, Department of Child and Adolescent Psychiatry/University Hospital, Medical University of Vienna, Vienna, Austria

MADELYN S. GOULD, PhD, MPH, Professor, Division of Child & Adolescent Psychiatry (College of Physicians & Surgeons) and Department of Epidemiology (School of Public Health), Columbia University; and Research Scientist, New York State Psychiatric Institute, New York, New York

BEVERLY J. INSEL, DrPH, Associate Research Scientist, Division of Child & Adolescent Psychiatry (College of Physicians & Surgeons), Columbia University; and Associate Research Scientist, New York State Psychiatric Institute, New York, New York

TIM KLEMPAN, PhD, Postdoctoral Fellow, Department of Psychiatry, McGill Group for Suicide Studies, Montreal, Québec, Canada

TOMER LEVY, MD, Sackler School of Medicine, Tel Aviv University, Tel Aviv; and Geha Mental Health Center, Tel Aviv University, Petach Tiqwa, Israel

ROSELIND LIEB, PhD, Professor, Institute of Psychology, Epidemiology and Health Psychology, University of Basel, Basel, Switzerland

J. JOHN MANN, MD, The Paul Janssen Professor of Translational Neuroscience in Psychiatry and Radiology; Vice Chair for Research; Scientific Director, Kreitchman PET Center, Columbia University; and Chief, Division of Molecular Imaging and Neuropathology, New York State Psychiatric Institute, New York, New York

NADINE MELHEM, PhD, Assistant Professor of Psychiatry, Western Psychiatric Institute & Clinic, Pittsburgh, Pennsylvania

ELLENOR MITTENDORFER-RUTZ, PhD, MSc, Epidemiologist and Researcher, Swedish National Suicide Prevention and Prevention of Mental Ill-Health (NASP), Department of Public Health Sciences, Karolinska Institutet, Solna, Stockholm, Sweden

MARIA A. OQUENDO, MD, Professor of Clinical Psychiatry, Division of Molecular Imaging and Neuropathology, New York State Psychiatric Institute and Columbia University; Vice Chair for Education, Department of Psychiatry, Columbia University; and Director, Clinical Evaluation Core, Silvio O. Conte Center for the Neurobiology of Mental Disorders, Division of Molecular Imaging and Neuropathology, New York State Psychiatric Institute, New York, New York

M. MERCEDES PEREZ-RODRIGUEZ, MD, Clinical Researcher in Psychiatry, Department of Psychiatry, Ramon y Cajal University Hospital, Madrid, Spain

GAL SHOVAL, MD, Sackler School of Medicine, Tel Aviv University, Tel Aviv; and Child and Adolescent Department, Geha Mental Health Center, Tel Aviv University, Petach Tiqwa, Israel

BARBARA STANLEY, PhD, Lecturer, Department of Psychiatry, College of Physicians & Surgeons, Columbia University; and Director, Suicide Intervention Center, New York State Psychiatric Institute, New York, New York

CAITLIN THOMPSON, PhD, Senior Instructor, University of Rochester School of Medicine; and Co-Director, University of Rochester Center for the Study and Prevention of Suicide (CSPS), Rochester, New York

GUSTAVO TURECKI, MD, PhD, Associate Professor, Department of Psychiatry, McGill Group for Suicide Studies, Montreal, Québec, Canada

DANUTA WASSERMAN, MD, PhD, Professor of Psychiatry and Suicidology, Karolinska Institutet; Chair, Swedish National Suicide Prevention and Prevention of Mental Ill-Health (NASP), Karolinska Institutet; Head of the Department of Public Health Sciences, Karolinska Institutet; and Director of the WHO Lead Collaborating Centre of Mental Health Problems and Suicide Across Europe, Karolinska Institutet, Solna, Stockholm, Sweden

GIL ZALSMAN, MD, Sackler School of Medicine, Tel Aviv University, Tel Aviv; Director, Child and Adolescent Department, Geha Mental Health Center, Tel Aviv University, Petach Tiqwa, Israel; and Neuroscience Division, Columbia University, New York, New York

PSYCHIATRIC CLINICS
OF NORTH AMERICA

Suicidal Behavior: A Developmental Perspective

Adoption and twin studies show that familial transmission of suicidal behavior is partly attributable to genetic factors. Transmission of suicidal behavior is mediated by transmission of impulsive aggression or neuroticism and neurocognitive deficits. The most plausible explanations for nongenetic familial transmission are the intergenerational transmission of abuse and adverse familial environments. Bereavement and relationship disruption contribute to suicidal risk via the development of complicated grief, although long-term effects may be mediated by a complex chain of interrelated events. Imitation may contribute to suicidal risk, at least in attempted suicide. However, so-called family environmental factors often are related to risk factors that are heritable. Conversely, genetic factors exert their impact on depression and suicidal behavior via interaction with a stressful environment.

Genetic epidemiology research has shown that genes contribute to suicide risk. Unfortunately, the first 30 years of candidate-based association studies have provided little information about the specific genetic contributors. This article reviews genetic association studies of suicidal phenotypes published to date. Possible theoretical, methodological, and operational challenges accounting for the modest success of association studies in the field are also discussed. The authors conclude that future research may benefit from using a more systematic and comprehensive selection of candidate genes and variants, examining gene–environment and gene–gene interactions, and investigating higher-order moderators.

Besides the well-known risk factors for youth suicidal behavior, recent evidence suggests that risk for youth suicidal behavior can be determined even very early in life, during the prenatal and perinatal period. Low birth weight and short birth length adjusted for gestational age were found to increase the risk for suicidal behavior, particularly by violent means. Several parental factors like low parental socioeconomic status, teenage and single parenthood, multiparity and parental psychopathology, substance abuse and suicidal behavior have been linked to an increase in youth suicidal behavior. Effective collaboration among the sectors within health care and social services is crucial for early detection and adequate intervention.

A considerable number of studies linking family history and high risk for suicide have reported that suicidality runs in families. Community studies that avoid a selection effect confirm these findings. These results seem independent of comorbidities such as depression, anxiety, substance use, and personality disorders. Furthermore, the results are stable over treatment settings, different age groups, and gender. Community studies interviewing families directly (family interview method) are primarily focused on maternal suicidality and suicidality in offspring. Two studies observed some indications for suicide attempts in young offspring of mothers (and fathers) who had attempted suicide compared with offspring of mothers who had no suicidality.

Early experiences of physical and sexual abuse and parental neglect are risk factors for suicidal behavior in adolescence and adulthood. This article reviews the correlational, retrospective findings, emphasizing the more recent prospective and familial transmission studies that explore the factors mediating the relationship between childhood abuse/neglect and suicidal behavior. Related areas of research such as protective factors and the personality traits that are possible risk factors that mediate this relationship are reviewed. Research on the neurobiologic correlates of trauma that might have implications for understanding suicidal behavior is discussed, and several models for the study of the relationship between childhood adverse experiences and suicidal behavior are described.

According to the Centers for Disease Control and Prevention, suicide is the third leading cause of death in adolescence in the United States. Nonfatal forms of suicidal behavior are the most common reasons for the psychiatric hospitalization of adolescents in many countries. The risk for suicide attempt among offspring of suicide completers is multifactorial, challenging experts to develop a strategy that includes assessment and management that consider these factors. Although treatment of depression is necessary, antisuicide treatment strategies that solely target depression may not be sufficient to reduce suicidal risk. Other factors, such as impulsive aggression and parental history of sexual abuse, also contribute to suicidal risk.

Suicidal behavior is partly heritable. Studies seeking the responsible candidate genes have examined genes involved in neurotransmitter systems shown to have altered function in suicide and attempted suicide. These neurotransmitter systems include the serotonergic, noradrenergic, and dopaminergic systems and the hypothalamic-pituitary-adrenal axis. With some exceptions, most notably the serotonin transporter gene promoter polymorphism (HTTLPR), replication of candidate gene association studies findings has been difficult. This article reviews current knowledge of specific gene effects and gene–environment interactions that influence risk for suicidal behavior. Effects of childhood stress on development and how it influences adult responses to current stress are shown to be relevant for mood disorders, aggressive/impulsive traits, and suicidal behavior.

Suicide in children and young adolescents up to 14 years of age has increased in many countries, warranting research and clinical awareness. International reported suicide rates per 100,000 in this young population vary between 3.1 and 0 (mean rate worldwide, approximately 0.6/100.000; male–female ratio, 2:1). Suicide occurs only in vulnerable children; this vulnerability begins with parental mood disorder and impulsive aggression, and family history of suicide. Childhood affective and disruptive disorders and abuse are the most often reported psychiatric risk factors. Suicide becomes increasingly common after puberty, most probably because of pubertal onset of depression and substance abuse, which substantially aggravate suicide risk. Biologic findings are scarce; however, serotonergic dysfunction is assumed. The most common precipitants are school and family problems and may include actual/anticipated transitions in these environments. Suicides in children and young adolescents up to 14 years of age often follow a brief period of stress. Cognitive immaturity/misjudgment, age-related impulsivity, and availability of suicide methods play an important role. Psychologic autopsy studies that focus on suicides in this age group are needed.

The evidence to date suggests that suicide modeling is a real phenomenon, although of a smaller effect size than other psychiatric and psychosocial risk factors for adolescent suicide. Multiple lines of inquiry provide converging evidence, including studies on suicide clusters, media influence on suicide (particularly coverage of nonfictional suicides), and peer influence on suicidality. Despite variations in study setting and methodology, the body of literature is consistent with a modeling hypothesis. Although advances in documentation of suicide modeling have been made over the past decade, we are still confronted by unresolved issues regarding the underlying mechanisms. Prevention and postvention strategies can be optimized to avert modeling of suicidal behavior only once research addresses the complexities and uncertainties of this phenomenon.

This article provides an update on suicidal behaviors in young women. The rates of completed suicide and suicide attempts among young women are reviewed, and the impact of race and ethnicity on these rates is described. The risk and protective factors associated with suicidal behaviors in young women are discussed, including stressful life events, mental disorders, and hormonal factors. Finally, some considerations for treating suicidal young women are included.

Suicide is a major public health concern for older adults, who have higher rates of completed suicide than any other age group in most countries of the world. Older men are at greatest risk. Reduction of suicide-related morbidity and mortality in this age group hinges on systematic study at each point in the suicide preventive intervention research cycle. Improvements in systems for surveillance of late-life suicidal behavior, particularly attempted suicide, are needed to further develop the foundation on which to evaluate differences in the elderly subgroup, over time, and in different locations, and to better assess changes in response to interventions. This article provides an overview of suicide in later life and a foundation on which to base decisions about the design and implementation of preventive interventions.

PSYCHIATRIC CLINICS
OF NORTH AMERICA

Psychiatr Clin N Am 31 (2008) xiii–xvi

PSYCHIATRIC CLINICS
OF NORTH AMERICA

Suicidal Behavior: A Developmental Perspective

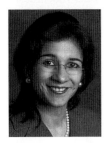 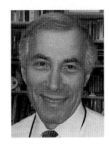

Maria A. Oquendo, MD
J. John Mann, MD

Guest Editors

I t has long been known that suicidal behavior varies strikingly across the life span. One example is the ratio of nonfatal to fatal suicide attempts, which goes from about 20:1 in youth to 4:1 in the elderly. In this issue, we have asked leading investigators in suicidology to produce a set of critical reviews of the scientific literature on suicidal behavior across the lifespan. This issue gives the reader a bird's eye view of the field with special emphasis on unanswered research questions that are relevant for clinical care. The issue is organized to cover different spectra of risk at major developmental stages: familial effects on suicidal behavior; the effect of early childhood experiences on later suicidal risk; phenomenology of child and adolescent suicidal behavior; and suicidal behavior in adulthood focused on two higher risk groups, nonfatal attempts in young women and suicide in elders.

FAMILIAL EFFECTS ON SUICIDAL BEHAVIOR

Because improved understanding of the mechanisms, such as heritability, involved in familial transmission of suicidal behavior can shed light on etiology, identify high-risk individuals, and frame targets for intervention and prevention, the article by Brent and Melhem presents the evidence supporting the familial transmission of suicidal behavior. The authors identify possible genetic and environmental explanations for this phenomenon. They describe putative intermediate phenotypes and discuss the contributions of early child-rearing and concurrent familial environmental stressors to suicidal risk.

Brezo, Klempan, and Turecki, in "The Genetics of Suicide: A Critical Review of Molecular Studies," provide an in-depth review of genetic association

0193-953X/08/$ – see front matter
doi:10.1016/j.psc.2008.03.001

studies of suicidal phenotypes, accompanied by a thoughtful discussion of possible theoretic and methodologic challenges that may explain the limited success of association studies thus far. As a potential solution, they propose more systematic and comprehensive studies of genes and variants, examination of gene–environment and gene–gene interactions, and investigation of higher-order moderators.

In "Pregnancies in High Psychosocial Risk Groups: Research Findings and Implications for Early Intervention," Mittendorfer-Rutz and Wasserman describe prenatal and perinatal period effects that may affect the risk for suicide in youth and adults. Low weight and short length at birth, adjusted for gestational age, seem to increase risk for suicidal behavior, and particularly violent suicide attempts. The authors suggest that associations between pre- and perinatal complications and subsequent suicidal acts could be mediated by neurodevelopmental impairment and by modifications in programming of neuroendocrine systems. Early intervention for low birth weight infants, preterm birth infants, or infants born and raised in families at high psychosocial risk may mitigate future suicide risk, indicating the relative importance of the pre- and perinatal environment.

Bronisch and Lieb examine another perspective in their article "Maternal Suicidality and Suicide Risk in Offspring." Age at first suicide attempt of offspring of parents (mothers and fathers) who have attempted suicide is on average younger than the parents' age of first suicide attempt and younger than onset of suicidal behavior in offspring of parents who do not have suicidality. Understanding this phenomenon can help understand causes of suicidal behavior and guide the timing and target of prevention. Together, these four articles provide evidence for the heritability of suicidal behavior from the perspective of genetics, pre- and perinatal environmental effects, and parental psychopathologic antecedents to suicidal behavior.

THE EFFECT OF EARLY EXPERIENCES ON LATER SUICIDAL RISK

In "Adverse Childhood Experiences and Suicidal Behavior" Brodsky and Stanley review factors mediating the relationship between suicidal behavior and childhood abuse/neglect. In describing (1) those personality traits that may be risk factors mediating this relationship, (2) protective factors, and (3) neurobiologic abnormalities, they describe the chain of events leading from childhood abuse or neglect to suicidal acts.

Zalsman, Levy, and Shoval describe the key observation that in pediatric populations, not all suicidal ideation or behavior is directly attributable to depression in their article, "Interaction of Child and Family Psychopathology Leading to Suicidal Behavior." A major survey found 12-month prevalences among high school students nationwide as follows: 28.6% felt sad or hopeless almost every day for at least 2 weeks in a row so that they stopped doing some of their usual activities, 16.9% of the students had seriously considered attempting suicide, 16.5% of students had planned a suicide attempt, 8.5% of students had actually attempted suicide one or more times, and 2.9% of students nationwide had made a suicide attempt requiring medical care. These high rates suggest the need for acute attention for these high-risk children.

"Stress, Genes, and the Biology of Suicidal Behavior," by Currier and Mann, reviews the genetic underpinnings of suicidal behavior. Genetic studies have mainly focused on genes involved in candidate neurotransmitter systems reported to be altered in completed and attempted suicide, including the serotonergic, noradrenergic and dopaminergic systems and the hypothalamic-pituitary-adrenal (HPA) axis. For the most part, replication of candidate gene association studies has been unsuccessful, with the notable exception of the serotonin transporter promotor HTTLPR polymorphism. In a review of specific gene effects and gene–environment interactions and their influence risk on suicidal behavior, the authors note that developmental effects of childhood stress and their influence on adult responses to current stress are clearly relevant not only for mood disorders but also for the development of aggressive/impulsive traits and later suicidal behavior.

CHILD AND ADOLESCENT SUICIDAL BEHAVIOR

Dervic, Brent, and Oquendo describe, in "Completed Suicide in Childhood," the alarming trend for more suicides in children aged 14 and younger. Childhood mood and disruptive disorders and childhood abuse are the most commonly reported psychiatric risk factors. Suicide becomes increasingly common after puberty, likely because of new onset of mood disorders and substance abuse, increasing suicide risk. Common precipitants include school and family problems and actual or anticipated transitions in these environments. Sadly, suicides in children may follow only a brief period of stress, creating a challenge for prevention. Cognitive immaturity, lack of judgment, impulsivity, and method availability may play a pivotal role.

As adolescents grow, other factors come into play. In "Impact of Modeling on Adolescent Suicidal Behavior," Insel and Gould note the mounting evidence for a role for imitation and modeling in completed suicide. The evidence emerges from three areas of research: (1) clusters of suicide occurring in temporal-spatial proximity, (2) individual exposure to the suicidal behavior of teen peers, and (3) media effects on subsequent suicidal behavior. A more complete picture of risk in young people requires consideration of family psychopathology and environmental effects, including contagion.

SUICIDAL BEHAVIOR IN ADULTHOOD

In "Suicidal Behavior in Young Women," Baca-Garcia, Perez-Rodriguez, Mann, and Oquendo provide an update on suicidal behaviors in young women. Young women are the demographic group with the highest risk for nonfatal suicide attempts. Rates of completed and attempted suicide among young females are presented with a special emphasis on the impact of race and ethnicity on these rates. Risk and protective factors are associated with suicidal behaviors in young females, including stressful life events, mental disorders, and hormonal factors and the treatment options for suicidal young females.

Conwell and Thompson describe the disturbing rates of suicide among older adults compared with other age groups in "Suicidal Behavior in Elders." They provide a foundation for decision making concerning design and implementation of preventive interventions. Risk and protective factors suggest potential pathogenic mechanisms and indicate the need for efficient methods to reach older adults at risk. With this information those interventions can be designed and preliminary testing conducted for their refinement before implementation at a larger scale. They emphasize the usefulness of effective surveillance tools to evaluate the impact of interventions in guiding the next steps for improvement. Nonetheless, the special challenges of suicide prevention among older adults remain considerable because of social isolation and assumptions that depression and nihilism are "understandable" in late life.

This issue strives to present a comprehensive review and incisive synthesis of the data regarding suicidal behavior across the lifespan.

Maria A. Oquendo, MD
Columbia University
NYSPI Unit #42
1051 Riverside Drive
New York, NY 10032

E-mail address: mao4@columbia.edu

J. John Mann, MD
New York State Psychiatric Institute
and Columbia University
NYSPI Unit #42
1051 Riverside Drive
New York, NY 10032

E-mail address: jjm@columbia.edu

Psychiatr Clin N Am 31 (2008) 157–177

PSYCHIATRIC CLINICS
OF NORTH AMERICA

Familial Transmission of Suicidal Behavior

David A. Brent, MD*, Nadine Melhem, PhD

Western Psychiatric Institute & Clinic, 3811 O'Hara Street, Pittsburgh, PA 15213, USA

Suicide and suicidal behavior is highly familial, and appears to be familially transmitted independently from the familial transmission of psychiatric disorder per se [1]. Adoption, twin, and family studies support the view that the etiology of the familial transmission of suicidal behavior is at least in part genetic, and may be mediated by the transmission of intermediate phenotypes, such as impulsive aggression. In addition, there may be environmental causes for familial transmission, including imitation, and the intergenerational transmission of family adversity. In this article, we cover the evidence supporting the familial transmission of suicidal behavior, possible genetic and environmental explanations for this phenomenon, describe putative intermediate phenotypes, and discuss the contributory roles of early child-rearing and concurrent familial environmental stressors to suicidal risk. A better understanding of the mechanisms for the familial transmission of suicidal behavior can help to shed light on etiology, identify individuals at high risk for the development of incident suicidal behavior, and frame targets for intervention and prevention.

ADOPTION STUDIES

Three adoption studies have been conducted, all using the same Danish adoption registry (Table 1). Kety and colleagues [2], in a study designed to examine the genetics of schizophrenia and mood disorders, found a nonsignificant trend toward higher concordance for suicide in biological, compared with adoptive relatives of adoptees who committed suicide. Subsequently, a second study compared the rates of suicide among the biological and adoptive relatives of adoptees who committed suicide versus biological and adoptive relatives of a matched living adoptee control group in Denmark [3]. This study found a sixfold higher rate of suicide in the biological relatives of the suicide versus those of the control adoptees, and an absence of suicide among the adopted relatives of the suicide versus control adoptees supporting a genetic rather

This work was supported by NIMH grants MH 43366, 55123, 6612, 56390, 66371, 62185, and 77930. The expert assistance of Beverly Sughrue in preparation of the manuscript is appreciated.

*Corresponding author. E-mail address: brentda@upmc.edu (D.A. Brent).

0193-953X/08/$ – see front matter
doi:10.1016/j.psc.2008.02.001

Table 1
Schulsinger et al. (1979) adoption study: rates of suicide in biological versus adoptive relatives of adoptees who committed suicide and of live adoptee controls

Adopted	Index cases	Suicide/biological relatives	Suicide/adopted relatives
Suicide	57	12/269*	0/148
Controls	57	2/269	0/150

*P<.01.
Data from Schulsinger F, Kety SS, Rosenthal D, et al. A family study of suicide. In: Schou M, Stromgren E, editors. Origin, prevention and treatment of affective disorders. London: Academic Press; 1979. p. 277–87.

than environmental etiology (see Table 1). The rate of suicide was higher in the biologic relatives of suicide adoptees regardless of whether the adoptees were psychiatric patients or not. However, it was not possible to determine if the genetic liability to suicide was attributable to the transmission of major psychiatric disorders or to a suicide diathesis per se.

A third adoption study using this registry (a comparison of biological and adoptive relatives of adult adoptees with mood disorder and matched unaffected adoptees were examined [4]) revealed a 15-fold increase in suicide among the biological relatives of the mood-disordered adoptees versus those of the unaffected adoptees [4]. This finding supports the role of mood disorder in the genetics of suicide. However, the greatest increased risk for suicidal behavior was found in the relatives of those probands with "affect reaction," a diagnosis akin to borderline personality disorder, suggesting that impulsive-aggressive personality traits may play a role in familial aggregation of suicidal behavior (Table 2).

Taken together, these studies support a strong role for genetics in explaining the familial concordance of completed suicide. Limitations of these studies include restriction to data gathered through routine medical records, and lack of systematic assessment of suicide attempts as well as completions. Thus, while these studies show there are genetic factors explaining the familial aggregation of suicide, they do not shed a great deal of light on *what factors* might be involved in familial transmission.

Table 2
Incidence of suicide in biological relatives of depressive and control adoptees

Diagnosis in adoptee	Incidence of suicide in biological relative (%)	OR	P
Affective reaction	5/62 (8.1)	30.3	<.0001
Bipolar depression	4/71 (5.6)	20.6	.003
Neurotic depression	3/122 (2.5)	8.7	.056
Unipolar depression	3/132 (2.3)	8.0	.066
No mental illness	1/346 (0.3)	—	—

Data from Wender PH, Kety SS, Rosenthal D, et al. Psychiatric disorders in the biological and adoptive families of adopted individuals with affective disorders. Arch Gen Psychiatry 1986;43:923–9.

TWIN STUDIES

In their review of twin case reports for suicide, Roy and Segal [5] found an increased concordance for suicide in monozygotic (MZ) versus dizygotic twins (DZ) (14.9% versus 0.7%), consistent with Tsuang's [6] original observations (Tables 3 and 4). Roy and colleagues [5,7] found an even higher concordance rate for *suicide attempt* in the surviving monozygotic twin of the co-twin's suicide in MZ versus DZ twins (38% versus 0%), supporting the view that the clinical phenotype for concordance included *both completed suicide and suicide attempts*. Because these meta-analyses use reported case series, they are not necessarily representative of all twin pairs affected by suicide. The differential concordance rate for suicide for MZ versus DZ twins does not appear to be due to greater bereavement reactions in MZ twins [8], since the risk of suicide attempt after the nonsuicide death of a co-twin is similar in MZ versus DZ twins (1.4% versus 3.3%).

Three twin studies demonstrate familial transmission for suicidal behavior that cannot be explained by the transmission of other psychopathology [9–11]. The heritability of suicidal behavior ranging from ideation to attempts ranged between 38% and 55%. While there appears to be overlap between the heritability of suicidal ideation and of actual suicidal behavior, there is a distinct heritable component of suicide attempts demonstrated in two of these studies [9,10]. In one study, the heritability of suicidal behavior was demonstrated, even after controlling for the heritability of psychiatric disorders [10]. Twin studies generally provide more detailed assessment than adoption studies, and allow for an assessment of environmental and genetic contributors to concordance. However, unless twin studies are combined with adoption studies (ie, comparison of twins adopted away to different parents), it is difficult to definitively differentiate shared environmental from genetic effects. For example, in a twins-adopted away design, components of maternal behavior previously considered "environment" were explained by genetic concordance of MZ twins eliciting similar maternal responses from unrelated mothers [12].

Table 3
Twins studies in which one twin has committed suicide

| Study | No. of twins (%) concordant for suicide behavior | | |
	MZ	DZ	P
Haberlandt [1967]	14/51 (17.6)[a]	0/98 (0)	<.001
Juel-Nielsen [1970]	4/19 (21.1)	0/58 (0)	<.003
Zair [1981]	1/1 (100)	0/0 (0)	NS
Roy et al [1991]	7/62 (11.3)	2/114 (0)	<.01
Roy et al [7]	10/26 (38.5)[b]	0/9 (1.7)	<.04
Roy and Segal [5]	4/13 (30.7)[c]	0/15 (0)	<.04
Total	40/172 (23.0)	2/294 (0.7)	<.00001

[a]Five pairs, co-twin attempted suicide.
[b]Ten pairs, co-twin attempted suicide.
[c]Three pairs, co-twin attempted suicide.
Data from Brent DA, Mann JJ. Family genetic studies, suicide, and suicidal behavior. Am J Psychiatry 2005;133C:13–24.

Table 4
Twin studies of the genetic epidemiology of suicidal behavior

Study	N	Gender	Concordance, % MZ	Concordance, % DZ	AOR MZ	DZ	Heritability % Ideation	Attempt
Statham et al [9]	5995	Both	23.1	0	3.8	—	43	55
Glowinski et al [11]	3416	Female	25	12.8	5.6	4.0	—	48
Fu et al [10]	7744	Male	—	—	12.1	7.4	43	30
							36	17[a]

Abbreviations: AOR, adjusted odds ratio; DZ, dizygotic; MZ, monozygotic; —, cannot be calculated.
[a]Adjusted for heritability of other risk factors.
Data from Brent DA, Mann JJ. Family genetic studies, suicide, and suicidal behavior. Am J Psychiatry 2005;133C:13–24.

A second limitation is that MZ versus DZ concordance may be differentially affected by shared or distinct perinatal experiences [13].

FAMILY STUDIES

Family studies compare the rate of suicide or suicidal behavior in the relatives of a proband with suicidality to the rate of suicide or suicidal behavior in the relatives of probands without suicidality. Studies have varied in outcome (family history of completed suicide, attempted suicide, or both), choice of proband (either completed or attempted suicide), choice of comparison group (community or psychiatric control), and method of assessment of family loading (record review, family history, or direct interview) [14–40]. Among the most convincing of these studies have been those based on large population registries, which have shown concordance in death by suicide between parents and children, even after controlling for psychiatric diagnosis and treatment [37,38,41].

Despite variations in methodology, the results are remarkably similar across studies, consistently showing that suicidal behavior aggregates within families. Those studies that adjusted statistically for the familial transmission of psychiatric disorder and other risk factors generally found a familial effect for suicidal behavior that still persisted even after statistical adjustment with effects ranging from a 2- to 12-fold elevation in rates after adjustment [23,24,26,28]. These studies support the view that the clinical phenotype of suicidal behavior that is familially transmitted includes both suicide attempt and suicide completion, since the rate of suicide is elevated in the families of attempters, and the rate of attempted suicide is elevated in the families of suicide completers.

STUDIES OF THE RISK OF SUICIDE IN PROBANDS WITH COMPLETED SUICIDE

In studies that examined the familial rates of completed suicide in the relatives of probands who committed suicide, all show an elevated rate of completed suicide in the relatives of completers versus relatives of a comparison group, regardless of whether that comparison group consists of psychiatric, general medical, and community controls (Table 5). Also, these findings are consistent, regardless of whether the probands were drawn from large community pedigrees [14], diagnostically heterogeneous inpatients [29,42], community samples [27], or bipolar suicides versus living bipolar controls [36]. Two of the studies showed a significant association between family history of suicide and familial suicide after controlling for other risk factors, stressing the unique contribution of the familial transmission of suicidal behavior to suicidal risk.

POPULATION REGISTRY STUDIES

Four studies using Scandinavian registries report an increased risk of suicide conveyed to a first-degree relative, even after controlling for parental and personal history of inpatient psychiatric treatment (Table 6) [35,37,38,41]. In one study, family history of suicide was associated with an increased rate of suicide even compared with those who have had a first-degree relative die from either accidents or homicides, supporting the view that the familial transmission of suicidal behavior is not strongly mediated by bereavement [38]. One study found an impact of parental suicide on children aged 10 to 21 for both maternal and paternal suicide, with an increased risk for suicide in offspring even for maternal loss from other causes; however, the effect of maternal suicide was greater than maternal loss due to other causes (adjusted odds ratio [AOR's] 4.8 versus 2.06). While such studies have the advantage of large, representative databases, they are limited to the information available in medical records, and assessment of psychiatric disorder is limited to those who received treatment. However, in Scandinavian countries, where access to health care has fewer barriers than in the United States, a treated sample is likely to be more representative than it would be in an American study.

FAMILY STUDIES OF SUICIDE PROBANDS AND FAMILIAL RATES OF SUICIDAL BEHAVIOR

Four studies have examined rates of attempted and completed suicide in the families of suicide probands versus the relatives of community controls

Table 5
Studies of the risk of familial suicide in the relatives of suicide probands

Study	Probands	Controls	Sample size proband/control	OR
Tsuang [42]	Patient suicides	Patient nonsuicides	29/491	3.8
Egeland [14]	Suicides in Amish studies	Comparison pedigree	N/A	4.6
Foster [27]	Irish suicides	Attendees in same general practice	118/118	3.0 (NS)[a]
Powell [29]	Inpatient suicides	Inpatient nonsuicides	112/112	4.6[a]
Tsai [36]	Bipolar suicides	Bipolar controls	41/41	15.1[a]

[a]Adjusted odds ratio (OR).
   Data from Brent DA, Mann JJ. Family genetic studies, suicide, and suicidal behavior. Am J Psychiatry 2005;133C:13–24.

Table 6
Studies of suicide based on registries and record linkage

Study	Country	Proband	Control	Sample size proband/controls	AOR
Qin [35]	Denmark	Suicides, 9–45	Matched community control	4262/80,238	2.6[a,b]
Agerbo [41]	Denmark	Suicides, 10–21	Matched community controls	496/24,800	2.3–4.8[a,b,c]
Qin [37]	Denmark	Suicides, all ages	Matched community controls	21,169/423,128	2.1[a,b]
Runeson [38]	Sweden	Suicides, all ages	Matched nonsuicide deaths	8396/7568	2.0[b]

Abbreviation: AOR, adjusted odds ratio.
[a]Adjusted for previous psychiatric admission/care.
[b]Adjusted for relative's previous psychiatric admission.
[c]Odds ratio for suicide in father/mother.
Data from Brent DA, Mann JJ. Family genetic studies, suicide, and suicidal behavior. Am J Psychiatry 2005;133C:13–24.

(Table 7) [23,24,28,40]. Two studies focused on adolescents [23,24], and two on adults [28], one of which focused exclusively on males [40]. All found an increased rate of suicidal behavior in the relatives of completers compared with relatives of community controls, even after controlling for differences in rates of psychiatric disorder in probands [23,28,40], parent-child discord [24], and rates of psychiatric disorder in family members [23,24,40]. Two studies

Table 7
Family studies of rates of suicidal behavior in relatives of suicide versus control probands

Study	Proband	Control	Number of probands/ number of controls	AOR[a,b]
Brent [23]	Adolescent suicides	Matched community controls	58/55	4.3
Gould [24]	Adolescent suicides	Matched community controls	120/147	5.1
Cheng [28]	Adult suicides	Matched community controls	113/226	5.2
Kim [40]	Adult male suicides	Matched community controls	217/171	10.6

Abbreviation: AOR, adjusted odds ratio.
[a]Chart review.
[b]Family history attempt/completion.
Data from Brent DA, Mann JJ. Family genetic studies, suicide, and suicidal behavior. Am J Psychiatry 2005;133C:13–24.

found that the rates of familial suicidal behavior were most significantly increased in the relatives of the probands with increased levels of aggression or Cluster B personality disorder in probands [23,40], supporting a relationship between the familial transmission of aggression and of suicidal behavior. An increased rate of suicide attempts in the relatives of suicide probands supports the definition of a clinical phenotype of suicidal behavior that includes both attempts and completions. In contrast, suicidal ideation was not increased in relatives of completers after adjusting for rates of psychiatric disorder in relatives [23,40], indicating that suicidal ideation is transmitted along with psychiatric disorder, whereas the tendency to translate that ideation into an actual attempt is co-transmitted with impulsivity and aggression.

FAMILY HISTORY OF SUICIDAL BEHAVIOR IN SUICIDE ATTEMPTING PROBANDS

Table 8 lists 12 studies that have examined the rate of suicidal behavior in the families of suicide attempter probands, using a family history method. The findings are very consistent across studies, finding an increased rate of both completed and attempted suicide in the relatives of suicide attempters compared with the family members of controls. These findings are robust across a wide range of conditions: age of attempters (adolescents and adults), sampling frame (community samples, inpatients, outpatients), and diagnostic category (mixed, depression, bipolar, alcohol abuse, substance abuse). Greater lethality and violence of the attempt was associated with increased family loading in two studies [15,18]. Loss of parent in childhood (under age of 11) either due to suicide [43] or due to any cause [22] was associated with an increased risk of attempt. Greater familial loading for suicidal behavior was associated with proband neuroticism, history of abuse or neglect, increased lifetime aggression, and, in those probands with mood disorder, an earlier age of onset of mood disorder [32–34,44,45]. Moreover, a history of abuse, increased lifetime aggression, and earlier age of onset of mood disorder were interrelated [44]. In one population study, significant relationships between parental and offspring ideation and attempt were reported [46]. However, after adjustment for comorbidity, the strongest relationships were between parental and offspring attempt.

FAMILY STUDIES OF SUICIDE-ATTEMPTING PROBANDS

Three family studies of child or adolescent suicide-attempting probands have been conducted, finding an increased risk of suicide attempt in the relatives of suicide-attempting probands (Table 9) [21,25,26]. These studies also support a definition of the clinical phenotype that includes suicidal behavior, but does not include suicidal ideation, insofar as Pfeffer and colleagues [21] found that a family history of attempts was increased only in the relatives of proband attempters but not in the relatives of proband ideators. A relationship between familial transmission of suicidal behavior and of impulsive aggression was also supported, since a higher rate of assaultive behavior was reported in the

Table 8
Family history studies of attempted suicide probands

Study	Proband	Control	Number of proband/control	Odds ratio
Garfinkel [15][a]	Adolescent attempters in ER	ER nonattempters	505/505	5.4
Roy [16][a]	Adult inpatient attempters	Adult inpatient nonattempts	243/5,602	3.4
Linkowski [18]	Adult inpatient attempters	Adult inpatient nonattempters	239/474	2.0–3.5
Mitterauer [19]	Manic-depressive attempters	Manic depressive nonattempters	342/80	3.3
Sorenson [20]	Suicide attempters	Nonattempters	93/2,211	5.8
Malone [22]	Depressed attempters	Depressed nonattempters	100/100	7.6
Roy [30]	Alcoholic attempters	Alcoholic nonattempters	124/209	2.4/4.0[b]
Roy [31]	Cocaine-dependent attempters	Cocaine-defendant non-attempters	84/130	4.5/5.9[b]
Roy [34]	Opiate-dependent attempters	Opiate-dependant nonattempters	105/171	2.9/6.0[b]
Roy [39]	Substance-dependent attempters	Substance dependent nonattempters	175/274	3.2/5.9[b]
Mann [44]	Mood disordered attempters	Mood-disordered nonattempters	234/223	2.0/2.1[b]
Goodwin [46]	Community sample (attempters)	Community sample (nonattempters)	165/1209	4.6

[a]Chart review.
[b]Family history of attempters/completions.
Data from Brent DA, Mann JJ. Family genetic studies, suicide, and suicidal behavior. Am J Psychiatry 2005;133C:13–24.

relatives of proband suicide attempters [21], and conversely, a higher rate of suicidal behavior in relatives was reported in the relatives of those proband attempters with higher levels of impulsive aggression [26].

HIGH-RISK STUDIES

A variant of the family study, the high-risk study, has been used to prospectively examine the risks and processes associated with the familial transmission of suicidal behavior. In three studies that have taken this strategy, results are consistent–offspring of adult mood-disordered suicide attempters have a much higher risk of suicide attempt than offspring of mood-disordered probands who have never made a suicide attempt (Fig. 1). Greater familial loading for suicidal behavior is associated with a higher risk and earlier age of onset of suicidal behavior in offspring (Fig. 2), as well as higher levels of impulsive aggression in both parent and offspring [46–50]. In one study, it was demonstrated that the familial transmission of suicidal behavior was in part mediated by the familial transmission of impulsive aggression [48]. Furthermore, in

Table 9
Family studies of child or adolescent suicide-attempting probands

Study	Proband	Control	Number of proband/control	OR
Pfeffer [21]	Prepubertal attempter	Ideator/clinical control community controls	25/28/16/54	4.3–8.3[a]
Johnson [26]	Adolescent inpatient attempters	Adolescent inpatient nonattempters	62/70	2.1[b]
Bridge [25]	Community attempters	Community controls	3/55	12.1[b]

Abbreviation: OR, odds ratio.
[a]Attempter/control; OR = 8.3, attempter/clinical control.
[b]Adjusted OR.
Data from Brent DA, Mann JJ. Family genetic studies, suicide, and suicidal behavior. Am J Psychiatry 2005;133C:13–24.

prospective follow-up of high-risk offspring, high levels of impulsive aggression, along with early-onset depression, predicted earlier onset and higher risk of suicidal behavior [49].

High-risk, family-genetic studies may also shed some light on some family-environmental factors that may contribute to the familial transmission of suicidal behavior. Most notably, the risk of suicide attempt in offspring of adult suicide attempters was greatly heightened if the parents themselves had a reported history of sexual abuse [47,49]. Using a high-risk design (top-down), this relationship between parental sexual abuse and offspring attempt appears to be mediated through two pathways [1]: parental history of abuse that leads to an increased risk of offspring abuse, which in turn increases the risk for mood and anxiety disorder and suicide attempt; and [2] parental history of

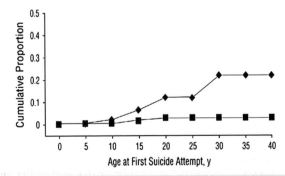

Fig. 1. Risk of suicide attempt in the offspring of attempters (*diamond*) compared with offspring of nonattempters (*square*). (*From* Brent DA, Oquendo M, Birmaher B, et al. Familial pathways to early-onset suicide attempt: Risk for suicidal behavior in offspring of mood-disordered suicide attempters. Arch Gen Psychiatry 2002;59:801–7; with permission.)

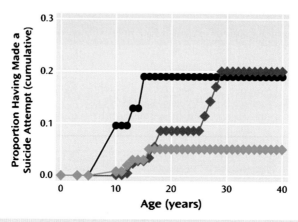

Fig. 2. Suicide attempts over time among offspring of mood disorder probands from sibling pairs concordant or discordant for suicidal behavior. Black circle, offspring of sibling-concordant suicidal probands; red diamond, offspring of sibling-discordant suicidal probands; green diamond, offspring of nonsuicidal probands. (*From* Brent DA, Oquendo M, Birmaher B, et al. Peripubertal suicide attempts in offspring of suicide attempters with siblings concordant for suicidal behavior. Am J Psychiatry 2003;160:1486–93; with permission. Copyright © 2003, American Psychiatric Association.)

abuse that is associated with higher offspring impulsive aggression, which in turn increases the risk for early onset mood disorder and suicide attempt [51,52]. Similar interrelationships among parental history of abuse, offspring early-onset mood disorder and impulsive aggression, and suicide attempt were found in a "bottom-up" family history study [44]. Taken together, these studies suggest that early abuse in childhood could account for some, but not all of the familial clustering of suicidal behavior because of the familial transmission of liability to abuse.

POSSIBLE MECHANISMS BY WHICH FAMILIAL TRANSMISSION OF SUICIDAL BEHAVIOR MAY OCCUR

Some possible intermediate phenotypes have emerged from family genetic studies. An intermediate phenotype according to Gottesman and Gould [53], must be related to the clinical phenotype, must be heritable, must predict the onset of the condition in offspring, and show evidence of mediation when controlling for the relationship between parent and offspring transmission of the overall clinical phenotype. The intermediate phenotype with the most convergent evidence is impulsive aggression, ie, the propensity to react with aggression or hostility to frustration or provocation. This construct has been shown to be related to risk for suicide attempt [54], to predict onset of suicide attempt [49], to be heritable [55], and to mediate the transmission of suicidal behavior [48]. Other possible intermediate phenotypes include neuroticism, which is heritable, and is related both to onset of attempt, and to family loading for suicidal behavior [56]. Impaired working memory and executive function, which may form the neurocognitive substrate for impulsive aggression and for poor interpersonal problem solving, has been shown to be altered in adult attempters, offspring of adult attempters, and to be heritable [57,58].

In addition to genetic transmission, familial transmission of suicidal behavior could be explained in a number of other ways, such as familial transmission of adverse family environment, imitation, or bereavement.

Intergenerational Transmission of Adverse Family Rearing Environments

As noted above, the familial transmission of suicidal behavior is confounded by the familial transmission of abuse. The interrelationship between the transmission of abuse and of suicidal behavior is complex, in part because parents who abuse their children are also at higher risk for psychiatric conditions that predispose to suicidal behavior, including depression, substance abuse, and suicidal behavior [59,60]. Furthermore, impulsive aggression in a parent may predispose that parent to be abusive, but also may be transmitted to that child as a heritable trait. In fact, the relationship between parental abuse and offspring suicidal behavior is mediated in part by the transmission of impulsivity and aggression [51,52]. Further complicating an understanding of this interrelationship between the child abuse and impulsive aggression are the longstanding neurobiological changes that have been reported in maltreated children that may account for increased impulsivity and aggression [61].

Imitation

The familial transmission of suicidal behavior could in theory be explained by imitation. This is plausible given evidence that youth suicide occurs in time-space clusters, and that exposure to print and electronic media publicity about suicidal behavior has been consistently been shown to be associated with an increase in suicidal behavior [62]. However, in youth exposed to a sibling's or a friend's suicide, there is no evidence of imitation [63,64]. In both high-risk and twin studies that have examined the temporal relationship between attempts in relatives, no relationship consistent with imitation could be found [9,47]. While imitation is difficult to disprove, these prospective case-control studies, taken with those of adoption studies, suggest that imitation is not a clinically significant contributor to the familial transmission of suicidal behavior.

Interestingly, exposure to a friend's suicide *attempt*, but not to a friend's *completed* suicide, appears to be associated with an increased risk for suicidal behavior [64,65]. Knowing a person who has attempted suicide, whether a relative or not, has also been reported to be a risk factor for suicidal behavior in mid-life [66]. It is possible, though, that exposure to suicidal behavior is the result of "assortative friendships," insofar as friends of individuals with psychologic difficulties are more likely to have mental disorder themselves. Peers with health-risk behaviors, including suicidal behavior, are much more likely to have friends with increased rates of these behaviors [67]. Moreover, the concordance among peers' health-risk behaviors is much higher in the face of family dysfunction [67]. Conversely, the deleterious impact of an adverse rearing environment can be buffered by a pro-social peer group [68].

Parental Bereavement

Retrospective, record linkage, and prospective longitudinal studies have found that bereavement conveys an increased risk for depression and suicide [69–73]. There seems to be a more deleterious effect of parental bereavement when the child who has lost a parent is younger than the age of 12 [33,65,74]. Record linkage studies indicate that parental loss by suicide is most strongly associated with suicide risk in offspring, but that so is maternal loss from any cause [41]. The relationship between early parental loss and suicidal behavior may be mediated by an increased risk for depression [71,72]. Other factors that may contribute further to suicidal risk are premorbid parental psychopathology [49], traumatic exposure predisposing to posttraumatic stress disorder (PTSD), and the development of complicated grief (prolonged negative affect and rumination about the loss), which in turn has been shown to predispose to suicidal ideation in young adults [75]. However, empiric data do not support a specific relationship between parent loss due to suicide and suicidal behavior in the child, compared with parent loss due to other causes [76–79]. Moreover, the association between child completed suicide and parental attempted suicide suggests that, while bereavement and loss may play a small role in the overall effect of familial transmission, the majority of the familial effect is due to some other mechanism.

OTHER FAMILY-ENVIRONMENTAL FACTORS THAT MAY INTERACT WITH GENETIC RISK FACTORS FOR SUICIDAL BEHAVIOR

Parental Divorce and Separation

There is a large literature documenting a higher risk for suicidal behavior and suicide in children from non-intact families. However, divorce per se is unlikely to lead to suicidal behavior [41,80,81]. For example, marital disruption is more common in parents with psychiatric disorder. In studies that have examined the three-way relationships among divorce, parental and child psychiatric disorder, and child suicidal behavior, the relationship between divorce and child suicidal behavior is markedly attenuated after controlling for higher rates of parental psychiatric disorder [82–84]. Young maternal age is another correlate of divorce that also predicts onset of suicidal behavior in adolescents [65]. It is likely that the processes that ensue subsequent to the divorce predict child adjustment. For example, Tousignant and colleagues [85] showed a dose-response relationship between the number of parental figures (and subsequent disruptions) and the risk for adolescent suicidal behavior. A cascade of processes and predisposing factors mediate the relationship between divorce and eventual suicidal behavior [86]. The relationship between parental divorce and child mental health disorders is mediated by the quality of the child's relationship with the caretaking parent, the caretaking parent's mental health, and the degree to which the child engages in active and problem-based coping.

Marital Break-Up and Conjugal Bereavement in Adult Life

Marital break-up is a frequent precipitant for suicide attempts and completed suicide, particularly in those with alcohol and substance abuse problems [87]. There is evidence that the relationship rupture in alcoholics often follows domestic violence [88]. In midlife and older individuals, particular males, conjugal bereavement is a risk factor for suicidal ideation and behavior, especially in concert with other psychiatric risk factors [89,90]. Among women, having a child was protective against conjugal bereavement's impact on suicide risk [91]. Complicated grief has been shown to increase the risk for suicidal ideation above and beyond psychiatric disorder [75]. Conversely, suicide, particularly in the geriatric age group is less likely to occur in those with a strong support network, eg, confiding friendships, children nearby, or living with children [92,93].

Quality of Family Relationships

Family discord, including high expressed emotion have consistently been shown to be both correlates and predictors of adolescent suicidal behavior [94], although the relationship between discord and suicide attempt is somewhat attenuated after controlling for parental and child psychiatric disorder [84]. Parent-child discord is the single most common precipitant for completed suicide in adolescents younger than 16 [95]. Other characteristics of parent-child relationships that have characterized suicidal adolescents have been lack of perceived support and poor communication, particularly between children and fathers [24,85,96]. In older individuals, marital conflict is often associated with depression and substance abuse, although it is difficult to disentangle the extent to which the psychiatric illness is a source of the discord, or a consequence. Nevertheless, marital therapy aimed at reducing discord and increasing support has been shown to relieve depression when discord is a prominent part of the presentation [97–100]. Moral objections to suicide have also been shown to protect against suicidal behavior, and such attitudes can also be familially transmitted [101,102].

Family Protective Factors

High parent-child warmth, parental monitoring, consistent parental discipline, and family cohesion have been shown to be protective against youthful suicidal behavior [103]. High levels of protective factors lower the risk for suicide attempt in adolescents even in the presence of other high-risk behaviors and predisposing factors [67,103].

Adult suicide attempters, in general, report lower perceived family support, and concern about the impact on family is one of the most common reasons given by depressed individuals for not engaging in suicidal behavior [104,105]. A much lower proportion of adults who commit suicide are in a stable relationship compared with living controls [76], suggesting that the continuation of a strong pair-bond is protective. As noted above, other factors protective against suicide in older individuals are a strong network of support, including living with children (if the individual is female) or having them nearby.

Childhood Experience of Abuse

Physical and sexual abuse, particularly sexual abuse that involves genital or anal penetration, are strongly associated with suicide attempts and completions. According to some epidemiologic studies, sexual abuse has a population-attributable risk of nearly 20%, meaning that the rate of suicidal behavior in adolescents could be decreased by 20% if sexual abuse could be eliminated [106–108]. The mechanism by which abuse increases risk for suicidal behavior is complex, as child maltreatment usually takes place against a background of family discord, parental psychopathology, including a parental history of suicidal behavior, all of which can also increase the risk for suicidal behavior in children [59,60]. However, while it is clear that abuse increases the risk for a wide array of psychiatric disorders, some studies show that even after controlling for the increased risk of psychiatric disorder, abuse increases the risk and decreases the age of onset for suicidal behavior [109,110].

Sexual abuse in parent and child appear to increase the risk for transmission of suicidal behavior through several possible mechanisms. As noted above, sexual abuse in a parent increases the likelihood of sexual abuse in the child, which in turn increases the likelihood for a mood or anxiety disorder, and for suicide attempt [33,48,51,111]. Second, parents who abuse their children are more likely to also attempt suicide as well as have mood and substance disorders, so that the liability for suicide attempt in the child may come from both genetic and environmental manifestations of a common diathesis [59,60]. Third, sexual abuse may increase the likelihood of expression of traits related to suicidal risk, like neuroticism, anxiety, depression, and impulsive aggression [32,47,51,110,112–114]. Also, abuse and other adverse circumstances could be familially transmitted by shared environmental rather than by genetic mechanisms. Fu and colleagues [10] found that shared environment explained as much of the variance in suicide attempts as did heritability. Dinwiddie and colleagues, in an analysis of the Australian twin registry reported in Statham and colleagues [9], found that the negative impact of sexual abuse on mental health outcomes was explained by shared environment, rather than genetic factors [115].

There is growing evidence of long-lasting neurobiological changes as a result of neglectful or abusive rearing environments. In mice, pups that are exposed to low levels of maternal grooming show changes in cortisol response to stress, cognitive impairment, and lower persistence in the face of frustrating tasks than those exposed to high levels of grooming [116–118]. Moreover, the specific maternal behavior (grooming) appears to be familially transmitted from mother to daughter. However, this transmission is not due to genetic factors because cross-fostering experiments show that it is exposure to grooming rather than the grooming style of the biological mother that determines grooming behavior in the offspring [116]. Neuroendocrine studies of children with a history of maltreatment show alternations in the hypothalamic pituitary adrenal axis (HPA), although some studies have reported lower than expected response to stress, and some, higher than expected response [119]. Neuroimaging studies in children exposed to maltreatment also show changes in corpus collusum and hippocampus volume that may account for some of the cognitive findings associated with a history of maltreatment [61]. Abuse and adverse rearing environments result in a decrease in central serotonergic function, a biological system that has been linked to impulsive aggression and suicidal behavior [120–124].

Interactions Between Genes and Environment

In the debate between about the relative contributions of nature and nurture, there is a "nature to nurture" [125], meaning that adverse family environments do not occur at random, and may arise due to parental or child genetic contributors to these adverse environments. Parental psychiatric illness is a risk factor for premature parental death, which in turn puts their offspring at higher risk for psychiatric disorder [49]. Parents who abuse their children are more likely to have psychiatric disorders such as depression, substance abuse, and a history of suicidal behavior, so that their children are at risk because of their genetic diathesis as well as because of the exposure to abuse [60,126]. Children who are at risk for depression may follow a stochastic pathway [1]: genes that predispose to anxiety also predispose to the occurrence of certain depressogenic life events, that, in the face of a genetic diathesis to anxiety, lead to depression [127]. Finally, studies of twins reared apart show that dimensions of maternal behavior such as parental warmth are actually heritable, being induced by the behavior of the twin offspring [12].

Second, it is important to recognize that environmental factors are most likely to affect those with a genetic diathesis. This was most elegantly demonstrated by Caspi and colleagues [112], who showed that the likelihood of depression and suicidal behavior was greatest when there was a history of stressful life events (including abuse) and a less functional allelic form of the serotonin transporter promoter gene. This finding has been replicated several times [71,128–130]. Kaufman and colleagues found that the risk for depression was greatest in abused children who also had a family history of depression.

Third, these different family-environmental stressors rarely occur in isolation. For example, it is more common for a child with a background of maltreatment to have been also exposed to multiple parental figures, parental criminality and psychiatric disorder, witnessing domestic violence, and economic instability [96,131,132]. Nevertheless, there is evidence that there are factors that are protective against suicidal behavior even in the face of substantial other risk factors [103].

SUMMARY

It is well recognized that suicidal behavior runs in families. Adoption and twin studies together make a compelling case that familial transmission of suicidal behavior is in part attributable to genetic factors. There is some evidence that the transmission of suicidal behavior is mediated by the transmission of impulsive aggression. Other, less thoroughly investigated possible mediators include neuroticism and neurocognitive deficits. However, given that at best, around 50% of the variance is explained by genes, there is a significant role for environmental factors as well. The most plausible explanations for nongenetic familial transmission are the intergenerational transmission of abuse and of adverse familial environments. Bereavement and relationship disruption may make a specific contribution to suicidal risk via the development of complicated grief although the long-term effects are likely to be mediated by complex chain of interrelated events. Imitation may also make a contribution to suicidal risk, at least with regard to attempted suicide. However, so-called family environmental factors often are related to risk factors that are heritable. Conversely, most genetic factors exert their impact on depression and suicidal behavior via an interaction with a stressful environment.

References

[1] Brent DA, Mann JJ. Family genetic studies of suicide and suicidal behavior. Am J Med Genet C Semin Med Genet 2005;133:13–24.

[2] Kety SS, Rosenthal D, Wender PH, et al. The types and prevalence of mental illness in the biological and adoptive families of adopted schizophrenia. J Psychiatr Res 1968;6:345–62.

[3] Schulsinger F, Kety SS, Rosenthal D, et al. A family study of suicide. In: Schou M, Stromgren E, editors. Origin, prevention and treatment of affective disorders. London: Academic Press; 1979. p. 277–87.

[4] Wender PH, Kety SS, Rosenthal D, et al. Psychiatric disorders in the biological and adoptive families of adopted individuals with affective disorders. Arch Gen Psychiatry 1986;43:923–9.

[5] Roy A, Segal NL. Suicidal behavior in twins: a replication. J Affect Disord 2001;66:71–4.

[6] Tsuang MT. Genetic factors in suicide. Dis Nerv Syst 1977;38:498–501.

[7] Roy A, Segal NL, Sarchiapone M. Attempted suicide among living co-twins of twin suicide victims. Am J Psychiatry 1995;152:1075–6.

[8] Segal NL, Roy A. Suicidal attempts and ideation in twins whose co-twins' deaths were non-suicides: replication and elaboration. Pers Individ Dif 2001;31:445–52.

[9] Statham DJ, Heath AC, Madden PAF, et al. Suicidal behaviour: an epidemiological and genetic study. Psychol Med 1998;28:839–55.

[10] Fu Q, Heath AC, Bucholz KK, et al. A twin study of genetic and environmental influences on suicidality in men. Psychol Med 2002;32:11–24.

[11] Glowinski A, Bucholz KK, Nelson EC, et al. Suicide attempts in an adolescent female twin sample. J Am Acad Child Adolesc Psychiatry 2001;40:1300–7.

[12] Plomin R, Reiss D, Hetherington EM, et al. Nature and nurture: genetic contributions to measures of the family environment. Dev Psychol 1994;30(1):32–43.

[13] Devlin B, Daniels M, Roeder K. The heritability of IQ. Nature 1997;388:468–71.

[14] Egeland JA, Sussex JN. Suicide and family loading for affective disorders. J Am Med Assoc 1985;254:915–8.

[15] Garfinkel BD, Froese A, Hood J. Suicide attempts in children and adolescents. Am J Psychiatry 1982;139:1257–61.

[16] Roy A. Family history of suicide. Arch Gen Psychiatry 1983;40:971–4.

[17] Tsuang MT. Risk of suicide in the relatives of schizophrenics, manics, depressives, and controls. J Clin Psychiatry 1983;44:396–400.

[18] Linkowski P, de Maertelaer V, Mendlewicz J. Suicidal behaviour in major depressive illness. Acta Psychiatr Scand 1985;72:233–8.

[19] Mitterauer B. A contribution to the discussion of the role of the genetic factor in suicide, based on five studies in an epidemiologically defined area (Province of Salzburg, Austria). Compr Psychiatry 1990;31:557–65.

[20] Sorenson SB, Rutter CM. Transgenerational patterns of suicide attempt. J Consult Clin Psychol 1991;59:861–6.

[21] Pfeffer CR, Normandin L, Tatsuyuki K. Suicidal children grow up: suicidal behavior and psychiatric disorders among relatives. J Am Acad Child Psychiatry 1994;33:1087–97.

[22] Malone KM, Haas GL, Sweeney JA, et al. Major depression and the risk of attempted suicide. J Affect Disord 1995;34:173–85.

[23] Brent DA, Bridge J, Johnson BA, et al. Suicidal behavior runs in families: a controlled family study of adolescent suicide victims. Arch Gen Psychiatry 1996;53:1145–52.

[24] Gould MS, Fisher P, Parides M, et al. Psychosocial risk factors of child and adolescent completed suicide. Arch Gen Psychiatry 1996;53:1155–62.

[25] Bridge JA, Brent DA, Johnson B, et al. Familial aggregation of psychiatric disorders in a community sample of adolescents. J Am Acad Child Adolesc Psychiatry 1997;36:628–36.

[26] Johnson BA, Brent DA, Bridge J, et al. The familial aggregation of adolescent suicide attempts. Acta Psychiatr Scand 1998;97:18–24.

[27] Foster T, Gillespie K, McClelland R, et al. Risk factors for suicide independent of DSM-III-R Axis I disorder: case control psychological autopsy study in Northern Ireland. Br J Psychiatry 1999;175:175–9.

[28] Cheng AT, Chen THH, Chen CC, et al. Psychosocial and psychiatric risk factors for suicide: case-control psychological autopsy study. Br J Psychiatry 2000;177:360–5.

[29] Powell J, Geddes J, Deeks J, et al. Suicide in psychiatric hospital in-patients: risk factors and their predictive powers. Br J Psychiatry 2000;176:266–72.

[30] Roy A. Relation of family history of suicide to suicide attempts in alcoholics. Am J Psychiatry 2000;157:2050–1.

[31] Roy A. Characteristics of cocaine-dependent patients who attempt suicide. Am J Psychiatry 2001;158:1215–9.

[32] Roy A. Family history of suicide and neuroticism: a preliminary study. Psychiatry Res 2002;110:87–90.

[33] Roy A. Childhood trauma and neuroticism as an adult: possible implication for the development of the common psychiatric disorders and suicidal behaviour. Psychol Med 2002;32:1471–4.

[34] Roy A. Characteristics of opiate dependent patients who attempt suicide. J Clin Psychiatry 2002;63:403–7.

[35] Qin P, Agerbo E, Mortensen PB. Suicide risk in relation to family history of completed suicide and psychiatric disorders: a nested case-control study based on longitudinal registers. Lancet 2002;360:1126–30.

[36] Tsai SY, Kuo C, Chen CC, et al. Risk factors for completed suicide in bipolar disorder. J Clin Psychiatry 2002;63:469–76.

[37] Qin P, Agerbo E, Mortensen PB. Suicide risk in relation to socioeconomic, demographic, psychiatric, and familial factors: a national register-based study of all suicides in Denmark, 1981–1997. Am J Psychiatry 2003;160:765–72.

[38] Runeson B, Asberg M. Family history of suicide among suicide victims. Am J Psychiatry 2003;160:1525–6.

[39] Roy A. Characteristics of drug addicts who attempt suicide. Psychiatry Res 2003;121:99–103.

[40] Kim CD, Seguin M, Therrien N, et al. Familial aggregation of suicidal behavior: a family study of male suicide completers from the general population. Am J Psychiatry 2005;162:1017–9.

[41] Agerbo E, Nordentoft M, Mortensen PB. Familial, psychiatric, and socioeconomic risk factors for suicide in young people: nested case-controlled study. BMJ 2002;325:74–7.

[42] Tsuang MT, Simpson JC. Mortality studies in psychiatry: should they stop or proceed? Arch Gen Psychiatry 1985;42:98–103.

[43] Roy A. Early parental death and adult depression. Psychol Med 1983;13:861–5.

[44] Mann JJ, Bortinger J, Oquendo MA, et al. Family history of suicidal behavior and mood disorders in probands with mood disorders. Am J Psychiatry 2005;162:1672–9.

[45] Hawton K, Haw C, Houston K, et al. Family history of suicidal behaviour: prevalence and significance in deliberate self-harm patients. Acta Psychiatr Scand 2002;106:387–93.

[46] Goodwin RD, Beautrais AL, Fergusson DM. Familial transmission of suicidal ideation and suicide attempts: evidence from a general population sample. Psychiatry Res 2004;126: 159–65.

[47] Brent DA, Oquendo M, Birmaher B, et al. Familial pathways to early-onset suicide attempt: risk for suicidal behavior in offspring of mood-disordered suicide attempters. Arch Gen Psychiatry 2002;59:801–7.

[48] Brent DA, Oquendo MA, Birmaher B, et al. Peripubertal suicide attempts in offspring of suicide attempters with siblings concordant for suicidal behavior. Am J Psychiatry 2003;160:1486–93.

[49] Melhem NM, Brent DA, Ziegler M, et al. Familial pathways to early-onset suicidal behavior: familial and individual antecedents of suicidal behavior. Am J Psychiatry 2007;164: 1364–70.

[50] Lieb R, Bronisch T, Hofler M, et al. Maternal suicidality and risk of suicidality in offspring: findings from a community study. Am J Psychiatry 2005;162:1665–71.

[51] Brodsky BS, Mann JJ, Stanley B, et al. Familial transmission of suicidal behavior: factors mediating the relationship between abuse and offspring suicide attempts. J Clin Psychiatry, in press.

[52] Brent DA, Oquendo MA, Birmaher B, et al. Familial transmission of mood disorders: convergence and divergence with transmission of suicidal behavior. J Am Acad Child Adolesc Psychiatry 2004;43:1259–66.

[53] Gottesman II, Gould TD. The endophenotype concept in psychiatry: etymology and strategic intentions. Am J Psychiatry 2003;160:636–45.

[54] Mann JJ, Waternaux C, Haas GL, et al. Toward a clinical model of suicidal behavior in psychiatric patients. Am J Psychiatry 1999;156:181–9.

[55] Coccaro E, Bergeman CS, Kavoussi RJ, et al. Heritability of aggression and irritability: a twin study of the Buss-Durkee aggression scales in adult male subjects. Biol Psychiatry 1997;41:273–84.

[56] Beautrais A, Joyce PR, Mulder RT. Personality traits and cognitive styles as risk factors for serious suicide attempts among young people. Suicide Life Threat Behav 1999;29: 37–47.

[57] Beers SR, Keilp JG, Melhem NM, et al. Familial transmission of suicidal behavior: neuropsychological dysfunction in offspring of suicide attempters. Psychol Med, submitted.

[58] Jeglic EL, Sharp IR, Chapman JE, et al. History of family suicide behaviors and negative problem solving in multiple suicide attempters. Arch Suicide Res 2005;9:135–46.

[59] Roberts J, Hawton K. Child abuse and attempted suicide. Br J Psychiatry 1980;137: 319–23.

[60] Chaffin M, Kelleher KJ, Hollenberg J. Onset of physical abuse and neglect: psychiatric, substance abuse and social risk factors from prospective community data. Child Abuse Negl 1996;20:191–203.

[61] DeBellis MD, Thomas LA. Biologic findings of post-traumatic stress disorder and child maltreatment. Curr Psychiatry Rep 2003;5:108–17.

[62] Gould MS. Suicide and the media. Ann N Y Acad Sci 2001;932:200–24.

[63] Brent DA, Moritz G, Bridge J, et al. The impact of adolescent suicide on siblings and parents: a longitudinal follow-up. Suicide Life Threat Behav 1996;26:253–9.

[64] Brent DA, Moritz G, Bridge J, et al. Long-term impact of exposure to suicide: a three-year controlled follow-up. J Am Acad Child Adolesc Psychiatry 1996;35(5):646–53.

[65] Lewinsohn PM, Rohde P, Seeley JR. Adolescent suicidal ideation and attempts: prevalence, risk factors, and clinical implications. Clinical Psychology and Scientific Practice 1996;3:25–46.

[66] Conner KR, Duberstein PR. Predisposing and precipitating factors for suicide among alcoholics: empirical review and conceptual integration. Alcohol Clin Exp Res 2004;28:6S–17S.

[67] Prinstein MJ, Boergers J, Spirito A. Adolescents' and their friends' health-risk behavior: factors that alter or add to peer influence. J Pediatr Psychol 2001;26:287–98.

[68] Lynskey MT, Fergusson DM. Factors protecting against the development of adjustment difficulties in young adults exposed to childhood sexual abuse. Child Abuse Negl 1997;21:1177–90.

[69] Kendler KS, Neale MC, Kessler RC, et al. Childhood parental loss and adult psychopathology in women: a twin study perspective. Arch Gen Psychiatry 1992;49:109–16.

[70] Kendler KS, Gardner CO, Prescott CA. Toward a comprehensive development model for major depression in men. Am J Psychiatry 2006;163:115–24.

[71] Kendler KS, Sheth K, Gardner CO, et al. Childhood parental loss and risk for first-onset of major depression and alcohol dependence: the time-decay of risk and sex differences. Psychol Med 2002;32:1187–94.

[72] Reinherz HZ, Giaconia RM, Carmola Hauf AM, et al. Major depression in the transition to adulthood: risks and impairments. J Abnorm Psychol 1999;108:500–10.

[73] Tremblay GC, Israel AC. Children's adjustment to parental death. Clinical Psychology and Scientific Practice 1998;5:424–38.

[74] Roy A. Childhood trauma and attempted suicide in alcoholics. J Nerv Ment Dis 2001;189:120–1.

[75] Latham AE, Prigerson HG. Suicidality and bereavement: complicated grief as a psychiatric disorder presenting greatest risk for suicidality. Suicide Life Threat Behav 2004;34:350–62.

[76] Melhem N, Walker M, Moritz G, et al. Antecedents and sequelae of sudden parental death in children and surviving caregivers. Arch Pediatr Adolesc Med, in press.

[77] Jordan JR. Is suicide bereavement different? A reassessment of the literature. Suicide Life Threat Behav 2001;31:91–102.

[78] Cerel J, Fristad M, Verducci J, et al. Childhood bereavement: psychopathology in the 2 years postparental death. J Am Acad Child Adolesc Psychiatry 2006;45:681–90.

[79] Cerel J, Fristad MA, Weller EB, et al. Suicide-bereaved children and adolescents: a controlled longitudinal examination. J Am Acad Child Adolesc Psychiatry 1999;38:672–9.

[80] Goldney RD. Parental loss and reported childhood stress in young women who attempt suicide. Acta Psychiatr Scand 1981;64:34–59.

[81] Adam KS, Bouckoms A, Streiner DL. Parental loss and family stability in attempted suicide. Arch Gen Psychiatry 1982;39:1081–5.

[82] Gould MS, Shaffer D, Fisher P, et al. Separation/divorce and child and adolescent completed suicide. J Am Acad Child Adolesc Psychiatry 1998;37:155–62.

[83] Gould MS, Greenberg T, Velting DM, et al. Youth suicide risk and preventative interventions: a review of the past 10 years. J Am Acad Child Adolesc Psychiatry 2003;42:386–405.

[84] Brent DA, Perper JA, Moritz G, et al. Familial risk factors for adolescent suicide: a case-control study. Acta Psychiatr Scand 1994;89:52–8.

[85] Tousignant M, Bastien MF, Hamel S. Suicidal attempts and ideations among adolescents and young adults: the contribution of the father's and mother's care and of parental separation. Soc Psychiatry Psychiatr Epidemiol 1993;28:256–61.

[86] Sandler IN, Tein JY, Mehta P, et al. Coping efficacy and psychological problems of children of divorce. Child Development 2000;71:1099–118.

[87] Murphy GE, Wetzel RD, Robins E, et al. Multiple risk factors predict suicide in alcoholism. Arch Gen Psychiatry 1992;49:459–63.

[88] Conner KR, Duberstein P, Conwell Y. Domestic violence, separation, and suicide in young men with early onset alcoholism: reanalyses of Murphy's data. Suicide Life Threat Behav 2000;30:354–9.

[89] Kposowa AJ. Marital status and suicide in the National Longitudinal Mortality Study. J Epidemiol Community Health 2000;54:254–61.

[90] Li G. The interaction effect of bereavement and sex on the risk of suicide in the elderly: an historical cohort study. Soc Sci Med 1995;40:825–8.

[91] Agerbo E. Midlife suicide risk, partner's psychiatric illness, spouse and child bereavement by suicide or other modes of death: a gender specific study. J Epidemiol Community Health 2005;59:407–12.

[92] Rowe JL, Conwell Y, Schulberg H, et al. Social support and suicidal ideation in order adults using home healthcare services. Am J Geriatr Psychiatry 2006;14:758–66.

[93] Rowe JL, Bruce ML, Conwell Y. Correlates of suicide among home health care utilizers who died by suicide and community controls. Suicide Life Threat Behav 2006;36:65–75.

[94] Wagner BM. Family risk factors for child and adolescent suicidal behavior. Psychol Bull 1997;121:246–98.

[95] Brent DA, Baugher M, Bridge J, et al. Age and sex-related risk factors for adolescent suicide. J Am Acad Child Adolesc Psychiatry 1999;38:1497–505.

[96] Fergusson DM, Lynskey MT. Childhood circumstances, adolescent adjustment, and suicide attempts in a New Zealand birth cohort. J Am Acad Child Adolesc Psychiatry 1995;34:612–22.

[97] Jacobson NS, Dobson KS, Truax PA, et al. A component analysis of cognitive-behavioral treatment for depression. J Consult Clin Psychol 1996;64(2):295–304.

[98] Jacobson NS, Schamaling KB, Holtzworth-Munroe A. Component analysis of behavioral marital therapy: 2-year follow-up and prediction of relapse. J Marital Fam Ther 1987;13:187–95.

[99] Jacobson NS, Holtzworth-Munroe A, Schmaling KB. Marital therapy and spouse involvement in the treatment of depression, agoraphobia and alcoholism. J Consult Clin Psychol 1989;57:5–10.

[100] Jacobson NS, Dobson K, Frizzetti AE, et al. Marital therapy as a treatment for depression. J Consult Clin Psychol 1991;59:547–57.

[101] Dervic K, Oquendo MA, Currier D, et al. Moral objections to suicide: can they counteract suidiality in patients with cluster B psychopathology? J Clin Psychiatry 2006;67:620–5.

[102] Gur M, Miller L, Warner V, et al. Maternal depression and the intergenerational transmission of religion. J Nerv Ment Dis 2005;193:338–45.

[103] Borowsky IW, Ireland M, Resnick MD. Adolescent suicide attempts: risks and protectors. Pediatrics 2001;107:485–93.

[104] Oquendo MA, Dragatsi D, Harkavy-Friedman J, et al. Protective factors against suicidal behavior in Latinos. J Nerv Ment Dis 2005;193:438–43.

[105] Malone KM, Oquendo MA, Haas GL, et al. Protective factors against suicidal acts in major depression: reasons for living. Am J Psychiatry 2000;157:1084–8.

[106] Fergusson DM, Horwood L, Lynskey MT. Childhood sexual abuse and psychiatric disorder in young adulthood: II. Psychiatric outcomes of childhood sexual abuse. J Am Acad Child Adolesc Psychiatry 1996;35:1365–74.

[107] Fergusson DM, Lynskey MT, Horwood LJ. Childhood sexual abuse and psychiatric disorder in young adulthood: I. Prevalence of sexual abuse and factors associated with sexual abuse. J Am Acad Child Adolesc Psychiatry 1996;35:1355–64.

[108] Brown J, Cohen P, Johnson JG, et al. Childhood abuse and neglect: specificity of effects on adolescent and young adult depression and suicidality. J Am Acad Child Adolesc Psychiatry 1999;38:1490–6.

[109] Borowsky IW, Resnick MD, Ireland M, et al. Suicide attempts among American Indian and Alaska native youth: risk and protective factors. Arch Pediatr Adolesc Med 1999;153:573–80.

[110] Molnar BE, Buka SL, Kessler RC. Child sexual abuse and subsequent psychopathology: results from the National Comorbidity Survey. Am J Public Health 2001;91:753–60.

[111] Herrenkohl EC, Herrenkohl RC, Toedter LJ. Perspectives on the intergenerational transmission of abuse. In: Finkelhor D, Gelles RJ, Hotaling GT, et al, editors. The dark side of families: current family violence research. Beverly Hills (CA): Sage; 1983. p. 305–16.

[112] Caspi A, McClay J, Moffitt TE, et al. Role of genotype in the cycle of violence in maltreated children. Science 2002;297:851–4.

[113] Caspi A, Sugden K, Moffitt TE, et al. Influence of life stress on depression: moderation by a polymorphism in the 5-HT gene. Science 2003;301:386–9.

[114] Molnar BE, Berkman LF, Buka SL. Psychopathology, childhood sexual abuse and other childhood adversities: relative links to subsequent suicidal behavior in the U.S. Psychol Med 2001;31:965–77.

[115] Dinwiddie S, Heath AC, Dunne MP, et al. Early sexual abuse and lifetime psychopathology: a co-twin-control study. Psychol Med 2000;30:41–52.

[116] Francis D, Diorio J, Liu D, et al. Nongenomic transmission across generations of maternal behavior and stress responses in the rat. Science 1999;286:1155–8.

[117] Liu D, Diorio J, Day JC, et al. Maternal care, hippocampal synaptogenesis and cognitive development in rats. Nat Neurosci 2000;3:799–806.

[118] Anisman H, Zaharia M, Meaney M, et al. Do early-life events permanently alter behavioral and hormonal responses to stressors? Int J Dev Neurosci 1998;16:149–64.

[119] DeBellis MD. Developmental traumatology: the psychobiological development of maltreated children and its implications for research, treatment, and policy. Dev Psychopathol 2001;13:539–64.

[120] Manuck SB, Flory JD, McCaffery JM, et al. Aggression, impulsivity, and central nervous system serotonergic responsivity in a nonpatient sample. Neuropsychopharmacology 1998;19:287–99.

[121] Mann JJ. Neurobiology of suicidal behavior. Nat Rev Neurosci 2003;4:819–28.

[122] Champoux M, Bennett A, Shannon C, et al. Serotonin transporter gene polymorphism, differential early rearing, and behavior in rhesus monkey neonates. Mol Psychiatry 2002;7:1058–63.

[123] Pine DS, Coplan J, Wasserman GA, et al. Neuroendocrine response to fenfluramine challenge in boys. Associations with aggressive behavior and adverse rearing. Arch Gen Psychiatry 1997;54:839–46.

[124] Kaufman J, Birmaher B, Perel J, et al. Serotonergic functioning in depressed abused children: clinical and familial correlates. Biol Psychiatry 1998;44:973–81.

[125] Rutter M, Dunn J, Plomin R, et al. Integrating nature and nurture: implications of person-environment correlations and interactions for developmental psychopathology. Dev Psychopathol 1997;9:335–64.

[126] Kelleher K, Chaffin M, Hollenberg J, et al. Alcohol and drug disorders among physically abusive and neglectful parents in a community-based sample. Am J Public Health 1994;84:1586–90.

[127] Eaves L, Silberg J, Erkanli A. Resolving multiple epigenetic pathways to adolescent depression. J Child Psychol Psychiatry 2003;44:1006–14.

[128] Kaufman J, Yang BZ, Douglas-Palumberi H, et al. Brain-derived neurotrophic factor-5-HTTLPR gene interactions and environmental modifiers of depression in children. Biol Psychiatry 2006;59:673–80.

[129] Zalsman G, Huang Y-Y, Oquendo MA, et al. Association of a triallelic serotonin transporter gene promoter polymorphism region (5-HTTLPR), with stressful life events and severity of depression. Am J Psychiatry 2006;163:1588–93.

[130] Kaufman J, Yang BZ, Douglas-Palumberi H, et al. Social supports and serotonin transporter gene moderate depression in maltreated children. Proc Natl Acad Sci U S A 2004;101:17316–21.

[131] Fergusson DM, Lynskey MT. Adolescent resiliency to family adversity. J Child Psychol Psychiatry 1996;37:281–92.

[132] Fergusson DM, Woodward LJ, Horwood LJ. Risk factors and life processes associated with the onset of suicidal behaviour during adolescence and early adulthood. Psychol Med 2000;30:23–39.

Psychiatr Clin N Am 31 (2008) 179–203

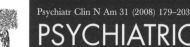

PSYCHIATRIC CLINICS
OF NORTH AMERICA

The Genetics of Suicide: A Critical Review of Molecular Studies

Jelena Brezo, PhD, Tim Klempan, PhD,
Gustavo Turecki, MD, PhD*

Department of Psychiatry, McGill Group for Suicide Studies,
6875 La Salle Boulevard, Montreal, Quebec, H4H 1R3, Canada

S uicidal behaviors (SBs), which include completed and attempted suicide and suicidal ideation, are associated with considerable challenges for individuals, families, and public health systems. The multifactorial character of SBs is evident in the diversity of associated correlates and risk factors. In addition to family and personal histories of psychopathology, proximal and distal environmental factors, including stressful life events and childhood abuse, may contribute as vulnerability or precipitating factors to various forms of SBs. Researchers are increasingly recognizing that these typically unshared environmental inputs may not be exclusively additive in character, but instead may be moderated by genetic factors, as in other complex diseases.

Genetic epidemiology studies suggest that genetic contribution is quantitatively somewhat weaker than the environmental one. The association-based quest for specific candidate genes and variants participating in the genetic diathesis for SBs has had a decidedly mixed success. This article reviews genetic association studies of suicidal phenotypes published to date; discusses relevant theoretical, methodological, and operational challenges; and suggests future avenues for research.

GENETIC EPIDEMIOLOGY

Over the past 30 years, indirect evidence for the existence of a genetic component in the suicidal diathesis has come largely from family, twin, and adoption studies. An adjusted meta-analysis of 21 family studies [1] estimated that close relatives of suicidal probands have a three times higher risk for engaging in suicidal acts compared with controls, irrespective of psychiatric history. A substantial familial component was confirmed by Kim and colleagues [2] who compared SBs in relatives of suicide completers with community controls. After adjusting for psychopathology, they found relatives of suicide completers to

This work was supported by the Canadian Institutes of Health Research: Grant MOP 151060.

*Corresponding author. E-mail address: gustavo.turecki@mcgill.ca (G. Turecki).

have a ten times greater risk for suicide and suicide attempts and more severe suicidal ideation than controls.

Familial predisposition to SBs was also shown in a large-scale, population-based Swedish study focusing on individuals hospitalized for suicide attempts between 1968 and 1980. Investigators reported that suicide attempts or completions in parents and suicide attempts in siblings increased the risk for proband suicide attempts between two and three times. Furthermore, family history of suicide was strongly associated with earlier onset suicide attempts and male gender [3]. Overall, family studies have indicated that heritability may be lowest for suicidal ideation, somewhat higher for suicide attempts, and highest for suicide completions [1,4].

Unlike family-based designs, twin studies allow for a better control of the influences of the shared environment. After pooling published twin studies, Baldessarini and colleagues [1] found a 175 times higher relative risk among monozygotic twins (MZTs) than dizygotic twins (DZTs). However, the authors urged caution in interpreting these results, given the low prevalence of SBs in twins and lack of control of postnatal environmental influences. Specifically regarding suicidal ideation, a recent twin study found only a statistical trend for its concordance in MZTs compared with DZTs [5].

Adoption studies have been scarce and based primarily on Danish public health records. These investigations suggested a 7 to 13 times higher risk for suicidality among biologic relatives of adoptees than among adopted relatives, and stronger heritability for suicide completions than attempts [6,7]. These estimates must be considered in light of several limitations, including low number of adoption studies, poor control of psychiatric confounders, lack of more recent adoption data, and shortage of data from other countries.

MOLECULAR GENETICS OF SUICIDE
Neurotransmitter Systems
Guided by the twin-, adoption-, and family-based evidence suggesting the existence of genetic diathesis for SBs, molecular studies began to look for specific genetic components of this diathesis. The candidate-based association approach has been the dominant strategy, and close to 50 candidate genes have been investigated. Spurred by the wealth of neurobiologic knowledge, molecular geneticists focused primarily on neurotransmitter systems and less on genes outside of these systems. The following sections review evidence from genetic association studies of SBs, and Tables 1 and 2 provide additional information on statistically significant studies.

Serotonergic candidates
Association studies have investigated variation in serotonergic genes involved in the transport (serotonin transporter), transmission (nine receptor genes), catabolism (tryptophan hydroxylase genes), and anabolism (monoamino oxidase A) of serotonin (see Table 1). The intense focus on this system is not surprising given the scope of its action, especially its roles in brain development and

mood and behavior regulation. Several lines of evidence have shown reduced serotonergic activity in individuals who have histories of SBs. Suicidal individuals seem to have reduced cerebrospinal fluid levels of 5-hydroxyindole acetic acid (5-HIAA), one of the main serotonergic metabolites [8]. Plasma levels of serotonin correlate negatively with the severity of SBs among suicidal adolescents [9]. Also, pharmacologic challenge tests using serotonergic agonists show a blunted prolactin response in suicide attempters, a potential marker of the lethality of the method [10]. Additional biochemical studies indicate alterations in the binding and density of the transporter and receptors, especially in the ventral prefrontal cortex (PFC) [11].

Serotonin transporter (SLC6A4). Of the 12 genes responsible for serotonergic turnover and transmission examined to date, SLC6A4 has received the most research attention. Its product regulates the duration of the serotonergic signal [12]. All molecular genetic studies focused exclusively on two of its variants, the 44-base promoter deletion/insertion (LPR) and its associated S/L alleles, respectively, and a VNTR polymorphism in intron 2. Of the 44 studies, approximately 20 have linked the former variant to predisposition to suicide attempts, finding S allele carriers to have an elevation in risk ranging between 1.7 and 6.5 times.

An early meta-analysis of 12 studies confirmed the association between this promoter variant and suicide attempts but not completions [13]. A subsequent meta-analysis found an overrepresentation of S genotypes in suicide attempters ($P = .004$) and violent suicides ($P = .0001$) relative to controls [14]. In the most recent meta-analysis, association with this locus was confirmed in 39 studies conducted in European and Asian populations [14].

Only a few studies have reported statistically significant association of VNTR-2 and suicide. Its 10-repeat allele was associated with suicidal outcomes in patients who had depression [15] and with suicide attempts in those who had schizophrenia [16]. Furthermore, close to a half of all association studies investigating SLC6A4 across diverse populations have found no association of its two variants with suicide [17,18] or suicide attempts [19–24].

Serotonin receptor genes. Other serotonergic genes, such as those coding for serotonin receptors and catabolizing enzymes, have been studied less often and with mixed success, as illustrated in Table 1. Only limited support was found for the involvement of receptor HTR1A [25–27]. Similarly, only one small study showed an association with HTR1B; the remaining investigations found no association with either suicide or suicide attempts [27–30]. Variants in other receptors from this class (HTR1D, 1E, and 1F) were not associated with suicide completions in French Canadian [31] and Slovenian study samples [30]. Finally, examination of HTR2C, HTR5A, and HTR6 receptor gene polymorphisms yielded no significant results in relation to suicide risk [26,31,32].

The HTR2A receptor gene may be the most promising serotonergic receptor gene. Its protein product is present at an increased density in some brain areas of suicide victims [11]. In a postmortem and genetic study, carriers of the

Table 1
Significant associations between serotonergic genes and suicidal behaviors

Gene (total number of studies)	Suicidal behavior	Sample (age mean ± SD)
SLC6A4 (44)	High-lethality suicide attempts	Attempters (20 ± 2 y) [147]
	Suicide attempts	Women, 33 ± 14 y; men, 34 ± 16 y [148]
	Suicide attempts	Schizophrenic (41 ± 11 y) [16]
	Impulsive suicide attempts	Obsessive–compulsive (39 ± 12 y)/impulsive (34 ± 13 y) women [149]
	Suicide attempts	Alcohol-dependent men (44 ± 10 y) [150]
	Repeated suicide attempts	MDD/schizophrenia RSAs (34 ± 12 y), nonRSAs (38 ± 14) [151]
	Suicide attempts	Major depression or schizophrenia [152]
	Suicide attempts	Schizophrenia or schizoaffective [153]
	Violent suicide attempts	Attempters, women (32 ± 9 y) [154]
	Suicide attempts	Alcohol dependence (43 ± 20 y) [155]
	Suicide attempts	Violent attempters (42 ± 8 y) [156]
	Violent suicide attempts	Unipolar/bipolar disorder (39 ± 13 y) [157]
	Violent suicide attempts	Alcoholic men [158]
	Suicide attempts	Healthy volunteers (44 ± 11 y) [159]
	Suicide attempts	Depressed completers who had family history of suicide attempts [160]
	Suicide	Completers (41 ± 17 y) [161]
	Suicide	Completers (46 ± 16 y) [162]
	Suicide	Depressed completers (51 ± 20 y) [163]
	Suicide	Depressed completers (42 ± 15 y) [15]
	Suicide	Completers (52 ± 19 y) [144]
	Suicide	Completers (51 ± 19 y) [164]
	Suicide attempts and ideation	Birth cohort (26 y) [132]
	Suicide attempts	Psychiatric patients (SS/SL: 37 ± 11 y; LL: 35 ± 12 y) [133]
5HT1A (5)	Suicide	Mood-disordered, Ontario Caucasians (43 ± 11 y) [165]
5HT1B (10)	Suicide attempts	Personality disordered, White (38 ± 10 y) [166]
5HT2A (23)	Nonviolent/ impulsive attempts	German (40 ± 13 y) [167]
	Suicide attempts	Major depression, Spanish (55 ± 16 y) [168]
	Suicide attempts	Major depression, Caucasian (39 ± 9 y) [169]
	Suicide attempts	Bipolar depression I, Caucasian (45 ± 14 y) [170]

(continued on next page)

Table 1
(continued)

Gene (total number of studies)	Suicidal behavior	Sample (age mean ± SD)
MAOA (9)	Violent suicide attempts	West European, Caucasian men (38 ± 14 y) [171]
	Suicide	Hungarian, Caucasian men (48 ± 14 y) [172]
	Suicide attempts	Depressed patients, English, Caucasian [48]
TPH2 (8)	Suicide attempts	Depressed patients, Han Chinese (33 ± 12 y) [173]
	Suicide	Southern German (47 ± 18 y) [174]
	Suicide attempts	Bipolar probands (35 ± 10 y) [175]
	Suicide	Depressed French Canadian (41.8 ± 14.7 y) [47]
TPH1 (33)	Repeated (suicide) attempts	Alcoholic offenders, Finnish Caucasian [176]
	Suicide attempts (violent)	Women, 36 ± 14 y; men, 36 ± 13 y [177]
	Suicide attempts	Han Chinese (46 ± 13 y) [178]
	Suicide attempts	Major depression, Chinese [179]
	Suicide	Completers, men (74 of 247 > 65 y) [141]
	Suicide	Completers (32 ± 9 y) [180]
	Suicide attempts	Patients who had schizophrenia, Korean (30 ± 9 y) [181]
	Suicide attempts (impulsive)	Alcoholic violent offenders, men of mixed ethnicities [182]
	Suicide attempts (impulsive)	Violent offenders, men (31 ± 1 y) [183]
	Suicide attempts	Major depression, Caucasian, European origin (35 ± 14 y) [184]
	Suicide attempts	Borderline–disordered, Stockholm, female (31 ± 8 y) [185]
	Suicide	Co-twins of completers, Swedish (69 ± 9 y) [186]

Abbreviation: MDD, major depressive disorder.

HRT2A 102T allele had a higher receptor density than those who had its C102 allele [33]. Genetic association studies in HTR2A implicated primarily the T102C polymorphism. However, subsequent meta-analyses based on 9, and more recently 25, studies failed to confirm its involvement [13,34]. The latter study suggested a significant role for the allele A of the A1438G variant, however. Given the high proportion of negative studies [33,35–38], more research is necessary, especially considering the possible mechanisms of HTR2A action, which may involve genetic imprinting [39,40].

Supporting genes.
   Tryptophan hydroxylase. Tryptophan hydroxylase 1 (*TPH1*) was the first serotonergic gene to be studied and the subject of more than 30 studies. Supportive evidence for completed suicide and repeated, impulsive, and violent suicide

Table 2
Significant associations between nonserotonergic genes and suicidal behaviors

Gene (total number of studies)	Suicidal behavior	Sample (age mean ± SD)
Noradrenergic/dopaminergic genes		
COMT (8)	Violent suicide attempts	German (40 ± 13 y) [187]
	Violent suicide attempts	Finish/non-Saami men (42 y), USA White/Hispanic men (43 y) [188]
	Suicide	Japanese men (47 ± 20 y) [189]
DRD2 (2)	Suicide attempts and ideation	Alcoholic inpatients, Caucasian German (43 ± 10 y) [190]
	Suicide attempts	Alcoholic patients, Caucasian German (43 ± 9 y) [191]
TH (4)	Suicide attempts	Adjustment-disordered patients, Swedish (41 y) [192]
Neurotrophic genes		
BDNF (3)	Violent suicide attempts	Caucasian (39.8 + 12.9 y) [81]
Other candidates genes		
PC 1 Duarte (1)	Suicide	Neurologic diseases [193]
ACE (2)	Suicide	Japanese (women:48 ± 16 y; men: 49 ± 20 y) [89]
YWHAE (1)	Suicide	Japanese (48 ± 18 y) [194]
SCN8A	Suicide attempts	Ukrainian (exploration: 23 ± 7 y; validation: 25 ± 8 y) [94]
VAMP4 (1)	Suicide attempts	Ukrainian (exploration: 23 ± 7 y; validation: 25 ± 8 y) [94]
RABAC1 (1)	Suicide attempts	Ukrainian (exploration: 23 ± 7 y; validation: 25 ± 8 y) [94]
CCK (1)	Suicide	Japanese men (age range: 17–92 y) [195]
WSF1 (3)	Suicide	French Canadian (32 ± 9 y) [196]
APOE4 (2)	Suicide attempts	Geriatric depressed, Chinese (75 ± 5 y) [142]
CREB1 (1)	Suicidal ideas	Men who had MDD treated with citalopram, USA (42.5 ± 13.4 y) [95]
RGS2 (1)	Suicide	Japanese: 189 (47.8 ± 17.5 y) [96]
NOS-I (1)	Suicide attempts	German (39.9 ± 13.9 y) [116]
NOS-III (2)	Suicide	Suicide attempters, German (39.9 ± 13.9 y) [116]
TBX19	Suicide attempts	Individuals with high angry/hostility scores, Ukrainian [85]
CRHR2	Suicide attempt severity	Bipolar families, Toronto (35.4 ± 10.4 y) [75]

Abbreviation: MDD, major depressive disorder.

attempts has been offered by approximately 37% of these studies (see Table 1). Much like the individual investigations, however, meta-analyses have disagreed about the significance of the variation in this gene. The earliest meta-analysis found no association with SBs [41]. Another showed increased risk in carriers of the A218 allele in Caucasian suicide attempters and victims [42]. A more recent meta-analysis indicated that A218C polymorphism confers a 60% increased risk for SBs [43]. The most recent investigation of TPH1 effects examined results from 22 studies, finding strong genotypic and allelic evidence for A779C/A218C but not the A6526G single nucleotide polymorphism (SNP) [44].

These positive findings have, however, been criticized because *TPH1* is primarily expressed in the periphery, its significantly associated SNPs are intronic and unrelated to splicing or exon skipping, and it exhibits high exonic homology with *TPH2* [45]. *TPH2* is a recently identified gene, found to be preferentially expressed in the brain stem and relevant to several psychiatric phenotypes through its involvement in amygdala-mediated responses to emotional stimuli [46]. This gene also seems to have significant allelic, genotypic, and haplotypic relationships with suicidal acts (see Table 1). For example, in a sample of 114 individuals who had depression and committed suicide, homozygosity for T and G alleles in its rs4448371 and rs4641527 variants, respectively, was associated with a fivefold increase in suicide risk, even after adjustment for confounders [47].

Similar to other candidate genes, attempts to replicate *TPH1* and *TPH2* associations have been unsuccessful, encompassing study populations with different psychiatric diagnoses, such as mood disorders [48], schizophrenia [49], and alcohol dependence [50], and ethnic membership: Brazilian [51], German [52], Jewish [53], Swedish [54], and Japanese [55].

Monoamine oxidase A. Monoamine oxidase A (*MAOA*) is an X-linked gene (Xp11.23) responsible for oxidative deamination of bioamines, such as central and peripheral serotonin and noradrenaline. Of the 9 studies examining *MAOA* variation, 6 focused exclusively on a promoter VNTR (variable number of tandem repeats). This variant was linked to suicide and violent suicide attempts in men and violent suicide attempts in depressed patients (see Table 1). A recent study investigated Fnu4I, finding its I/I genotypes of relevance in women who had depression [48]. Other studies failed to showed allelic, haplotypic, or epistatic effects of MAOA variants on suicide attempts [55–59].

Noradrenergic and dopaminergic genes

Because SBs are often precipitated by stressful events, systems involved in stress response regulation, such as noradrenergic and dopaminergic systems, are important targets for genetic research [60]. Neurobiologic findings indicate that noradrenaline levels and noradrenergic neurons may be reduced and alpha 2-adrenoceptor binding elevated in the brain stem of suicide victims [61]. Moreover, the byproducts of dopamine metabolism, homovanillic acid and 3-methoxy-4-hydroxyphenylglycol, seem to be higher in individuals who commit violent suicides [62].

In contrast, brain stem levels of tyrosine hydroxylase (TH), the rate limiting-enzyme in the synthesis of noradrenaline and dopamine, are reduced [63]. Specifically, immunoreactivity of TH is decreased in the locus coeruleus of suicide completers [64]. Genetic evidence shows that the TH-K3 allele of the *TH* gene may be related to the risk for suicide attempts in a Swedish Caucasian sample with adjustment disorders (see Table 2). Supportive evidence for its Val81Met and Val468Met association with suicide, however, has not been found in a comparison of 189 suicide victims and 187 controls [65].

DRD2 was, nevertheless, the only dopamine-specific gene to be linked to nonfatal SBs, with its 141Cdel allele conferring a 30% and its E8 allele a 70% increased risk in patients who had alcohol dependence. Neither *DRD2* nor *TH* gene variation mattered in a sample of English suicide attempters who had depressive disorders [48]. Nonsignificant findings have been reported for several variants: microsatellites in exon III of DRD4 [66,67]; an exon 15 VNTR of the dopamine transporter gene (SLC6A3) [68]; G1800T, C1291G, G261A, and N251K variants in the ADRA2A gene [69]; and G1287A SNP found in SLC6A2 [70].

The most studied supporting enzyme in adrenergic and dopaminergic systems has been the catechol-O-methyltransferase (COMT), responsible for metabolizing the breakdown of levodopa into 3-O-methyldopa. Genetic studies examined exclusively its Val158Met SNP, reporting a positive relationship between the low-activity Met allele and violent suicide attempts in two European samples and a negative association between Val/Val genotypes and suicide risk in Japanese individuals (see Table 2). No association was otherwise found between this variant and suicide in patients who have schizophrenia [56] or depression [71,72].

Hypothalamic-pituitary-adrenal axis genes
Altered hypothalamic-pituitary-adrenal (HPA) axis activity may be related to the risk of SBs. The cerebrospinal fluid of suicidal individuals has elevated levels of corticotropin-releasing factor and corticotropin-releasing hormone [73]. The frontal cortex has fewer binding sites for corticotropin-releasing hormone and reduced plasma adrenocorticotropin and cortisol responsiveness [74]. Variation in only one HPA gene seems to have been studied in relation to suicide risk; the CRCH2 gene's haplotype 5-2-3 was positively associated with the severity of SBs (see Table 2) [75].

Neurotrophic, GABAergic, and glutamatergic genes
Brain-derived neurotrophic factor (BDNF), the most abundant neurotrophin in the brain, may be lower in the plasma of patients who are suicidal than in those who are nonsuicidal and depressed, although it seems to be unrelated to the lethality of suicide attempts [76]. Its mRNA was, however, reduced in the hippocampus and PFC of individuals who committed suicide [76].

Association studies have examined three neurotrophic genes (*NOTCH4*, *NGFR*, and *BDNF*). None exhibited main effects [77–80]. In a sample of 813 Caucasian suicide attempters, however, *BDNF* was implicated if considered in the context of environment; only Val/Val genotype conferred risk for violent suicide attempts in individuals reporting childhood sexual abuse. Furthermore, maltreatment severity was significantly associated with the number and age of onset of suicide attempts [81].

Although expression data suggest alterations in γ-aminobutyric acid (GABA) and glutamate system neurotransmission [82], very few association studies have examined their genetic variation. None of the four published studies investigating GABAergic and glutamatergic gene variation showed support for its relevance to SBs. Genes examined include glutamate decarboxylase 1 and 2 [83] and GABA receptor alpha-3 [84] and alpha-5 genes [85], each subject of one study.

Other Candidate Genes

Since 1979, approximately 20 genes outside the major systems reviewed earlier were studied for association with SBs in diverse ethnic samples. Most of these candidates are involved in signaling and transport, with a few participating in lipid metabolism, deoxidation, and gene transcription.

Both adenylyl cyclase and phosphoinositide signaling systems and their components may contribute to vulnerability to SBs. The cyclic AMP response element-binding protein (CREB), a transcription factor shared by both systems and important to genes expressed in neurons, is one such component [86]. Its mRNA and protein products may be significantly decreased in the PFC, although not in the hippocampus of adolescent individuals who commit suicide [87].

The renin-angiotensin system may also be involved in suicidal diathesis through affecting the HPA axis by way of corticotropin-releasing hormone [88]. The angiotensin-converting enzyme (*ACE*) gene is one of its key components. The presence of one or two 287-bp Alu repeat sequences in intron 16 of this gene confers an increased suicide risk of 50% and 80%, respectively [89]. Homozygosity for this allele also correlates negatively with serum ACE levels [90].

Nitric oxide synthase (NOS) 1 and 3 genes were recently investigated in suicide risk. Selected haplotypes and single-SNP alleles in NOS 1 may be related to suicide attempts, and to suicide completions in NOS 3 (see Table 2).

As many as eight genes involved in lipid and cholesterol metabolism have been investigated as candidates for SBs (see Table 2). This exploration is not surprising, given that lower cholesterol has been found in the orbitofrontal and ventral PFC of individuals who commit violent suicide compared with those who commit nonviolent suicides [91]. Deficiency in the 7-dehydrocholesterol reductase (DHCR7) enzyme involved in cholesterol biosynthesis, which underlies the Smith-Lemli-Opitz syndrome, may also be responsible for a fourfold increase in suicidal acts in relatives of carriers of this syndrome compared with controls [92]. Gene association study of this and related cholesterol-metabolizing genes (HMGCR, DHCR7, LPL, LDLR, and APOE) could not relate variation to the increased risk for suicide in French Canadian completers [93].

Nevertheless, apolipoprotein E4 (*APOE4*) and cholecystokinin (*CCK*) genes were linked to risk for suicide attempts in geriatric patients who had depression and to the risk for suicide in Japanese men, respectively (see Table 2). Other promising candidates awaiting independent replications are *SCN8A* and *VAMP4* [94]; *CREB1* [95]; the regulator of G-protein signaling 2 [96]; and renin–angiotensin system genes [89]. *ABCG1* [97], *MNSOD* [98], and *ESR1* [99] gene investigations yielded negative findings.

Conclusions

Knowing which genes and polymorphisms influence susceptibility or severity of SBs may be useful in preventing and managing this important public health problem. The first 30 years of candidate-based association studies, unfortunately, provided little information about specific gene contributors.

The most studied system focused on the serotonin transporter and *TPH* genes, with suggestive evidence for these genes and MAOA. Adrenergic and dopaminergic genes, particularly *DRD2*, *TH*, and *COMT*, deserve more attention before firm conclusions can be made. Genetic candidates outside these major neurotransmitter systems require independent replications before preliminary positive results can be further considered. The modest success of candidate-based association studies can be attributed to theoretical, operational, and methodological challenges addressed in the next section.

THEORETICAL ISSUES
Lack of a Unified Theory and Working Hypotheses

Over the years, suicidologists studying SBs from different perspectives have developed discipline-specific models to guide their research. Little effort has been spent on building a unified, cross-disciplinary theory necessary to integrate the many seemingly disparate risk factors and guide the selection of candidate genes. This model would need to recognize that contribution of individual genes to multifactorial phenotypes such as SBs must be understood in the context of internal (gene–gene interactions) and external environments (precipitating stressful and traumatic events). It should also help explain the relationship between genes and SBs through identifying relevant mediating endophenotypes along with demographic and other moderators of this relationship (Fig. 1).

Past theoretical models have had a somewhat narrow and static focus, giving priority exclusively to one or only a few components implicated in the risk for SBs, such as possible neuropsychologic endophenotypes [100]. Other models have recognized the interactive relationship between suicide-precipitating stressors and trait-like diathesis [101], but failed to hypothesize on the specific components of that diathesis. The same omission is characteristic of the "top-down" models attempting to understand interrelationships among SBs in terms of their severity and natural history [102].

Regarding genetic diathesis, these theories have limited value, except to suggest that the more serious the phenotype, the stronger its heritability, making it more amenable to detecting small genetic effects. Unfortunately, they do not allow hypotheses to be made about specific genes. This lack of more targeted, suicidality-specific hypotheses has been a major hurdle in the field. So far, gene and SNP candidates have been the same ones studied across several psychiatric phenotypes. In addition to the traditionally used neurobiologic evidence, generation of new, more targeted hypotheses necessitates new approaches, such as genome-wide association, linkage, and microarray gene expression studies.

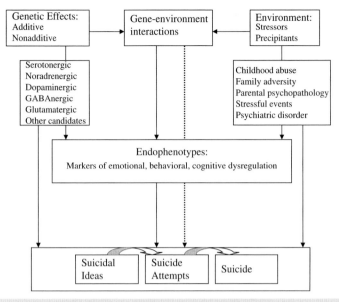

Fig. 1. Integrating risk factors and correlates of suicidal behaviors.

Microarray Studies

Gene expression microarrays allow the evaluation of tens of thousands of mRNA transcripts on a single chip, permitting the identification of gene expression patterns characterizing clinical phenotypes of interest and providing the potential for focus on specific gene systems. Used most widely in cancer research, microarray approaches are now becoming commonplace in psychiatric studies, where notable advantages include the non–hypothesis-directed nature of the design, the high throughput capabilities of the approach, and the more direct connection to biologic changes than pure genetic approaches. More recently, a few studies have investigated the suicide phenotype using microarray expression platforms [82,103]. An interesting lead from these studies concerns alterations in the cortical expression of spermidine/spermine N^1-acetyltransferase [104], a finding that is consistent with expression data from animal models of depression [105]. Independent replications [106] of this finding suggest that alterations in the polyamine system may be involved in the neurobiology of major depression or suicide.

Microarray studies may also be useful in elucidating biologic processes and relevant gene–gene interactions. A good example is a recent German study implicating molecules involved in cell adhesion and proliferation in the context of suicide with and without a history of depression [107].

Linkage Studies

The first linkage efforts used families ascertained through psychiatric phenotypes with comorbid SBs. Since 2004, acyl-CoA binding protein and protein kinase C loci were found to be linked to suicide attempts in families with histories of alcohol dependence [108]. Two bipolar pedigrees showed linkage to completed and attempted suicide [109], singling out two candidate genes (*TACR1* and *TGOLN2*) for suicide attempts [110]. An early linkage study in families with major depressive disorder identified six loci for suicide risk, none of which contained known candidate genes [111].

Similar to the dominant, case-control–based approach in candidate gene studies of SBs, samples used in linkage studies are clinical and heterogeneous. Disentangling susceptibility genes for suicidality from those for other psychiatric phenotypes is challenging and raises the following questions: how different are susceptibility genes/alleles across comorbid psychiatric phenotypes (ie, are suicides committed within the context of an Axis II disorder different from those comorbid with Axis I disorders); are there suicide-specific susceptibility genes or are pleiotropy and, consequently, phenomes present? More generally, can different alleles of the same gene be responsible for different psychiatric outcomes or, alternatively, is the ultimate psychiatric outcome of an allele determined by environment?

OPERATIONAL AND METHODOLOGICAL ISSUES
Refining the Phenotype

Adding to the challenge of identifying small-sized genetic effects underlying multifactorial phenotypes are phenotypic complexity, imprecise terminology, and high degree of subjectivity associated with the ascertainment of SBs. The terminology in the field is ambiguous and entails a fair degree of subjective interpretation. Related problems include lack of operational definitions of suicidal intent and lethality and of universally accepted classification schemes [112]. For example, a review of family studies [1] found risk estimates to be heavily affected by the definitions of suicidal phenotypes and methods of case ascertainment.

Identifying moderators

Phenotypic refinement should extend beyond considerations of subphenotypes of SBs proper. Stratification based on demographic moderators (sex, age, and ethnicity) could help more easily identify distinct, possibly more homogeneous subgroups and associated genetic factors. Studies have mainly done this with sex and much less with age and ethnicity. Careful characterization of ethnic composition [112] crucial for addressing population stratification and preventing spurious findings is, unfortunately, still missing in many association studies. Similar to other research fields, often only national origin may be reported, or ambiguous and diverse labels such as *Caucasian* or *West European*. Reliable self-reports would at a minimum require information on participants' nationality, native language, and ethnic membership at least up to the second-generation ancestors.

Identifying mediators: endophenotypes

SBs must be refined not only using moderators but also using possible mediators, ie, endophenotypes. Association of endophenotypes with genes may be easier to detect because they are, by definition, more proximal to genetic factors than the typically later-onset phenotypes such as SBs. Additionally, endophenotypes may indicate mechanisms of action and intermediate steps and processes [113].

Personality traits as endophenotypes. Personality traits are useful markers of maladaptive behaviors (impulsive aggression, dissocial behavior, and stimulus/novelty-seeking), emotions (neuroticism, harm avoidance, anxiousness, and affective instability), and cognitions (cognitive rigidity, perfectionism, and impaired decision making). Impulsivity, aggression, and impulsive aggression, traits that seem to segregate with SBs (i.e., aggressive relatives of suicide completers have a higher risk for suicide than their nonaggressive counterparts) may be especially useful endophenotypes for SBs [4]. Impulsive-aggressive behaviors in adolescents and their parents increase the risk for suicide in adolescents [114]. Suicide attempters and completers are more impulsive than controls [115].

Evidence linking genes and these personality traits has been accumulating. Level of aggression was linked to variation in *NOS III* [116], *ABCG1* [117], *SLC6A3* [68], and *SLC6A4* genes [118], and 5-HIAA levels [119]. Perhaps the best supported is the relationship of *MAOA* gene and aggressive behaviors. In humans, low MAOA activity has been associated with impulsivity and aggression. A study of a large family showed male members who had a nonsense mutation in exon 8 of this gene to display, among other symptoms, impulsive aggression [120]. Community-sample men who had low-activity MAOA alleles exhibited significantly lower aggressiveness and impulsivity than men who had the more efficient alleles [121]. Similar associations were found in animal models [122].

With emotional dysregulation, research has implicated the traits of anger and anxiety. Anxious traits are one of the earliest markers of emotional dysregulation to be linked to the serotonergic system and particularly *SLC6A4* [123], *HTR2A* [124], and *TPH2* genes [125]. Anxiety traits have also been linked to *BDNF* [126]. *ABCG1* [117] and *CREB* [87] genes, however, have been linked to anger.

Suicidal individuals exhibit multiple cognitive deficits. In addition to impaired decision making and problem solving, they seem to have lower general intellectual functioning; autobiographical memory and executive function deficits; attention biases; inability to anticipate problems and positive events; and cognitive rigidity [127]. Research into genetic correlates of cognitive deficits is limited. One study has identified a G703T polymorphism effect of the *TPH2* gene on attention performance, excluding the involvement of the Val158Met variant in *COMT* [125].

Exploring the nonadditive effects. With a handful of exceptions, association studies in the field have largely investigated additive effects. Given that genetic and environmental factors contribute substantially to psychiatric risk and exceed additive and linear effects, understanding gene–environment and gene–gene interactions is fundamental [128]. Gene–gene interactions are especially poorly understood, but potentially important in understanding how other loci affect phenotypic expression at the locus of interest. As for gene–environment interactions, genetic polymorphisms can affect the level, type, and intensity of sensitivity to environmental stressors, and the direction and strength of their relationship with psychiatric outcomes [128]. Consequently, a given allele or genotype may render individuals or subpopulations more or less susceptible to SBs only in the presence of a specific environmental stressor, presumably through altering their sensitivity to the impact of that stressor. These types of interactions may explain inconsistent genetic associations and developmental differences in the correlates and risk factors for SBs. For example, distinctiveness of a person's genetic background and environmental context [129] may explain why, depending on the study, S and L alleles of the 5HTLPR polymorphism behave as risk factors for SBs.

Gene-environment interactions. Nonhuman primate studies have shown that suboptimal early environments lead to abnormalities in neuroendocrine stress axis [130]. With human psychopathology, gene–environment interaction has been most convincingly shown to be associated with major depressive disorder [129]. Both positive and negative environmental factors, including family adversity, negative life events, and social support, have been studied as plausible targets of moderation by genes [129], primarily *SLC6A4* [131,132].

Association studies of SBs exploring gene–environment interactions have been rare. Caspi and colleagues [132] showed that having at least one short allele of the SLC6A4-LPR variant doubles the risk for nonfatal SBs in the presence of negative life events. Gibb and colleagues [133] found the same variant to moderate the relationship of childhood sexual and physical, but not emotional, abuse with suicide attempts. As discussed earlier, the most recent gene–environment interaction study found *BDNF* Val/Val genotype to moderate the effect of childhood sexual abuse on violent suicide attempts [81].

The authors' findings have suggested a moderating role for *HTR2A* in the context of childhood sexual abuse and suicide attempts [134]. Their longitudinal, population-based design affords one major advantage over similar studies investigating gene–environment interactions in SBs: the possibility of understanding developmental trends in these interactions that affect final suicidal outcomes and candidate endophenotypes [135,136]. This function is important because genetic effects vary across developmental stages [137], resulting in variable estimates of heritability across age [138]. Genetically determined modulation of environmental impact may plausibly involve gene products involved in behavioral and mood responses to stress across developmental stages [139], which may then explain quantitative and qualitative differences in SBs across ages. For example, younger suicide attempters and completers are more impulsive, whereas older suicides use more violent or lethal methods and plans [115,140]. Younger suicidal individuals may also display a different pattern of serotonergic abnormality than adults, as shown for HTR1A or HTR2A receptor responsiveness [119]. However, despite this evidence, genetic association studies have been primarily cross-sectional, focusing mostly on individuals between ages 30 and 50 years (see Tables 1 and 2); very few examined candidate genes in older suicides [141,142] or suicidal children and adolescents [85,143].

Progress in research depends on recognizing that statistical gene–environment interaction does not automatically equal biologic interaction [129] and that preliminary investigations must be followed by studies investigating mechanisms and consequences of gene–environment interaction, such as epigenetic modification at the DNA level, changes in neurotransmission at the cellular level, or behavioral or mood dysregulation at the level of organism. Second, environmental factors must be measured as comprehensively as possible, to include micro-, meso-, and even macroenvironments. Third, their assessment, much like the assessment of candidate endophenotypes, requires standardized measures to ensure interstudy comparability.

Epistasis. Given the number of systems that have been implicated in SBs, it is necessary to understand whether and to what degree genetic interactions between and within these systems contribute to suicidal diathesis. One association study examined intrasystem interactions indirectly, concluding that the concurrence of low-activity variants in *SLC6A4* and *TPH* genes contributes to suicide risk [144].

Intersystem interactions also deserve more attention. De Luca and colleagues [71] were unable to find evidence for gene–gene interactions between *MAO* and *COMT* in patients who were bipolar and had schizophrenia [56] and had suicide attempt histories. Neurobiologic evidence suggests, however, that interactions are plausible among a number of genes, such as between *HTR2A* or *HTR1A* genes and HPA system components [145] and between serotonergic genes and *BDNF* variants [81]. Examining interactions among key system components, such as rate-limiting enzymes, across systems would also be interesting.

Future research

In addition to the ability to generate targeted hypotheses regarding candidate genes, making adequate and comprehensive selection of candidate polymorphisms is also important. A systematic effort to identify functional variants could greatly improve progress in the field because these variants may play a more direct role in susceptibility to SBs.

A more effective search for specific genes and variants contributing to suicidal diathesis also necessitates a cross-disciplinary approach and consideration of interacting genes and environments. Furthermore, given the complexity of SBs and consistent evidence of moderation by demographic variables, future hypotheses should also focus on testing second-order moderation. For example, serotonergic transmission and personality endophenotypes may be affected by sex hormones or HPA axis hyperactivity [5,146], which would necessitate investigation of how gender and other higher-level moderators affect identified epistatic and gene–environment interactions and endophenotypes in suitably sized samples.

References

[1] Baldessarini RJ, Hennen J. Genetics of suicide: an overview. Harv Rev Psychiatry 2004;12: 1–13.

[2] Kim CD, Seguin M, Therrien N, et al. Familial aggregation of suicidal behavior: a family study of male suicide completers from the general population. Am J Psychiatry 2005;162: 1017–9.

[3] Mittendorfer-Rutz E, Rasmussen F, Wasserman D. Familial clustering of suicidal behaviour and psychopathology in young suicide attempters: a register-based nested case control study. Soc Psychiatry Psychiatr Epidemiol 2007;43:28–36.

[4] Brent DA, Bridge J, Johnson BA, et al. Suicidal behavior runs in families. A controlled family study of adolescent suicide victims. Arch Gen Psychiatry 1996;53:1145–52.

[5] Cho H, Guo G, Iritani BJ, et al. Genetic contribution to suicidal behaviors and associated risk factors among adolescents in the U.S. Prev Sci 2006;7:303–11.

[6] Wender PH, Kety SS, Rosenthal D, et al. Psychiatric disorders in the biological and adoptive families of adopted individuals with affective disorders. Arch Gen Psychiatry 1986;43:923–9.

[7] Schulsinger F, Key SS, Reoshental D, et al. A family study of suicide. In: Schou M, Stromgren E, editors. Origins, prevention, and treatment of affective disorders. New York: Academic; 1979. p. 277–87.

[8] Asberg M. Neurotransmitters and suicidal behavior. The evidence from cerebrospinal fluid studies. Ann N Y Acad Sci 1997;836:158–81.

[9] Zalsman G, Braun M, Arendt M, et al. A comparison of the medical lethality of suicide attempts in bipolar and major depressive disorders. Bipolar Disord 2006;8:558–65.

[10] Oquendo MA, Friend JM, Halberstam B, et al. Association of comorbid posttraumatic stress disorder and major depression with greater risk for suicidal behavior. Am J Psychiatry 2003;160:580–2.

[11] Pandey GN, Dwivedi Y, Rizavi HS, et al. Higher expression of serotonin 5-HT(2A) receptors in the postmortem brains of teenage suicide victims. Am J Psychiatry 2002;159: 419–29.

[12] Patkar AA, Berrettini WH, Hoehe M, et al. Serotonin transporter polymorphisms and measures of impulsivity, aggression, and sensation seeking among African-American cocaine-dependent individuals. Psychiatry Res 2002;110:103–15.

[13] Anguelova M, Benkelfat C, Turecki G. A systematic review of association studies investigating genes coding for serotonin receptors and the serotonin transporter: II. Suicidal behavior. Mol Psychiatry 2003;8:646–53.

[14] Li D, He L. Meta-analysis supports association between serotonin transporter (5-HTT) and suicidal behavior. Mol Psychiatry 2007;12:47–54.

[15] Lopez de Lara C, Dumais A, Rouleau G, et al. STin2 variant and family history of suicide as significant predictors of suicide completion in major depression. Biol Psychiatry 2006;59: 114–20.

[16] De Luca V, Zai G, Tharmalingam S, et al. Association study between the novel functional polymorphism of the serotonin transporter gene and suicidal behaviour in schizophrenia. Eur Neuropsychopharmacol 2006;16:268–71.

[17] Pungercic G, Videtic A, Pestotnik A, et al. Serotonin transporter gene promoter (5-HTTLPR) and intron 2 (VNTR) polymorphisms: a study on Slovenian population of suicide victims. Psychiatr Genet 2006;16:187–91.

[18] Helbecque N, Sparks DL, Hunsaker JC III, et al. The serotonin transporter promoter polymorphism and suicide. Neurosci Lett 2006;400:13–5.

[19] Rujescu D, Giegling I, Sato T, et al. A polymorphism in the promoter of the serotonin transporter gene is not associated with suicidal behavior. Psychiatr Genet 2001;11:169–72.

[20] Segal J, Pujol C, Birck A, et al. Association between suicide attempts in south Brazilian depressed patients with the serotonin transporter polymorphism. Psychiatry Res 2006;143: 289–91.

[21] Zalsman G, Frisch A, Bromberg M, et al. Family-based association study of serotonin transporter promoter in suicidal adolescents: no association with suicidality but possible role in violence traits. Am J Med Genet 2001;105:239–45.

[22] Shen Y, Li H, Gu N, et al. Relationship between suicidal behavior of psychotic inpatients and serotonin transporter gene in Han Chinese. Neurosci Lett 2004;372:94–8.

[23] Courtet P, Buresi C, Abbar M, et al. No association between non-violent suicidal behavior and the serotonin transporter promoter polymorphism. Am J Med Genet B Neuropsychiatr Genet 2003;116:72–6.

[24] Yen FC, Hong CJ, Hou SJ, et al. Association study of serotonin transporter gene VNTR polymorphism and mood disorders, onset age and suicide attempts in a Chinese sample. Neuropsychobiology 2003;48:5–9.

[25] Ohtani M, Shindo S, Yoshioka N. Polymorphisms of the tryptophan hydroxylase gene and serotonin 1A receptor gene in suicide victims among Japanese. Tohoku J Exp Med 2004;202:123–33.

[26] Serretti A, Mandelli L, Giegling I, et al. HTR2C and HTR1A gene variants in German and Italian suicide attempters and completers. Am J Med Genet B Neuropsychiatr Genet 2007;144:291–9.

[27] Nishiguchi N, Shirakawa O, Ono H, et al. Lack of an association between 5-HT1A receptor gene structural polymorphisms and suicide victims. Am J Med Genet 2002;114:423–5.

[28] Tsai SJ, Hong CJ, Yu YW, et al. Association study of serotonin 1B receptor (A-161T) genetic polymorphism and suicidal behaviors and response to fluoxetine in major depressive disorder. Neuropsychobiology 2004;50:235–8.

[29] Hong CJ, Pan GM, Tsai SJ. Association study of onset age, attempted suicide, aggressive behavior, and schizophrenia with a serotonin 1B receptor (A-161T) genetic polymorphism. Neuropsychobiology 2004;49:1–4.

[30] Videtic A, Pungercic G, Pajnic IZ, et al. Association study of seven polymorphisms in four serotonin receptor genes on suicide victims. Am J Med Genet B Neuropsychiatr Genet 2006;141:669–72.

[31] Turecki G, Sequeira A, Gingras Y, et al. Suicide and serotonin: study of variation at seven serotonin receptor genes in suicide completers. Am J Med Genet B Neuropsychiatr Genet 2003;118:36–40.

[32] Okamura K, Shirakawa O, Nishiguchi N, et al. Lack of an association between 5-HT receptor gene polymorphisms and suicide victims. Psychiatry Clin Neurosci 2005;59:345–9.

[33] Turecki G, Briere R, Dewar K, et al. Prediction of level of serotonin 2A receptor binding by serotonin receptor 2A genetic variation in postmortem brain samples from subjects who did or did not commit suicide. Am J Psychiatry 1999;156:1456–8.

[34] Li D, Duan Y, He L. Association study of serotonin 2A receptor (5-HT2A) gene with schizophrenia and suicidal behavior using systematic meta-analysis. Biochem Biophys Res Commun 2006;340:1006–15.

[35] Correa H, De ML, Boson W, et al. Association study of T102C 5-HT(2A) polymorphism in schizophrenic patients: diagnosis, psychopathology, and suicidal behavior. Dialogues Clin Neurosci 2007;9:97–101.

[36] Correa H, De ML, Boson W, et al. Analysis of T102C 5HT2A polymorphism in Brazilian psychiatric inpatients: relationship with suicidal behavior. Cell Mol Neurobiol 2002;22:813–7.

[37] Preuss UW, Koller G, Bahlmann M, et al. No association between suicidal behavior and 5-HT2A-T102C polymorphism in alcohol dependents. Am J Med Genet 2000;96:877–8.

[38] Crawford J, Sutherland GR, Goldney RD. No evidence for association of 5-HT2A receptor polymorphism with suicide. Am J Med Genet 2000;96:879–80.

[39] Polesskaya OO, Sokolov BP. Differential expression of the "C" and "T" alleles of the 5-HT2A receptor gene in the temporal cortex of normal individuals and schizophrenics. J Neurosci Res 2002;67:812–22.

[40] De Luca V, Likhodi O, Kennedy JL, et al. Differential expression and parent-of-origin effect of the 5-HT2A receptor gene C102T polymorphism: analysis of suicidality in schizophrenia and bipolar disorder. Am J Med Genet B Neuropsychiatr Genet 2007;144:370–4.

[41] Lalovic A, Turecki G. Meta-analysis of the association between tryptophan hydroxylase and suicidal behavior. Am J Med Genet 2002;114:533–40.

[42] Rujescu D, Giegling I, Sato T, et al. Genetic variations in tryptophan hydroxylase in suicidal behavior: analysis and meta-analysis. Biol Psychiatry 2003;54:465–73.

[43] Bellivier F, Chaste P, Malafosse A. Association between the TPH gene A218C polymorphism and suicidal behavior: a meta-analysis. Am J Med Genet B Neuropsychiatr Genet 2004;124:87–91.

[44] Li D, He L. Further clarification of the contribution of the tryptophan hydroxylase (TPH) gene to suicidal behavior using systematic allelic and genotypic meta-analyses. Hum Genet 2006;119:233–40.

[45] Shaltiel G, Shamir A, Agam G, et al. Only tryptophan hydroxylase (TPH)-2 is relevant to the CNS. Am J Med Genet B Neuropsychiatr Genet 2005;136:106.

[46] Canli T, Congdon E, Gutknecht L, et al. Amygdala responsiveness is modulated by tryptophan hydroxylase-2 gene variation. J Neural Transm 2005;112:1479–85.

[47] Lopez de Lara C, Brezo J, Rouleau G, et al. Effect of tryptophan hydroxylase-2 gene variants on suicide risk in major depression. Biol Psychiatry 2007;62:72–80.

[48] Ho LW, Furlong RA, Rubinsztein JS, et al. Genetic associations with clinical characteristics in bipolar affective disorder and recurrent unipolar depressive disorder. Am J Med Genet 2000;96:36–42.

[49] De Luca V, Voineskos D, Wong GW, et al. Promoter polymorphism of second tryptophan hydroxylase isoform (TPH2) in schizophrenia and suicidality. Psychiatry Res 2005;134:195–8.

[50] Zill P, Preuss UW, Koller G, et al. SNP- and haplotype analysis of the tryptophan hydroxylase 2 gene in alcohol-dependent patients and alcohol-related suicide. Neuropsychopharmacology 2007;32:1687–94.

[51] Viana MM, De Marco LA, Boson WL, et al. Investigation of A218C tryptophan hydroxylase polymorphism: association with familial suicide behavior and proband's suicide attempt characteristics. Genes Brain Behav 2006;5:340–5.

[52] Koller G, Engel RR, Preuss UW, et al. Tryptophan hydroxylase gene 1 polymorphisms are not associated with suicide attempts in alcohol-dependent individuals. Addict Biol 2005;10:269–73.

[53] Zalsman G, Frisch A, King RA, et al. Case control and family-based studies of tryptophan hydroxylase gene A218C polymorphism and suicidality in adolescents. Am J Med Genet 2001;105:451–7.

[54] Geijer T, Frisch A, Persson ML, et al. Search for association between suicide attempt and serotonergic polymorphisms. Psychiatr Genet 2000;10:19–26.

[55] Kunugi H, Ishida S, Kato T, et al. No evidence for an association of polymorphisms of the tryptophan hydroxylase gene with affective disorders or attempted suicide among Japanese patients. Am J Psychiatry 1999;156:774–6.

[56] De Luca V, Tharmalingam S, Muller DJ, et al. Gene-gene interaction between MAOA and COMT in suicidal behavior: analysis in schizophrenia. Brain Res 2006;1097:26–30.

[57] Gerra G, Garofano L, Bosari S, et al. Analysis of monoamine oxidase A (MAO-A) promoter polymorphism in male heroin-dependent subjects: behavioural and personality correlates. J Neural Transm 2004;111:611–21.

[58] Huang YY, Cate SP, Battistuzzi C, et al. An association between a functional polymorphism in the monoamine oxidase a gene promoter, impulsive traits and early abuse experiences. Neuropsychopharmacology 2004;29:1498–505.

[59] Ono H, Shirakawa O, Nishiguchi N, et al. No evidence of an association between a functional monoamine oxidase a gene polymorphism and completed suicides. Am J Med Genet 2002;114:340–2.

[60] Westrin A. Stress system alterations and mood disorders in suicidal patients. A review. Biomed Pharmacother 2000;54:142–5.

[61] Ordway GA, Widdowson PS, Smith KS, et al. Agonist binding to alpha 2-adrenoceptors is elevated in the locus coeruleus from victims of suicide. J Neurochem 1994;63:617–24.

[62] Maris RW. Suicide. Lancet 2002;360:319–26.

[63] Ordway GA, Smith KS, Haycock JW. Elevated tyrosine hydroxylase in the locus coeruleus of suicide victims. J Neurochem 1994;62:680–5.

[64] Biegon A, Fieldust S. Reduced tyrosine hydroxylase immunoreactivity in locus coeruleus of suicide victims. Synapse 1992;10:79–82.

[65] Hattori H, Shirakawa O, Nishiguchi N, et al. No evidence of an association between tyrosine hydroxylase gene polymorphisms and suicide victims. Kobe J Med Sci 2006;52:195–200.

[66] Zalsman G, Frisch A, Lewis R, et al. DRD4 receptor gene exon III polymorphism in inpatient suicidal adolescents. J Neural Transm 2004;111:1593–603.

[67] Persson ML, Geijer T, Wasserman D, et al. Lack of association between suicide attempt and a polymorphism at the dopamine receptor D4 locus. Psychiatr Genet 1999;9:97–100.

[68] Gerra G, Garofano L, Pellegrini C, et al. Allelic association of a dopamine transporter gene polymorphism with antisocial behaviour in heroin-dependent patients. Addict Biol 2005;10:275–81.

[69] Sequeira A, Mamdani F, Lalovic A, et al. Alpha 2A adrenergic receptor gene and suicide. Psychiatry Res 2004;125:87–93.

[70] Owen D, Du L, Bakish D, et al. Norepinephrine transporter gene polymorphism is not associated with susceptibility to major depression. Psychiatry Res 1999;87:1–5.

[71] De Luca V, Tharmalingam S, Sicard T, et al. Gene-gene interaction between MAOA and COMT in suicidal behavior. Neurosci Lett 2005;383:151–4.

[72] Ohara K, Nagai M, Suzuki Y, et al. Low activity allele of catechol-o-methyltransferase gene and Japanese unipolar depression. Neuroreport 1998;9:1305–8.

[73] Westrin A, Ekman R, Traskman-Bendz L. Alterations of corticotropin releasing hormone (CRH) and neuropeptide Y (NPY) plasma levels in mood disorder patients with a recent suicide attempt. Eur Neuropsychopharmacol 1999;9:205–11.

[74] Pfennig A, Kunzel HE, Kern N, et al. Hypothalamus-pituitary-adrenal system regulation and suicidal behavior in depression. Biol Psychiatry 2005;57:336–42.

[75] De Luca V, Tharmalingam S, Kennedy JL. Association study between the corticotropin-releasing hormone receptor 2 gene and suicidality in bipolar disorder. Eur Psychiatry 2007;22:282–7.

[76] Dwivedi Y, Rizavi HS, Conley RR, et al. Altered gene expression of brain-derived neurotrophic factor and receptor tyrosine kinase B in postmortem brain of suicide subjects. Arch Gen Psychiatry 2003;60:804–15.

[77] Carmine A, Chheda MG, Jonsson EG, et al. Two NOTCH4 polymorphisms and their relation to schizophrenia susceptibility and different personality traits. Psychiatr Genet 2003;13:23–8.

[78] Kunugi H, Hashimoto R, Yoshida M, et al. A missense polymorphism (S205L) of the low-affinity neurotrophin receptor p75NTR gene is associated with depressive disorder and attempted suicide. Am J Med Genet B Neuropsychiatr Genet 2004;129:44–6.

[79] Hong CJ, Huo SJ, Yen FC, et al. Association study of a brain-derived neurotrophic-factor genetic polymorphism and mood disorders, age of onset and suicidal behavior. Neuropsychobiology 2003;48:186–9.

[80] McGregor S, Strauss J, Bulgin N, et al. p75(NTR) gene and suicide attempts in young adults with a history of childhood-onset mood disorder. Am J Med Genet B Neuropsychiatr Genet 2007;144:696–700.

[81] Perroud N, Courtet P, Vincze I, et al. Interaction between BDNF Val66Met and childhood trauma on adult's violent suicide attempt. Genes Brain Behav 2007.

[82] Sequeira A, Klempan T, Canetti L, et al. Patterns of gene expression in the limbic system of suicides with and without major depression. Mol Psychiatry 2007;12:640–55.

[83] De Luca V, Muglia P, Masellis M, et al. Polymorphisms in glutamate decarboxylase genes: analysis in schizophrenia. Psychiatr Genet 2004;14:39–42.

[84] Baca-Garcia E, Vaquero C, Diaz-Sastre C, et al. Lack of association between polymorphic variations in the alpha 3 subunit GABA receptor gene (GABRA3) and suicide attempts. Prog Neuropsychopharmacol Biol Psychiatry 2004;28:409–12.

[85] Wasserman D, Geijer T, Sokolowski M, et al. Genetic variation in the hypothalamic-pituitary-adrenocortical axis regulatory factor, T-box 19, and the angry/hostility personality trait. Genes Brain Behav 2007;6:321–8.

[86] Dwivedi Y, Rizavi HS, Shukla PK, et al. Protein kinase A in postmortem brain of depressed suicide victims: altered expression of specific regulatory and catalytic subunits. Biol Psychiatry 2004;55:234–43.

[87] Pandey GN, Dwivedi Y, Ren X, et al. Cyclic AMP response element-binding protein in postmortem brain of teenage suicide victims: specific decrease in the prefrontal cortex but not the hippocampus. Int J Neuropsychopharmacol 2007;10:621–9.

[88] Saavedra JM, Ando H, Armando I, et al. Brain angiotensin II, an important stress hormone: regulatory sites and therapeutic opportunities. Ann N Y Acad Sci 2004;1018:76–84.

[89] Hishimoto A, Shirakawa O, Nishiguchi N, et al. Association between a functional polymorphism in the renin-angiotensin system and completed suicide. J Neural Transm 2006;113:1915–20.

[90] Tiret L, Rigat B, Visvikis S, et al. Evidence, from combined segregation and linkage analysis, that a variant of the angiotensin I-converting enzyme (ACE) gene controls plasma ACE levels. Am J Hum Genet 1992;51:197–205.

[91] Lalovic A, Levy E, Luheshi G, et al. Cholesterol content in brains of suicide completers. Int J Neuropsychopharmacol 2007;10:159–66.

[92] Lalovic A, Merkens L, Russell L, et al. Cholesterol metabolism and suicidality in Smith-Lemli-Opitz syndrome carriers. Am J Psychiatry 2004;161:2123–6.

[93] Lalovic A, Sequeira A, DeGuzman R, et al. Investigation of completed suicide and genes involved in cholesterol metabolism. J Affect Disord 2004;79:25–32.

[94] Wasserman D, Geijer T, Rozanov V, et al. Suicide attempt and basic mechanisms in neural conduction: relationships to the SCN8A and VAMP4 genes. Am J Med Genet B Neuropsychiatr Genet 2005;133:116–9.

[95] Perlis RH, Purcell S, Fava M, et al. Association between treatment-emergent suicidal ideation with citalopram and polymorphisms near cyclic adenosine monophosphate response element binding protein in the STAR*D study. Arch Gen Psychiatry 2007;64:689–97.

[96] Cui H, Nishiguchi N, Ivleva E, et al. Association of RGS2 gene polymorphisms with suicide and increased RGS2 immunoreactivity in the postmortem brain of suicide victims. Neuropsychopharmacology 2007.

[97] Rujescu D, Giegling I, Dahmen N, et al. Association study of suicidal behavior and affective disorders with a genetic polymorphism in ABCG1, a positional candidate on chromosome 21q22.3. Neuropsychobiology 2000;42(Suppl 1):22–5.

[98] Pae CU, Yoon SJ, Patkar A, et al. Manganese superoxide dismutase (MnSOD: Ala-9Val) gene polymorphism and mood disorders: a preliminary study. Prog Neuropsychopharmacol Biol Psychiatry 2006;30:1326–9.

[99] Tsai SJ, Wang YC, Hong CJ, et al. Association study of oestrogen receptor alpha gene polymorphism and suicidal behaviours in major depressive disorder. Psychiatr Genet 2003;13:19–22.

[100] Baumeister RF. Suicide as escape from self. Psychol Rev 1990;97:90–113.

[101] Rubinstein DH. A stress-diathesis theory of suicide. Suicide Life Threat Behav 1986;16:182–97.

[102] Runeson BS, Beskow J, Waern M. The suicidal process in suicides among young people. Acta Psychiatr Scand 1996;93:35–42.

[103] Klempan TA, Sequeira A, Canetti L, et al. Altered expression of genes involved in ATP bio-synthesis and GABAergic neurotransmission in the ventral prefrontal cortex of suicides with and without major depression. Mol Psychiatry, in press.

[104] Sequeira A, Gwadry FG, Ffrench-Mullen JM, et al. Implication of SSAT by gene expression and genetic variation in suicide and major depression. Arch Gen Psychiatry 2006;63: 35–48.

[105] Karssen AM, Her S, Li JZ, et al. Stress-induced changes in primate prefrontal profiles of gene expression. Mol Psychiatry 2007;12:1089–102.

[106] Klempan TA, Rujescu D, Mérette C, et al. Profiling spermidine/spermine N1-acetyltransfer-ase brain gene expression differences in depressed suicides. Mol Psychiatry, Submitted.

[107] Thalmeier A, Dickmann M, Giegling I, et al. Gene expression profiling of post-mortem orbitofrontal cortex in violent suicide victims. Int J Neuropsychopharmacol 2008;11: 217–28.

[108] Hesselbrock V, Dick D, Hesselbrock M, et al. The search for genetic risk factors associated with suicidal behavior. Alcohol Clin Exp Res 2004;28:70S–6S.

[109] Cheng R, Juo SH, Loth JE, et al. Genome-wide linkage scan in a large bipolar disorder sample from the National Institute of Mental Health genetics initiative suggests putative loci for bipolar disorder, psychosis, suicide, and panic disorder. Mol Psychiatry 2006;11: 252–60.

[110] Willour VL, Zandi PP, Badner JA, et al. Attempted suicide in bipolar disorder pedigrees: evidence for linkage to 2p12. Biol Psychiatry. 2007;61:725–7.

[111] Zubenko GS, Maher BS, Hughes HB III, et al. Genome-wide linkage survey for genetic loci that affect the risk of suicide attempts in families with recurrent, early-onset, major depres-sion. Am J Med Genet B Neuropsychiatr Genet 2004;129:47–54.

[112] Silverman MM. The language of suicidology. Suicide Life Threat Behav 2006;36: 519–32.

[113] Munafo MR. Candidate gene studies in the 21st century: meta-analysis, mediation, mod-eration. Genes Brain Behav 2006;5(Suppl 1):3–8.

[114] Pfeffer CR, Normandin L, Kakuma T. Suicidal children grow up: suicidal behavior and psychiatric disorders among relatives. J Am Acad Child Adolesc Psychiatry 1994;33: 1087–97.

[115] Oquendo MA, Galfalvy H, Russo S, et al. Prospective study of clinical predictors of suicidal acts after a major depressive episode in patients with major depressive disorder or bipolar disorder. Am J Psychiatry 2004;161:1433–41.

[116] Rujescu D, Giegling I, Mandelli L, et al. NOS-I and -III gene variants are differentially associated with facets of suicidal behavior and aggression-related traits. Am J Med Genet B Neuropsychiatr Genet 2007;147:42–8.

[117] Gietl A, Giegling I, Hartmann AM, et al. ABCG1 gene variants in suicidal behavior and aggression-related traits. Eur Neuropsychopharmacol 2007;17:410–6.

[118] Holmes A, Murphy DL, Crawley JN. Reduced aggression in mice lacking the serotonin transporter. Psychopharmacology (Berl) 2002;161:160–7.

[119] Zalsman G, Oquendo MA, Greenhill L, et al. Neurobiology of depression in children and adolescents. Child Adolesc Psychiatr Clin N Am 2006;15:843–68, vii–viii.

[120] Brunner HG, Nelen M, Breakefield XO, et al. Abnormal behavior associated with a point mutation in the structural gene for monoamine oxidase A. Science 1993;262:578–80.

[121] Manuck SB, Flory JD, Muldoon MF, et al. Central nervous system serotonergic responsivity and aggressive disposition in men. Physiol Behav 2002;77:705–9.

[122] Seif I, De Maeyer E. Knockout Corner: knockout mice for monoamine oxidase A. Int J Neu-ropsychopharmacol 1999;2:241–3.

[123] Zalsman G, Anderson GM, Peskin M, et al. Relationships between serotonin trans-porter promoter polymorphism, platelet serotonin transporter binding and clinical phe-notype in suicidal and non-suicidal adolescent inpatients. J Neural Transm 2005;112: 309–15.

[124] van Heeringen K. The neurobiology of suicide and suicidality. Can J Psychiatry 2003;48: 292–300.

[125] Reuter M, Kuepper Y, Hennig J. Association between a polymorphism in the promoter region of the TPH2 gene and the personality trait of harm avoidance. Int J Neuropsychopharmacol 2007;10:401–4.

[126] Lang UE, Hellweg R, Kalus P, et al. Association of a functional BDNF polymorphism and anxiety-related personality traits. Psychopharmacology (Berl) 2005;180:95–9.

[127] Jollant F, Bellivier F, Leboyer M, et al. Impaired decision making in suicide attempters. Am J Psychiatry 2005;162:304–10.

[128] Kendler KS. Genetic epidemiology in psychiatry. Taking both genes and environment seriously. Arch Gen Psychiatry 1995;52:895–9.

[129] Thapar A, Harold G, Rice F, et al. The contribution of gene-environment interaction to psychopathology. Dev Psychopathol 2007;19:989–1004.

[130] Bastian ML, Sponberg AC, Sponberg AC, et al. Long-term effects of infant rearing condition on the acquisition of dominance rank in juvenile and adult rhesus macaques (Macaca mulatta). Dev Psychobiol 2003;42:44–51.

[131] Kaufman J, Yang BZ, Douglas-Palumberi H, et al. Brain-derived neurotrophic factor-5-HTTLPR gene interactions and environmental modifiers of depression in children. Biol Psychiatry 2006;59:673–80.

[132] Caspi A, Sugden K, Moffitt TE, et al. Influence of life stress on depression: moderation by a polymorphism in the 5-HTT gene. Science 2003;301:386–9.

[133] Gibb BE, McGeary JE, Beevers CG, et al. Serotonin transporter (5-HTTLPR) genotype, childhood abuse, and suicide attempts in adult psychiatric inpatients. Suicide Life Threat Behav 2006;36:687–93.

[134] Brezo J, Bureau A, Barker ED, et al. Serotonergic variants as predictors and moderators of the risk for suicide attempts, in preparation, 2007.

[135] Caspi A, McClay J, Moffitt TE, et al. Role of genotype in the cycle of violence in maltreated children. Science 2002;297:851–4.

[136] Newman TK, Syagailo YV, Barr CS, et al. Monoamine oxidase A gene promoter variation and rearing experience influences aggressive behavior in rhesus monkeys. Biol Psychiatry 2005;57:167–72.

[137] Hansson SR, Mezey E, Hoffman BJ. Serotonin transporter messenger RNA in the developing rat brain: early expression in serotonergic neurons and transient expression in non-serotonergic neurons. Neuroscience 1998;83:1185–201.

[138] Lau JY, Eley TC. Gene-environment interactions and correlations in psychiatric disorders. Curr Psychiatry Rep 2004;6:119–24.

[139] Heim C, Nemeroff CB. The role of childhood trauma in the neurobiology of mood and anxiety disorders: preclinical and clinical studies. Biol Psychiatry 2001;49:1023–39.

[140] Conwell Y, Duberstein PR, Cox C, et al. Age differences in behaviors leading to completed suicide. Am J Geriatr Psychiatry 1998;6:122–6.

[141] Stefulj J, Kubat M, Balija M, et al. TPH gene polymorphism and aging: indication of combined effect on the predisposition to violent suicide. Am J Med Genet B Neuropsychiatr Genet 2006;141:139–41.

[142] Hwang JP, Yang CH, Hong CJ, et al. Association of APOE genetic polymorphism with cognitive function and suicide history in geriatric depression. Dement Geriatr Cogn Disord 2006;22:334–8.

[143] Zalsman G, Frisch A, Baruch-Movshovits R, et al. Family-based association study of 5-HT(2A) receptor T102C polymorphism and suicidal behavior in Ashkenazi inpatient adolescents. Int J Adolesc Med Health 2005;17:231–8.

[144] Jernej B, Stefulj J, Hranilovic D, et al. Intronic polymorphism of tryptophan hydroxylase and serotonin transporter: indication for combined effect in predisposition to suicide. J Neural Transm 2004;111:733–8.

[145] Van de Kar LD, Javed A, Zhang Y, et al. 5-HT2A receptors stimulate ACTH, corticosterone, oxytocin, renin, and prolactin release and activate hypothalamic CRF and oxytocin-expressing cells. J Neurosci 2001;21:3572–9.

[146] Bethea CL, Mirkes SJ, Su A, et al. Effects of oral estrogen, raloxifene and arzoxifene on gene expression in serotonin neurons of macaques. Psychoneuroendocrinology 2002;27: 431–45.

[147] Wasserman D, Geijer T, Sokolowski M, et al. Association of the serotonin transporter promotor polymorphism with suicide attempters with a high medical damage. Eur Neuropsychopharmacol 2007;17:230–3.

[148] Gaysina D, Zainullina A, Gabdulhakov R, et al. The serotonin transporter gene: polymorphism and haplotype analysis in Russian suicide attempters. Neuropsychobiology 2006;54:70–4.

[149] Baca-Garcia E, Salgado BR, Segal HD, et al. A pilot genetic study of the continuum between compulsivity and impulsivity in females: the serotonin transporter promoter polymorphism. Prog Neuropsychopharmacol Biol Psychiatry 2005;29:713–7.

[150] Limosin F, Loze JY, Boni C, et al. Male-specific association between the 5-HTTLPR S allele and suicide attempts in alcohol-dependent subjects. J Psychiatr Res 2005;39:179–82.

[151] Courtet P, Picot MC, Bellivier F, et al. Serotonin transporter gene may be involved in short-term risk of subsequent suicide attempts. Biol Psychiatry 2004;55:46–51.

[152] Correa H, Campi-Azevedo AC, De ML, et al. Familial suicide behaviour: association with probands suicide attempt characteristics and 5-HTTLPR polymorphism. Acta Psychiatr Scand 2004;110:459–64.

[153] Campi-Azevedo AC, Boson W, De ML, et al. Association of the serotonin transporter promoter polymorphism with suicidal behavior. Mol Psychiatry 2003;8:899–900.

[154] Bayle FJ, Leroy S, Gourion D, et al. 5HTTLPR polymorphism in schizophrenic patients: further support for association with violent suicide attempts. Am J Med Genet B Neuropsychiatr Genet 2003;119:13–7.

[155] Baca-Garcia E, Vaquero C, Diaz-Sastre C, et al. A gender-specific association between the serotonin transporter gene and suicide attempts. Neuropsychopharmacology 2002;26: 692–5.

[156] Preuss UW, Koller G, Soyka M, et al. Association between suicide attempts and 5-HTTLPR-S-allele in alcohol-dependent and control subjects: further evidence from a German alcohol-dependent inpatient sample. Biol Psychiatry 2001;50:636–9.

[157] Courtet P, Baud P, Abbar M, et al. Association between violent suicidal behavior and the low activity allele of the serotonin transporter gene. Mol Psychiatry 2001;6:338–41.

[158] Bellivier F, Szoke A, Henry C, et al. Possible association between serotonin transporter gene polymorphism and violent suicidal behavior in mood disorders. Biol Psychiatry 2000;48:319–22.

[159] Gorwood P, Batel P, Ades J, et al. Serotonin transporter gene polymorphisms, alcoholism, and suicidal behavior. Biol Psychiatry 2000;48:259–64.

[160] Joiner TE Jr, Johnson F, Soderstrom K. Association between serotonin transporter gene polymorphism and family history of attempted and completed suicide. Suicide Life Threat Behav 2002;32:329–32.

[161] Faludi G, Du L, Palkovits M, et al. Serotonin transporter, serotonin-2A receptor and tryptophan hydroxilase gene polymorphisms in depressed suicide victims. Neurobiology (Bp) 2000;8:269–71.

[162] Bondy B, Erfurth A, de JS, et al. Possible association of the short allele of the serotonin transporter promoter gene polymorphism (5-HTTLPR) with violent suicide. Mol Psychiatry 2000;5:193–5.

[163] Du L, Faludi G, Palkovits M, et al. Frequency of long allele in serotonin transporter gene is increased in depressed suicide victims. Biol Psychiatry 1999;46:196–201.

[164] Hranilovic D, Stefulj J, Furac I, et al. Serotonin transporter gene promoter (5-HTTLPR) and intron 2 (VNTR) polymorphisms in Croatian suicide victims. Biol Psychiatry 2003;54:884–9.

[165] Lemonde S, Turecki G, Bakish D, et al. Impaired repression at a 5-hydroxytryptamine 1A receptor gene polymorphism associated with major depression and suicide. J Neurosci 2003;23:8788–99.

[166] New AS, Gelernter J, Goodman M, et al. Suicide, impulsive aggression, and HTR1B genotype. Biol Psychiatry 2001;50:62–5.

[167] Giegling I, Hartmann AM, Moller HJ, et al. Anger- and aggression-related traits are associated with polymorphisms in the 5-HT-2A gene. J Affect Disord 2006;96:75–81.

[168] Arias B, Gasto C, Catalan R, et al. The 5-HT(2A) receptor gene 102T/C polymorphism is associated with suicidal behavior in depressed patients. Am J Med Genet 2001;105: 801–4.

[169] Du L, Bakish D, Lapierre YD, et al. Association of polymorphism of serotonin 2A receptor gene with suicidal ideation in major depressive disorder. Am J Med Genet 2000;96:56–60.

[170] Bonnier B, Gorwood P, Hamon M, et al. Association of 5-HT(2A) receptor gene polymorphism with major affective disorders: the case of a subgroup of bipolar disorder with low suicide risk. Biol Psychiatry 2002;51:762–5.

[171] Courtet P, Jollant F, Buresi C, et al. The monoamine oxidase A gene may influence the means used in suicide attempts. Psychiatr Genet 2005;15:189–93.

[172] Du L, Faludi G, Palkovits M, et al. High activity-related allele of MAO-A gene associated with depressed suicide in males. Neuroreport 2002;13:1195–8.

[173] Ke L, Qi ZY, Ping Y, et al. Effect of SNP at position 40237 in exon 7 of the TPH2 gene on susceptibility to suicide. Brain Res 2006;1122:24–6.

[174] Zill P, Buttner A, Eisenmenger W, et al. Single nucleotide polymorphism and haplotype analysis of a novel tryptophan hydroxylase isoform (TPH2) gene in suicide victims. Biol Psychiatry 2004;56:581–6.

[175] Lopez VA, tera-Wadleigh S, Cardona I, et al. Nested association between genetic variation in tryptophan hydroxylase II, bipolar affective disorder, and suicide attempts. Biol Psychiatry 2007;61:181–6.

[176] Nielsen DA, Goldman D, Virkkunen M, et al. Suicidality and 5-hydroxyindoleacetic acid concentration associated with a tryptophan hydroxylase polymorphism. Arch Gen Psychiatry 1994;51:34–8.

[177] Abbar M, Courtet P, Bellivier F, et al. Suicide attempts and the tryptophan hydroxylase gene. Mol Psychiatry 2001;6:268–73.

[178] Liu X, Li H, Qin W, et al. Association of TPH1 with suicidal behaviour and psychiatric disorders in the Chinese population. J Med Genet 2006;43:e4.

[179] Tsai SJ, Hong CJ, Wang YC. Tryptophan hydroxylase gene polymorphism (A218C) and suicidal behaviors. Neuroreport 1999;10:3773–5.

[180] Turecki G, Zhu Z, Tzenova J, et al. TPH and suicidal behavior: a study in suicide completers. Mol Psychiatry 2001;6:98–102.

[181] Paik I, Toh K, Kim J, et al. TPH gene may be associated with suicidal behavior, but not with schizophrenia in the Korean population. Hum Hered 2000;50:365–9.

[182] Rotondo A, Schuebel K, Bergen A, et al. Identification of four variants in the tryptophan hydroxylase promoter and association to behavior. Mol Psychiatry 1999;4:360–8.

[183] Nielsen DA, Virkkunen M, Lappalainen J, et al. A tryptophan hydroxylase gene marker for suicidality and alcoholism. Arch Gen Psychiatry 1998;55:593–602.

[184] Mann JJ, Malone KM, Nielsen DA, et al. Possible association of a polymorphism of the tryptophan hydroxylase gene with suicidal behavior in depressed patients. Am J Psychiatry 1997;154:1451–3.

[185] Zaboli G, Gizatullin R, Nilsonne A, et al. Tryptophan hydroxylase-1 gene variants associate with a group of suicidal borderline women. Neuropsychopharmacology 2006;31: 1982–90.

[186] Roy A, Rylander G, Forslund K, et al. Excess tryptophan hydroxylase 17 779C allele in surviving cotwins of monozygotic twin suicide victims. Neuropsychobiology 2001;43: 233–6.

[187] Rujescu D, Giegling I, Gietl A, et al. A functional single nucleotide polymorphism (V158M) in the COMT gene is associated with aggressive personality traits. Biol Psychiatry 2003;54: 34–9.

[188] Nolan KA, Volavka J, Czobor P, et al. Suicidal behavior in patients with schizophrenia is related to COMT polymorphism. Psychiatr Genet 2000;10:117–24.

[189] Ono H, Shirakawa O, Nushida H, et al. Association between catechol-O-methyltransferase functional polymorphism and male suicide completers. Neuropsychopharmacology 2004;29:1374–7.

[190] Johann M, Putzhammer A, Eichhammer P, et al. Association of the -141C Del variant of the dopamine D2 receptor (DRD2) with positive family history and suicidality in German alcoholics. Am J Med Genet B Neuropsychiatr Genet 2005;132:46–9.

[191] Finckh U, Rommelspacher H, Kuhn S, et al. Influence of the dopamine D2 receptor (DRD2) genotype on neuroadaptive effects of alcohol and the clinical outcome of alcoholism. Pharmacogenetics 1997;7:271–81.

[192] Persson ML, Wasserman D, Geijer T, et al. Tyrosine hydroxylase allelic distribution in suicide attempters. Psychiatry Res 1997;72:73–80.

[193] Comings DE. Pc 1 Duarte, a common polymorphism of a human brain protein, and its relationship to depressive disease and multiple sclerosis. Nature 1979;277:28–32.

[194] Yanagi M, Shirakawa O, Kitamura N, et al. Association of 14-3-3 epsilon gene haplotype with completed suicide in Japanese. J Hum Genet 2005;50:210–6.

[195] Shindo S, Yoshioka N. Polymorphisms of the cholecystokinin gene promoter region in suicide victims in Japan. Forensic Sci Int 2005;150:85–90.

[196] Sequeira A, Kim C, Seguin M, et al. Wolfram syndrome and suicide: Evidence for a role of WFS1 in suicidal and impulsive behavior. Am J Med Genet B Neuropsychiatr Genet 2003;119:108–13.

Psychiatr Clin N Am 31 (2008) 205–212

PSYCHIATRIC CLINICS
OF NORTH AMERICA

ELSEVIER
SAUNDERS

Pregnancies in High Psychosocial Risk Groups: Research Findings and Implications for Early Intervention

Ellenor Mittendorfer-Rutz, PhD, MSc[a,b],
Danuta Wasserman, MD, PhD[a,b],*

[a]Department of Public Health Sciences, Karolinska Institutet, Granits väg 4, Solna,
Stockholm, Sweden
[b]Swedish National Suicide Prevention and Prevention of Mental Ill-Health (NASP),
Karolinska Institute, 171 77 Stockholm, Sweden

SUICIDAL BEHAVIOR IN YOUNG PEOPLE

Based on a review of community surveys, the prevalence of youth suicide attempt in the general population ranges from 2% to 20% [1–5]. In interpreting these prevalence data, the variability in definitions used for suicide attempt has to be taken into account. As the proportion of adolescent suicide attempters receiving medical care ranges from 12% to 50% [2,3], the rates for youth suicide attempt based on hospital care data are much lower. Data from the WHO/EURO multicenter study using the same definition for suicide attempt, report mean suicide attempt rates per 100,000 in 15 European centers in 13 countries for female adolescents between 1989–1992 ranging from 99 in Guipuzcoa in Spain to 766 in Clergy-Pontoise in France [6]. Young females represent the only age group with increasing trends (17%) from 1989 till 1999 in 11 centers in 10 European countries with increasing trends in attempted suicide rates [7].

Youth suicide mortality varies also considerably internationally [8–10]. Based on latest available suicide mortality statistics from the WHO mortality database, suicide rates in adolescents (15–19 years) ranged from below 2 per 100,000 in some Southern European and Central American countries to rates above 20 in Lithuania, Russian Federation, and Sri Lanka [8–10]. On average, suicide accounted for 9.1% of deaths in adolescents in 90 countries worldwide. Suicide rates have been increasing in 15 of these countries on average in young males, accompanied by stable trends in young females [10].

*Corresponding author. Swedish National Suicide Prevention and Prevention of Mental Ill-Health (NASP), Karolinska Institute, 171 77 Stockholm, Sweden. *E-mail address*: danuta. wasserman@ki.se (D. Wasserman).

0193-953X/08/$ – see front matter
doi:10.1016/j.psc.2008.01.010

FAMILIAL MENTAL ILLNESS AND SUICIDAL BEHAVIOR

The overwhelming majority of the literature on parental risk factors increasing the risk of the offspring for suicidal behavior focuses on parental mental illness and suicidal behavior. Adolescent suicide attempters and completers have higher rates of familial psychopathology than community and clinical controls, mainly affective, substance abuse and personality disorders [11–15]. A history of hospital admission due to psychopathology in a first-degree relative was 2.3 to 3.7 times more common in youth suicide attempters than in community controls [14–16]. Familial clustering of suicidal behavior has also been reported for adolescent suicide attempters and completers [11,13–15,17,18]. Odds ratios for youth suicide attempt in the presence of a suicide attempt in a first-degree relative ranged from 2.9 to 5.7. There appears to be an independent effect of familial suicidal behavior as well as familial psychopathology on youth suicidal behavior beyond the transmission of mental illness. This effect can reflect transmission of impulsivity, imitation or the psychosocial consequences of parental mental illness. Nearly a quarter (21%) of all suicide attempts can be attributed to familial psychopathology (13%), family suicide attempt (7%), and suicide completion in the family (1%) [14].

PARENTAL SOCIOECONOMIC AND PSYCHOSOCIAL STATUS

Other determinants for mental illness include parental socioeconomic and psychosocial factors. Low parental socioeconomic status is a well-known risk factor for suicidal behavior in offspring [8,16]. However, this risk is considerably decreased once adjusted for parental mental illness [17]. Maternal teenage parenthood has been linked to an increased risk of suicide and suicide attempt in the offspring [8,19]. Adjusting teenage parenthood for the effect of a series of parental socioeconomic, psychopathological, and psychosocial determinants decreased this risk only to some extent [20].

It is possible that young motherhood is associated with an adverse psychosocial home environment, inadequate social support, inadequate child-rearing practices, the stress burden of single motherhood and consequently superimposed long-term socioeconomic problems. These conditions may exacerbate the risk of the offspring's mental ill-health and consequently the risk of suicidal behavior [21–23].

Women who are pregnant in their teens are more likely to have been exposed to parental separation, abuse or neglect, foster care and parental substance abuse than older childbearing women [21]. Teenage motherhood is also found with increased frequency in women suffering from a mental disorder, primarily personality disorder and substance abuse disorders [24]. Among adolescent mothers, those who had been victims of child physical abuse constitute a high-risk group for abusing their own children [25]. Child abuse and neglect appears to be one central part in the association of teenage mothers and later outcome of their offspring [22].

Single parenthood was also found to be linked to an increase in suicide mortality and morbidity in offspring, adjusted for a variety of psychosocial, psychopathological, and socioeconomic parental risk factors [26,27]. An association of disrupted family background and the risk for suicide has even been reported from psychologic autopsy studies [11,28]. Furthermore, results from aggregate level studies suggest a positive association of the divorce rate with the suicide rates in youth [29,30]. The increase in family break-up, often with the loss of the father to the family, was proposed to have affected boys to a greater extent than girls due to the loss of a role model [31–33].

PRE- AND PERINATAL FACTORS AND SUBSEQUENT MENTAL ILL-HEALTH AND SUICIDAL BEHAVIOR

Fetal Growth

Evidence of a relationship between obstetric and neonatal complications and mental disorder, primarily schizophrenia and depression, has been reported [34,35]. In addition, a number of studies found an association between small size at birth and minor neurologic abnormalities as well as subnormal psychologic performance and stress tolerance later in life [36–39]. Interesting in this context are the findings from the Dutch Hunger winter of 1944/45, where an association of maternal starvation during second trimester and affective disorder in the offspring was reported [40].

Concerning an association between adverse obstetric and neonatal conditions, and elevated risk of suicidal behavior in adolescents and young adults, sparse results have been reported. Salk and colleagues [41] pioneered in this field and found a substantially elevated frequency of obstetric, neonatal, and maternal complications among adolescents who committed suicide, compared with controls. Subsequently, Neugebauer and Reuss [42] and Barker and colleagues [43] failed to replicate such findings. Recent results from large cohort studies from Sweden and Scotland comprising several hundred thousands of individuals suggest an inverse association between specific perinatal factors and suicidal behavior in young adults [8,19].

Among all analyzed neonatal factors, low birth weight (below 2500 g) adjusted for gestational age was significantly associated with suicide and violent suicide attempt and short birth length was also found to be associated with an increase in risk of attempted suicide, particularly by violent means [8,14,19]. Preterm birth was particularly important for violent suicide attempt. The risk was increased fourfold for men born before the 34th week of gestation. Prematurity at birth has also been linked to an increased risk of depressive disorder, anorexia nervosa, and schizophrenia [44–46].

Relations between pre- and perinatal complications, and later suicidality, could be due to neurodevelopmental impairment, acquired increased vulnerability to environmental stressors [41] or confounding by maternal mental disorder, maternal life style—particularly smoking and alcohol abuse—or socioeconomic status. Future research should focus on investigating how maternal lifestyle (alcohol consumption and smoking) and mental illness would attenuate the relationship between restricted fetal growth and subsequent suicidal behavior.

Another hypothetical pathway underlying these associations is an alteration of the serotonin metabolism in fetal life [43]. The serotonin metabolism is hypothesized to be more specifically associated with the diathesis of suicidal behavior than with any underlying psychiatric morbidity [47].

The importance of serotonin metabolism for brain development as well as pre-and postnatal growth in animal models has been reported [48,49]. Children, born preterm, show damage in various parts of the brain, including the amygdaloid nuclear complex, hippocampus, and the prefrontal cortex [50]. The prefrontal cortex has been reported as a site of alterations in the serotonin metabolism in suicide completers [47]. It is also possible that serotonin function is altered by the hypoxia induced by preterm delivery [50,51]. Perinatal asphyxia is also known to negatively affect growth hormone release [48]. Serotonin metabolism is further affected by other factors leading to fetal growth restriction or preterm birth, like maternal prenatal alcohol, drug and nicotine abuse, stress, and malnutrition [49,50]. Additionally, impulsivity and aggression, which are well-known features of violent suicidal behavior and associated with low serotonin levels, have been reported for children born preterm [47,50].

A number of studies investigated whether catch-up growth during childhood and adolescence would alter the inverse association between fetal growth and mental ill-health and suicidality. Growth in childhood is often used as an indicator of nutrition and well-being and catch-up growth in low birth weight infants has been found to decrease the risk for subsequent subnormal intellectual and psychologic performance and for the development of schizophrenia, but not for the risk of attempting suicide [14,37,52].

Multiparity

Multiparity has been linked to subsequent depression, schizophrenia, suicide attempt, and suicide completion in young adulthood [8,19,35,53]. It seems plausible that stress and depressed mood perceived by multiparous mothers, as well as their lack of time for adequate child rearing, may adversely affect a child's psychosocial and socioeconomic environment [54] and hereby increasing the risk of mental disorder and suicidal behavior.

EARLY INTERVENTION

Based on these findings, early intervention in families in psychosocial risk with appropriate psychosocial and educational measures seems crucial. The importance of early intervention in families in psychosocial risk has also been highlighted during the World Health Organization Ministerial conference of mental health in Helsinki, Finland, in 2005 [55]. Among other strategies to prevent mental health problems and suicide, the document, which has been published following the conference and has been ratified by all health ministries in Europe, suggests that routine assessment of the mental health of new mothers by obstetricians and health visitors should be introduced and that they should provide intervention where necessary. Furthermore, the document states that for families at risk, home-based educational intervention should be provided to help proactively to improve parenting skills, health behavior, and interaction between parents and children. These ideas have been followed up by the "Green Paper" produced by the European Commission in Brussels, Belgium, in 2005 [56].

There are several programs in use internationally to improve the interaction between parents and children in parent groups, such as "right from the start" and "The International Child Development Program" [57,58]. With regard to programs focusing on individual counseling or treatment, three examples should be mentioned here, where short- and long-term effects could be achieved [59–61].

An early intervention for families at psychosocial risk, the "Linköping model," resulted in short-term improvements in mother-child relations [61]. In this study, parents at psychosocial risk were defined as parents with mental ill-health, substance abuse, teenage and single parents, multiparous mothers, parents who were unemployed long-term or on social welfare, or mothers with a jail sentence or with children previously placed at foster care. The 6-week intervention focused on supporting the mothers in their parenting, strengthening the mothers in their caregiving skills and improving the mother-child relationship and interaction. Mothers with psychosocial risk factors could be referred to the parent-baby clinics, where the treatment intervention was performed. The program actively facilitated collaboration among various agencies.

Another study, which targeted early intervention through a 5-year family counseling program by a psychiatric nurse, reported significantly fewer psychiatric symptoms in young adults in the counseling program after a 20-year follow-up [59]. Counseling through home visits and parent groups for families at psychosocial risk with children with low birth weight and preterm infants, proved to be effective for children's cognitive development and prevented both criminal behavior and socioeconomic difficulties [60]. Important in all these counseling and educational programs are both the educational level and motivation of the counselor and the motivation and involvement of both parents as well as the duration of the program.

SUMMARY

In summary, recent research suggests that the risk for suicidal behavior in young adults is associated with a wide range of pre-and perinatal and familial psychosocial risk factors interacting with but also independent of familial mental illness and suicidal behavior. Pregnancies in these high psychosocial risk groups are often associated with parenting stress that is likely to affect the parent-child relationship. Several examples of effective counseling and educational programs are available. Collaboration among the various sectors within health care and social services seems crucial for early detection and adequate intervention with regard to the psychosocial problems these children may have to face, and to the consequent prevention of suicidal behavior. This collaboration should include ante- and postnatal health care, social services, schools, and child and adult psychiatry services.

References

[1] Andrews JA, Lewinsohn PM. Suicidal attempts among older adolescents: prevalence and co-occurrence with psychiatric disorders. J Am Acad Child Adolesc Psychiatry 1992;31(4):655–62.

[2] Grossman DC, Milligan BC, Deyo RA. Risk factors for suicide attempts among Navajo adolescents. Am J Public Health 1991;81(7):870–4.

[3] Harkavy-Friedman JM, Asnis GM, Boeck M, et al. Prevalence of specific suicidal behaviors in a high school sample. Am J Psychiatry 1987;144(9):1203–6.

[4] Kienhorst CW, de Wilde EJ, van den Bout J, et al. Self-reported suicidal behavior in Dutch secondary education students. Suicide Life Threat Behav 1990;20(2):101–12.

[5] Rubenstein JL, Heeren T, Housman D, et al. Suicidal behavior in "normal" adolescents: risk and protective factors. Am J Orthopsychiatry 1989;59(1):59–71.

[6] Hawton K, Arensman E, Wasserman D, et al. Relation between attempted suicide and suicide rates among young people in Europe. J Epidemiol Community Health 1998;52(3):191–4.

[7] Schmidtke A, Weinacker C, Löhr U, et al. Suicide and suicide attempt in Europe—an overview. In: Schmidtke A, Bille-Brahe U, De Leo D, et al, editors. Suicidal behaviour in Europe, results from the WHO/EURO multicentre study on suicidal behaviour. Göttingen (Germany): Hogrefe & Huber, ISBN 0-88937-249-7; 2004.

[8] Mittendorfer-Rutz E, Rasmussen F, Wasserman D. Restricted foetal growth and mothers' adverse psychosocial and socioeconomic conditions as risk factors for offspring's suicidal behaviour. Cohort study of 713,370 adolescents and young adults in Sweden. Lancet 2004;364(9440):1135–40.

[9] Mittendorfer-Rutz E, Wasserman D. Trends in adolescent suicide mortality in the WHO European Region. Eur Child Adolesc Psychiatry 2004;13(5):321–31.

[10] Wasserman D, Cheng Q, Jiang GX. Global suicide rates among young people aged 15–19. World Psychiatry 2005;4(2):114–20.

[11] Brent DA, Perper JA, Moritz G, et al. Familial risk factors for adolescent suicide: a case-control study. Acta Psychiatr Scand 1994;89(1):52–8.

[12] Garfinkel BD, Froese A, Hood J. Suicide attempts in children and adolescents. Am J Psychiatry 1982;139:1257–61.

[13] Johnson BA, Brent DA, Bridge J, et al. The familial aggregation of adolescent suicide attempts. Acta Psychiatr Scand 1998;97(1):18–24.

[14] Mittendorfer-Rutz E. Perinatal and familial risk factors of youth suicidal behaviour [Doctoral thesis]. Karolinska Institutet, Stockholm, Sweden; 2005.

[15] Pfeffer CR, Normandin L, Kakuma T. Suicidal children grow up: suicidal behavior and psychiatric disorders among relatives. J Am Acad Child Adolesc Psychiatry 1994;33(8): 1087–97.

[16] Christoffersen MN, Poulsen HD, Nielsen A. Attempted suicide among young people: risk factors in a prospective register based study of Danish children born in 1966. Acta Psychiatr Scand 2003;108(5):350–8.

[17] Agerbo E, Nordentoft M, Mortensen PB. Familial psychiatric, and socioeconomic risk factors for suicide in young people: nested case-control study. BMJ 2002;323:74–9.

[18] Qin P, Agerbo E, Mortensen PB. Suicide risk in relation to family history of completed suicide and psychiatric disorders: a nested case-control study based on longitudinal registers. Lancet 2002;360:1126–30.

[19] Riordan DV, Sevaraj S, Stark C, et al. Perinatal circumstances and risk of offspring suicide. Birth cohort study. Br J Psychiatry 2006;189:502–7.

[20] Ekeus C. Teenage parenthood. Paternal characteristics and child health outcome. Stockholm (Sweden): Department of Public Health Sciences, Karolinska Institutet; 2004.

[21] Elster AB, Mc Anarney ER, Lamb ME. Parental behaviour of adolescent mothers. Pediatrics 1983;71:494–503.
[22] Fergusson DM, Woodward LJ. Maternal age and educational and psychosocial outcomes in early adulthood. Child Psychol Psychiatry 1999;40(3):479–89.
[23] Olausson PO, Haglund B, Weitoft GR, et al. Teenage childbearing and long-term socioeconomic consequences: a case study in Sweden. Fam Plann Perspect 2001;33(2):70–4.
[24] Lier L, Kastrup M, Rafaelsen OJ. Psychiatric illness in relation to pregnancy and child-birth. Nord Psykiatr Tidsskr 1989;43:535–42.
[25] de Paul J, Domenech L. Childhood history of abuse and child abuse potential in adolescent mothers: a longitudinal study. Child Abuse Negl 2000;24(5):701–13.
[26] Gilman SE, Kawachi I, Fitzmaurice GM, et al. Socio-economic status, family disruption and residential stability in childhood: relation to onset, recurrence and remission of major depression. Psychol Med 2003;33(8):1341–55.
[27] Ringbäck-Weitoft GR, Hjern A, Haglund B, et al. Mortality, severe morbidity, and injury in children living with single parents in Sweden: a population-based study. Lancet 2003;361(9354):289–95.
[28] Gould MS, Shaffer D, Fisher P, et al. Separation/divorce and child and adolescent completed suicide. J Am Acad Child Adolesc Psychiatry 1998;37(2):155–62.
[29] Johnson GR, Krug EG, Potter LB. Suicide among adolescents and young adults: a cross-national comparison of 34 countries. Suicide Life Threat Behav 2000;30(1):74–82.
[30] Lester D. Domestic integration and suicide in 21 nations, 1950–1985. Int J Comp Sociol 1994;35:132–7.
[31] Gould MS, Fisher P, Parides M, et al. Psychosocial risk factors of child and adolescent completed suicide. Arch Gen Psychiatry 1996;53:1155–62.
[32] Sauvola A, Rasanen PK, Joukamaa MI, et al. Mortality of young adults in relation to single-parent family background. A prospective study of the northern Finland 1966 birth cohort. Eur J Public Health 2001;11(3):284–6.
[33] Tucker JS, Friedman HS, Schwartz JE. Parental divorce: effects on individual behavior and longevity. J Pers Soc Psychol 1997;73(2):381–91.
[34] Gale CR, Martyn CN. Birth weight and later risk of depression in a national birth cohort. Br J Psychiatry 2004;184:28–33.
[35] Jones PB, Rantakallio P, Hartikainen AL, et al. Schizophrenia as a long-term outcome of pregnancy, delivery, and perinatal complications: a 28-year follow-up of the 1966 north Finland general population birth cohort. Am J Psychiatry 1998;155(3):355–64.
[36] Hadders-Algra M, Huisjes HJ, Touwen BC. Preterm or small-for-gestational-age infants. Neurological and behavioural development at the age of 6 years. Eur J Pediatr 1988;147:460–7.
[37] Lundgren EM, Cnattingius S, Jonsson B, et al. Intellectual and psychological performance in males born small for gestational age with and without catch-up growth. Pediatr Res 2001;50:91–6.
[38] Nilsson PM, Nilsson JA, Ostergren PO, et al. Foetal growth predicts stress susceptibility independent of parental education in 161991 adolescent Swedish male conscripts. J Epidemiol Community Health 2004;58(7):571–3.
[39] Pryor J, Silva PA, Brooke M. Growth, development and behaviour in adolescents born small-for-gestational-age. Paediatr Child Health 1995;31(5):403–7.
[40] Neugebauer R, Hoek HW, Susser E. Prenatal exposure to wartime famine and development of antisocial personality disorder in early adulthood. JAMA 1999;282(5):455–62.
[41] Salk L, Lipsitt LP, Sturner WQ, et al. Relationship of maternal and perinatal conditions to eventual adolescent suicide. Lancet 1985;1(8429):624–7.
[42] Neugebauer R, Reuss ML. Association of maternal, antenatal and perinatal complications with suicide in adolescence and young adulthood. Acta Psychiatr Scand 1998;97(6):412–8.
[43] Barker DJ, Osmond C, Rodin I, et al. Low weight gain in infancy and suicide in adult life. BMJ 1995;311:1203.

[44] Cnattingius S, Hultman CM, Dahl M, et al. Very preterm birth, birth trauma, and the risk of anorexia nervosa among girls. Arch Gen Psychiatry 1999;56(7):634–8.

[45] Dalman C, Allebeck P, Cullberg J, et al. Obstetric complications and the risk of schizophrenia: a longitudinal study of a national birth cohort. Arch Gen Psychiatry 1999;56(3): 234–40.

[46] Patton GC, Coffey C, Cardin JB, et al. Prematurity at birth and adolescent depressive disorder. Br J Psychiatry 2004;184:446–7.

[47] Mann JJ, Malone KM. Cerebrospinal fluid amines and higher-lethality suicide attempts in depressed inpatients. Biol Psychiatry 1997;41:162–71.

[48] Bercu BB, Diamond FB Jr. Regulation of growth hormone secretion. Relevance to the pediatrician. Pediatrician 1987;14:94–108.

[49] Sodhi MS, Sanders-Bush E. Serotonin and brain development. Int Rev Neurobiol 2004;59: 111–74.

[50] Luciana M. Cognitive development in children born preterm: implications for theories of brain plasticity following early injury. Dev Psychopathol 2003;15:1017–47.

[51] Kim CS, McNamara MC, Lauder JM, et al. Immunocytochemical detection of serotonin content in raphe neurons of newborn and young adult rabbits before and after acute hypoxia. Int J Dev Neurosci 1994;12:499–505.

[52] Gunnell D, Rasmussen F, Fouskakis D, et al. Patterns of foetal and childhood growth and the development of psychosis in young males: a cohort study. Am J Epidemiol 2003;158: 291–300.

[53] Kemppainen L, Makikyro T, Jokelainen J, et al. Is grand multiparity associated with offsprings' hospital-treated mental disorders? A 28-year follow-up of the North Finland 1966 birth cohort. Soc Psychiatry Psychiatr Epidemiol 2000;35(3):104–8.

[54] Gurel S, Gurel H. The evaluation of determinants of early postpartum low mood: the importance of parity and inter-pregnancy interval. Eur J Obstet Gynecol Reprod Biol 2000;91(1): 21–4.

[55] WHO/EURO. World Health Organization Ministerial Conference. Helsinki, Finland, November 2005.

[56] European Commission. Green Paper. Brussels (Belgium): European Commission; 2005.

[57] Niccols A, Mohammed S. Parent-child interaction skills training in groups: pilot study with parents of infants with developmental delay. Journal of Early Intervention 2000;23:59–69.

[58] ICDP. International Child Development Programme. Available at: www.icdp.info. Accessed November 1, 2007.

[59] Aronen ET, Arajarvi T. Effects of early intervention on psychiatric symptoms of young adults in low-risk and high-risk families. Am J Orthopsychiatry 2000;70(2):223–32.

[60] Haskins R. Beyond metaphor: the efficiency of early childhood education. Am Psychol 1989;44:274–82.

[61] Wadsby M, Sydsjö G, Svedin CG. Evaluation of an intervention programme to support mothers and babies at psychosocial risk: assessment of mother/child interaction and mother's perceptions of benefit. Health Soc Care Community 2001;9(3):125–33.

Psychiatr Clin N Am 31 (2008) 213–221

PSYCHIATRIC CLINICS
OF NORTH AMERICA

Maternal Suicidality and Suicide Risk in Offspring

Thomas Bronisch, MD[a],*, Roselind Lieb, PhD[b]

[a]Max-Planck-Institute of Psychiatry, Kraepelinstr. 10, D-80804 Munich, Germany
[b]Institute of Psychology, Epidemiology and Health Psychology, University of Basel, Missionsstrasse 60-62, S-4055 Basel, Switzerland

OCCURRENCE OF SUICIDALITY IN FAMILIES

A considerable number of studies examining family history and high risk for suicide have reported that suicidality runs in families [1–29]. Family studies of relatives of probands who completed or attempted suicide report a four- to sixfold greater risk for suicide or suicidal behavior compared with relatives of community or patient controls [4].

Individuals contacting suicide prevention centers, patients hospitalized for attempted suicide, and subjects assessed in epidemiologic studies [10,11,27] have reported family histories of completed and attempted suicides [12–17,23,26,29]. The studies involved adolescents [2–5,8,9,28], adults [6,7,14,16,17,21–24,29,30], and elderly individuals [1].

Familial loading is not restricted to suicides but also affects suicide attempts [1,4,9,11–13,17–19,23,25]. Therefore, different types of suicide attempt show a different familial loading of suicidality [12,18,25]. Patients who attempt violent suicides report a higher frequency of suicides and suicide attempts in their families than those who attempt nonviolent suicides. One study assessing patients attempting suicide using violent and nonviolent methods reported a significantly greater loading of ancestral secondary cases of suicide observed on the maternal side in the violent attempter group and on the paternal side in the nonviolent attempter group [18].

Furthermore, two studies found a familial loading for suicide in both men and women who commit suicide [27,31] and a study of male suicide completers observed a familial loading for suicide and suicide attempts [10]. One community study showed a familial loading for maternal suicidality among male and female offspring who attempted suicide [11]. Additionally, twin studies comparing the concordance rate between identical (monozygotic) and nonidentical (dizygotic) twins have consistently shown a higher concordance rate for suicides [30,32] and suicide attempts [33] among monozygotic twins.

*Corresponding author. E-mail address: bronisch@mpipsykl.mpg.de (T. Bronisch).

0193-953X/08/$ – see front matter
doi:10.1016/j.psc.2008.01.003

FAMILIAL AGGREGATION IN TREATMENT AND NONTREATMENT SAMPLES

For suicidal attempt and ideation, most studies included clinically referred samples. Only a few studies addressed the familial transmission of suicidality in nontreatment samples [11,21,27,34]. However, because the studies by Qin and colleagues [21] and Runeson and Asberg [27] used death registers, treatment and nontreatment samples were entangled. In contrast, the community sample of 3021 subjects used by Lieb and colleagues [11] indicated a strong effect of familial transmission, with offspring who had familial loading showing at least a four times higher risk for developing suicidal behavior compared with offspring who had no familial loading.

COMORBIDITY

Previous studies further suggest that familial transmission of suicidality is independent of comorbid mental disorders, because an elevated risk for suicidality was found even after controlling for familial aggregation of mental disorders [3,4,6,8,9,20,27,34,35], such as depression [3,4,6,9,20,27,34,35], anxiety disorders [3], substance use disorders [3,4,6,9,19,27,30,34,35], and personality disorders [9,19].

PERSONALITY TRAITS

Impulsiveness, aggressiveness, or irritability that might be directed inward or outward and is stable over time and generations has been suggested to be associated with familial clustering [36]. Brent and colleagues [3,4] investigated familial pathways to suicide in attempters in general, nonattempters [37], and early-age attempters [5]. Brent and colleagues [5] also examined siblings concordant and discordant for suicide attempts and their respective offspring groups. They observed that aggressiveness was significantly more frequent among the offspring of attempters compared with offspring of nonsuicidal individuals. Impulsive aggression in offspring was the most powerful predictor of familial transmission of suicidal behavior and early first attempt. Mann and colleagues [14] reported that risk for suicidal behavior in families of probands who have mood disorders seems to be related to early onset of mood disorders, aggressive/impulsive traits, and reported childhood abuse in probands.

CHILDHOOD TRAUMA

In their report on familial pathways to early-onset suicide attempt, Brent and colleagues [4] found that sexual abuse in both parent and child played an important role in transmission of suicidal behavior. Offspring of a parent who had a history of reported sexual abuse had an increased risk for suicide attempts, regardless of the offspring's reported abuse status. In addition, a history of sexual abuse in probands increased the likelihood that of offspring being sexually abused, which was then associated with increased probability of suicide attempt among offspring. In addition to family history, Roy and Janal [26] reported childhood trauma as an independent and noninteracting risk factor for suicidal behavior among abstinent substance-dependent patients. In addition to impulsive/aggressive traits, Mann and colleagues [14] found sexual abuse to be an independent risk factor for suicidal behavior in families of probands who had mood disorders.

FAMILIAL TRANSMISSION

Few data are available from representative samples concerning the effect of familial suicidality on the age of first manifestation of suicidality among offspring. This information, however, would be of major interest for areas such as prevention, because it would allow the identification of not only high-risk groups but also risk group–specific periods of high-risk for first manifestation of suicidality.

Lieb and colleagues [11] found some indications for suicide attempts occurring at an earlier age in offspring of mothers who attempted suicide than in those of mothers who had no suicidal tendencies (Fig. 1). These findings were not found when mothers reported suicidal ideation only.

Brent and colleagues [5] reported a comparable effect in a clinical sample specifically for offspring of probands who had mood disorders. Greater familial loading for suicidal behavior was associated with an earlier age at first suicide attempt in offspring.

METHODOLOGICAL ASPECTS

However, as consistent and powerful as the empiric evidence seems, some critical points require further exploration.

Most studies used the family history method; the subjects or patients were asked for suicidality and other variables concerning their immediate families or, in the case of psychologic autopsy studies, their relatives or significant others. Only few studies used the family interview approach, whereby family members of offspring were directly asked about suicidal behavior. This

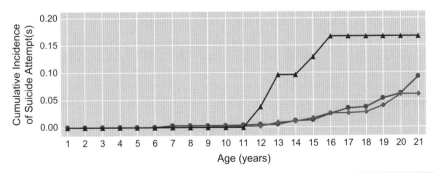

Fig. 1. The offspring's age-specific probability for first suicide attempt according to maternal suicidality status. Blue circle, no maternal suicidality; orange diamond, maternal suicidal ideation; purple triangle, maternal suicide attempts. (*From* Lieb R, Bronisch T, Höfler M, et al. Maternal suicidality and risk for suicidality in offspring: findings of a community study. Am J Psychiatry 2005;162:1665–71; with permission. Copyright © 2005, American Psychiatric Association.)

approach is obviously much less influenced by the incomplete information available to the subjects and patients. In clinical studies, only Pfeffer and colleagues [19] interviewed both parents, whereas Brent and colleagues [38], Bridge and colleagues [34], and Johnson and colleagues [9] interviewed only one family member (mostly mothers) and did not report on the frequency of mothers and fathers separately. Lieb and colleagues [11] interviewed primarily the mothers of offspring, and only fathers if mothers were not available. Besides the study by Pfeffer and colleagues [19], how frequent suicidal behavior was in fathers and how incomplete the information was on gender differences remain unclear.

For suicidal attempt and ideation, most of these studies included clinically referred samples. This fact may be crucial because familial aggregation in samples could be attributable to treatment bias and thus may be limited to a subgroup of patients undergoing treatment for severe psychiatric illness [39]. For preventive and early intervention, for example, showing that these effects can also be found in a representative community sample is important.

Until now, only few studies have addressed the familial transmission of suicidality in nontreatment samples [11,21,27,34]. Qin and colleagues [21] and Runeson and Asberg [27] used death registers, and therefore treatment and nontreatment samples are not disentangled. Although their results support the hypothesis of familial aggregation, uncertainty still exists about the strength of the familial risk in community samples. However, Lieb and colleagues [11] showed a strong effect for suicide attempts and a rather weak one for suicidal ideation.

Only one study stemming from a representative sample [11] investigates the effect of familial suicidality on the age of first manifestation in offspring. That study showed an earlier age of onset among offspring of mothers who had suicidal behavior compared with those of mothers who did not.

Furthermore, the subjects in all community studies did not yet complete the entire risk period for onset of suicidal behavior. Clinical samples show some indication that suicidal behavior also develops in older ages [5].

Finally, community studies focused on suicidal ideation and suicide attempts; the extent to which the results can be generalized for completed suicide remains to be explored.

DISCUSSION

A considerable number of studies on family history and high risk factors have reported that suicidality runs in families and is present in offspring of probands who completed or attempted suicide. These studies report a four to sixfold greater risk for suicide or suicidal behavior in the relatives of these probands compared with those of community or patient controls [4]. These results are also confirmed in community studies avoiding a selection effect, with at least a four times higher risk for developing suicidal behavior among relatives of probands. Considering the fact that the subjects passed only a limited time span (4 years), the risk should be even higher [11].

These results seem independent of comorbidity such as depression, anxiety disorders, substance abuse, and personality disorders. Furthermore, the results are stable over treatment settings, different age groups, and gender.

Regarding severity of suicide attempts and suicides, the results are generally similar to suicide and suicide attempts. However, patients who attempt a violent suicide report a higher frequency of suicides and suicide attempts in their families compared with patients who attempt nonviolent suicides One study assessing patients attempting suicide using violent and nonviolent methods reported a significantly greater loading of ancestral secondary cases of suicide observed on the maternal side in the violent attempter group and on the paternal side in the nonviolent attempter group [18]. Suicide ideas, however, do not significantly impact the development of suicidal behavior in offspring [3,11].

One community study [11] showed some indications for suicide attempt occurring at an earlier age in offspring of mothers who attempted suicide compared with offspring of mothers who had no suicidality (see Fig. 1). These findings are corroborated by a clinical study [3,4] reporting a comparable effect in a clinical sample of offspring of probands who had mood disorders. These results were not found when mothers reported suicidal ideation only [3,11].

Despite the postulated continuum from suicidal ideation to suicide attempts [40], this finding provides more support for a threshold model to explain the development of suicidal behavior generally and especially within families [41].

The mechanisms that may be involved in the familial transmission must be considered. Genetic mechanisms may partially explain the observed associations. Specifically, the findings of monozygotic and dizygotic twin studies conducted in this area of research support this hypothesis [33,35,42]. These results were further confirmed by the Danish Adoption Studies, in which the monozygotic twins were reared apart from each other very early in life, in either biologic or adoptive families. Heavy familial loading was present in the biologic families of origin but not in the adoptive families [43,44].

The familial transmission of suicidal behavior can also involve nongenetic mechanisms, such as exposure to family violence; hostility and discord; separation and loss; and low parental involvement, or imitation of parental suicidal behavior.

Furthermore, experts have suggested that familial clustering may be related to impulsiveness, aggressiveness, or irritability that might be directed inward or outward and is stable over time and generations [36,37,45–47]. This behavior seems to be strongly connected with a dysfunction of the serotonergic system [45–47]. Currently, the genetic basis of this dysfunction is unclear [48].

Brent and colleagues [3] observed that familial aggregation for suicidal behavior occurred even after controlling for impulsive aggressive personality disorders, assaultive behavior, and other measures of aggression, so that familial transmission of suicidal behavior seems to be at least partially independent of familial transmission of aggression. However, in a later study, these investigators [5] examined siblings concordant and discordant for suicide attempts or their respective offspring groups. They observed that aggressiveness was significantly more frequent among the offspring of attempters than in the off-spring of nonsuicidal individuals. The most powerful predictor of familial transmission of suicidal behavior and early first attempt in offspring was impulsive aggression in offspring. Mann and colleagues [14] found that early onset of mood disorder, aggressive/impulsive traits, and reported childhood abuse were risk factors for suicidal behavior in families of patients who had mood disorders and attempted suicide.

In their study of familial pathways to early-onset of suicide attempts, Brent and colleagues [4] reported that sexual abuse in both parent and child played an important role in transmission of suicidal behavior. In addition to family history of suicidal behavior, Roy and Janal [26] showed childhood trauma to be an independent and noninteracting risk factor in abstinent substance-dependent patients.

In addition, imitation or modeling could play an important role in transmission of suicidal behavior from parent to child [49–51]. Imitation might also explain the finding by Lieb and colleagues [11] that maternal suicidal ideation was not associated with suicidal behavior in offspring because suicidal thoughts are not specifically observable to others. However, studies addressing this issue directly do not support the imitation hypothesis as explanation for familial transmission. The data of Brent and colleagues [4] are not consistent with imitation as an explanation for parent–child transmission. The time difference between parent and child attempt was highly variable, with the child attempt preceding the parent attempt in some cases. Other studies of familial transmission of suicidal behavior are also inconsistent with imitation; studies of youth exposed to suicide, including siblings, did not find imitation of suicidal behavior [37,38]. Twins concordant for suicide attempt show great variability in timing of their suicide attempts [35]. The Danish adoption studies do not support a strong role for modeling of suicide within families [43,44].

FUTURE PROSPECTS

Studies are needed to overcome the methodological weaknesses. Community studies are lacking that are not restricted to younger age cohorts covering different age ranges. Additionally, prospective multiple longitudinal assessments would enable more accuracy in assessing suicidal thoughts and attempts. Furthermore, larger samples are needed for observing suicides in the offspring of mothers and fathers who have suicidal tendencies. Assessment of fathers together with mothers of offspring who have suicidal tendencies and those who do not seems especially urgent.

The combined assessment of suicidality, personality traits, and genetic variations in combination with stressful events could be a possible approach to investigating the development of suicidality within families [52]. Additionally, investigating psychologic and neuropsychological characteristics [53] combined with neurobiologic assessment (eg, using neuroimaging methods) and consideration of genetic variants would be important in understanding the interaction between nature and nurture within families [54].

References

[1] Batchelor I, Napler M. Attempted suicide in old age. Br Med J 1953;2:1186–90.

[2] Brent DA, Perper JA, Moritz G, et al. Familial risk factors for adolescent suicide: a case-control study. Acta Psychiatr Scand 1994;89:52–8.

[3] Brent DA, Bridge J, Johnson BA, et al. Suicidal behavior runs in families. A controlled family study of adolescent suicide victims. Arch Gen Psychiatry 1996;53:1145–52.

[4] Brent DA, Oquendo M, Birmaher B, et al. Familial pathways to early-onset suicide attempt: risk for suicidal behavior in offspring. Arch Gen Psychiatry 2002;59:801–7.

[5] Brent DA, Oquendo M, Birmaher B, et al. Peripubertal suicide attempts in offspring of suicide attempters with siblings concordant for suicidal behavior. Am J Psychiatry 2003; 160:1486–93.

[6] Cheng ATA, Chen TH, Chen C-C, et al. Psychosocial and psychiatric risk factors for suicide. Br J Psychiatry 2000;177:360–5.

[7] Farberow N, Simon M. Suicide in Los Angeles and Vienna: an intercultural study of two cities. Public Health Rep 1969;84:389–403.

[8] Gould MS, Fisher P, Parides M, et al. Psychosocial risk factors of child and adolescent completed suicide. Arch Gen Psychiatry 1996;53:1155–62.

[9] Johnson BA, Brent DA, Bridge J, et al. The familial aggregation of adolescent suicide attempts. Acta Psychiatr Scand 1998;97:18–24.

[10] Kim CD, Seguin M, Therrien N, et al. Familial aggregation of suicidal behaviour: a family study of male suicide completers from the general population. Am J Psychiatry 2005;162: 1017–9.

[11] Lieb R, Bronisch T, Höfler M, et al. Maternal suicidality and risk for suicidality in offspring: findings of a community study. Am J Psychiatry 2005;162:1665–71.

[12] Linkowski P, Maertelaere De V, Mendlewicz J. Suicidal behaviour in major depressive illness. Acta Psychiatr Scand 1985;72:233–8.

[13] Malone KM, Haas GL, Sweeney JA, et al. Major depression and the risk of attempted suicide. J Affect Disord 1995;34:173–85.

[14] Mann JJ, Bortinger J, Oquendo MA, et al. Family history of suicidal behaviour and mood disorders in probands with mood disorders. Am J Psychiatry 2005;162:1672–9.

[15] Mitterauer B. A contribution to the discussion of the role of the genetic factor in suicide based on five studies in an epidemiological defined area (province of Salzburg, Austria). Compr Psychiatry 1990;31:557–65.

[16] Murphy GE, Wetzel RD, Swallow CS, et al. Who calls the Suicide Prevention Centre: a study 55 persons calling on their own behalf. Am J Psychiatry 1969;126:314–24.

[17] Murphy GE, Wetzel RD. Family history of suicidal behavior among suicide attempters. J Nerv Ment Dis 1982;170:86–90.

[18] Papadimitriou GN, Linkowski P, Delarbre C, et al. Suicide on the paternal and maternal sides of depressed patients with a lifetime history of attempted suicide. Acta Psychiatr Scand 1991;83:417–9.

[19] Pfeffer CR, Normandin L, Kakuma T. Suicidal children grown up: suicidal behavior and psychiatric disorders among relatives. J Am Acad Child Adolesc Psychiatry 1994;33: 1087–97.

[20] Powell J, Geddes J, Deeks J, et al. Suicide in psychiatric hospital in-patients: risk factors and their predictive power. Br J Psychiatry 2000;176:266–72.

[21] Qin P, Agerbo E, Mortensen PB. Suicide risk in relation to family history of completed suicide and psychiatric disorders: a nested case control study based on longitudinal registers. Lancet 2002;360:1126–30.

[22] Qin P, Agerbo E, Mortensen PB. Suicide risk in relation to socioeconomic, demographic, psychiatric, and familial factors: a national register-based study of all suicides in Denmark, 1981–1997. Am J Psychiatry 2003;160:765–72.

[23] Robins E, Schmidt EH, O'Neal P. Some interrelations of social factors and clinical diagnosis in attempted suicide: a study of 109 patients. Am J Psychiatry 1957;40:971–4.

[24] Roy A. Family history of suicide. Arch Gen Psychiatry 1983;40:971–4.

[25] Roy A. Features associated with suicide attempts in depression: a partial replication. J Affec Disord 1993;27:35–8.

[26] Roy A, Janal M. Family history of suicide, female sex, and childhood trauma: separate or interacting risk factors for attempts at suicide? Acta Psychiatr Scand 2005;112:367–71.

[27] Runeson B, Asberg M. Family history of suicide among suicide victims. Am J Psychiatry 2003;160:1525–6.

[28] Shafii M, Carrigan S, Whittinghill JR, et al. Psychological autopsy of completed suicide in children and adolescents. Am J Psychiatry 1985;142:1061–4.

[29] Tsunag MT. Suicide in relatives of schizophrenics, manics depressives, and controls. J Clin Psychiatry 1983;44:396–400.

[30] Roy A, Segal NL, Centerwall B, et al. Suicide in twins. Arch Gen Psychiatry 1991;48: 29–32.

[31] Qin P, Mortensen PB. The impact of parental status on the risk of completed suicide. Arch Gen Psychiatry 2003b;60:797–802.

[32] Roy A, Segal NL. Suicidal behavior in twins: a replication. J Affect Disord 2001;66:71–4.

[33] Roy A, Segal NL, Sarchiapone M. Attempted suicide among living co-twins of twin suicide victims. Am J Psychiatry 1995;152:1075–6.

[34] Bridge JA, Brent DA, Johnson BA, et al. Familial aggregation of psychiatric disorders in a community sample of adolescents. J Am Acad Child Adolesc Psychiatry 1997;36: 628–36.

[35] Statham DJ, Heath AC, Madden PA, et al. Suicidal behaviour: an epidemiological and genetic study. Psychol Med 1998;28:839–55.

[36] Huesmann LR, Eron LD, Lefkowitz MM, et al. Stability of aggression over time and generations. Dev Psychol 1984;20:1120–34.

[37] Brent DA, Moritz G, Bridge J, et al. Long-term impact of exposure to suicide: a three-year controlled follow-up. J Am Acad Child Adolesc Psychiatry 1996;35:646–53.

[38] Brent DA, Moritz G, Bridge J, et al. The impact of adolescent suicide on siblings and parents: a longitudinal follow-up. Suicide Life Threat Behav 1996;26:253–9.

[39] Kendler KS. Is seeking treatment for depression predicted by a history of depression in relatives? Implications for family studies of affective disorder. Psychol Med 1995;25:807–14.

[40] Fergusson DM, Lynskey MT. Suicide attempts and suicidal ideation in a birth cohort of 16-year-old New Zealanders. J Am Acad Child Adolesc Psychiatry 1995;34:1308–17.

[41] Bronisch T. The relationship between suicidality and depression. Arch Suicide Res 1996;2: 235–54.

[42] Fu Q, Heath AC, Buchholz KK, et al. A twin study of genetic and environmental influences on suicidality in men. Psychol Med 2002;32:11–24.

[43] Schulsinger F, Kety SS, Rosenthal D, et al. A family study of suicide. In: Schou M, Stroemgren E, editors. Origin prevention and treatment of affective disorders. London: Academic press; 1979. p. 277–87.

[44] Wender PH, Kety SS, Rosenthal D, et al. Psychiatric disorders in the biological and adoptive families of adopted individuals with affective disorders. Arch Gen Psychiatry 1986;43: 923–9.

[45] Davidson RJ, Putnam KM, Larson CL. Dysfunction in the neural circuitry of emotion regulation—a possible prelude in violence. Science 2000;289:591–4.

[46] Mann JJ. The neurobiology of suicide. Nat Med 1998;4:25–30.

[47] Mann JJ, Brent DA, Arango V. The neurobiology and genetics of suicide and attempted suicide: a focus on the serotonergic system. Neuropsychopharmacology 2001;24:467–77.

[48] Arango V, Huang Y, Underwood MD, et al. Genetics of the serotonergic system in suicidal behavior. J Psychiatr Res 2003;37:375–86.

[49] Bandura A, Mischel W. Modification of self-imposed delay of reward through exposure to life and symbolic models. J Pers Soc Psychol 1965;2:698–705.

[50] Bandura A. Social learning theory of aggression. J Commun 1978;28:12–29.

[51] Schmidtke A, Schaller S. The role of mass media in suicide prevention. In: Hawton K, van Heeringen K, editors. The international handbook of suicide and attempted suicide. Chichester: Wiley; 2000. p. 675–97.

[52] Caspi A, Sudgen K, Moffitt TE, et al. Influence of life stress on depression: moderation by a polymorphism in the 5-HT gene. Science 2003;301:386–9.

[53] Keilp JG, Sackheim HA, Brodsky BS, et al. Neuropsychological dysfunction in suicide attempters. Am J Psychiatry 2001;158:735–41.

[54] Hariri AR, Mttay VS, Tessitore A, et al. Serotonin transporter genetic variation and the response of the human amygdala. Science 2002;297:400–3.

Psychiatr Clin N Am 31 (2008) 223–235

PSYCHIATRIC CLINICS
OF NORTH AMERICA

Adverse Childhood Experiences and Suicidal Behavior

Beth S. Brodsky, PhD[a], Barbara Stanley, PhD[a,b],*

[a]Department of Psychiatry, College of Physicians & Surgeons, Columbia University, NY, USA
[b]New York State Psychiatric Institute, Unit 42, 1051 Riverside Drive, New York, NY 10032, USA

E arly experiences of physical and sexual abuse and parental neglect are well-documented risk factors for suicidal behavior in adolescence and adulthood [1–20]. Until recently, much of what was known about the relationship between adverse experiences in childhood and suicidal behavior was based on correlational studies with retrospective reporting. Therefore, little was understood about the mechanisms by which trauma in childhood results in self-destructive behavior later in life.

Childhood abuse and neglect are among the many etiologic factors in the development of suicidal behavior. Childhood abuse and neglect are more likely to occur in families characterized by a range of adversities that might also contribute to the development of psychopathology, such as familial conflict, parental psychopathology, and suicide attempts in abusing parents. There is strong evidence for a robust relationship between childhood abuse/neglect and suicide, even when controlling for other environmental variables [21,22].

Methodologic limitations in the study of this relationship have included inconsistencies in the definition and measure of abuse, self-injury, and suicidal behavior across studies. Many studies focus exclusively on sexual abuse, whereas others define abuse more broadly. Specific dimensions of the abuse, such as type, duration, and severity, are addressed in varying degrees from one study to the next. Fewer studies measure neglect in relation to suicidal behavior. Similar limitations exist with regard to the distinction between suicidal behavior and self-harm. Some studies have not distinguished between self-injurious behaviors with and without intent to die, and use the term "parasuicidal behavior" to refer to all nonlethal self-injury.

Retrospective reporting of childhood abuse is another major limitation in many existing studies. Although there is some evidence that reporting error tends to underestimate the prevalence of childhood abuse, Fergusson and colleagues [23] and Maughan and Rutter [24] emphasized the susceptibility of memory of early

*Corresponding author. New York State Psychiatric Institute, Unit 42, 1051 Riverside Drive, New York, NY 10032. *E-mail address*: bhs2@columbia.edu (B. Stanley).

0193-953X/08/$ – see front matter
doi:10.1016/j.psc.2008.02.002

trauma to distortion and recommended that retrospective methods be supplemented by corroborative evidence whenever possible. In addition, subjective reports of abuse can result in inconsistencies in the definition of abuse. For example, individuals may have different thresholds for physical punishment, with some calling it abuse and others considering it within the normal limits of discipline.

The measurements of childhood physical and sexual abuse and parental neglect are becoming more standardized [25], as are the classifications of suicidal behavior [26,27]. More recent prospective and familial transmission studies have shed further light on risk factors that mediate the relationship between childhood abuse/neglect and suicidal behavior [21,28–30]. These factors include mood disorders, personality traits, and comorbid psychiatric conditions. Genetic and biologic studies of the relationship between adverse childhood experiences and the serotonergic system, which is implicated in suicidal behavior, are beginning to identify links between biologic and environmental vulnerabilities to suicide [31–33]. Studies of posttraumatic stress disorder (PTSD) [34,35] and the hypothalamic-pituitary-adrenal axis [36,37] also shed light on a possible biologic pathway to suicidal behavior that is related to having experienced childhood abuse and neglect.

This article briefly reviews the correlational, retrospective findings while giving emphasis to the more recent prospective and familial transmission studies that explore the factors mediating the relationship between childhood abuse/neglect and suicidal behavior. In addition, related areas of research such as protective factors and the personality traits that are possible risk factors that mediate this relationship are reviewed. Research on the neurobiologic correlates of trauma that might have implications for understanding suicidal behavior is also discussed. Several models for the study of the relationship between childhood adverse experiences and suicidal behavior are described.

DEFINITIONS OF EARLY ADVERSE EXPERIENCES

Measurement of childhood abuse and neglect has varied widely between studies. For example, measures of abuse range from chart reviews to self-reports or semistructured interviews to independently verified reports (eg, police records) [38]. Self-reports and semistructured interviews vary in their definitions of abuse and its severity. The age that is considered the cutoff between childhood and adulthood ranges from 15 to 18 years [25,38,39]. The age difference between the perpetrator and the child, if defined at all, has been set typically at 5 years. Some measures do not specify the age difference, merely asking whether the perpetrator was an adult or someone older than the child. Some measures define objective criteria for physical and sexual abuse [38–40], whereas others rely on more subjective reports. A variety of self-reports and semistructured interviews have been used over the course of the past 20 years. In the past decade, the Childhood Trauma Questionnaire self-report has become one of the most widely used measures to determine the presence or absence of physical or sexual abuse, emotional or physical neglect, or emotional abuse [25]. This 28-item self-report form asks the subject to rate how often various feelings or experiences were true for them when they were growing up. These items cover instances of physical neglect, physical abuse, sexual abuse, and psychologic/emotional abuse. The measure does not specifically define physical abuse, sexual abuse, or neglect and does not specify an age range or assess duration, severity of abuse, or relationship of the perpetrator. As investigators reach consensus and as the measure of adverse childhood experiences narrows to a smaller number of validated measures, the field is moving toward increased consistency in the definition of childhood abuse/neglect across studies. In the authors' studies, they have operationally defined childhood physical abuse as deliberate infliction of physical harm that results in bruising by an adult who is at least 5 years older than a child aged 0 to 18 years. The authors' definition of sexual abuse is sexual contact (from genital fondling to penetration) by an adult who is at least 5 years older than a child aged 0 to 18 years. Childhood neglect can be physical (failure of primary caregivers to provide adequate shelter, food, and clothing) or emotional (indicated by inattention to emotional needs or severe denigation and invalidation of feelings).

CORRELATES OF ABUSE AND SUICIDAL BEHAVIOR

Although the relationship between childhood abuse/neglect and suicidal behavior has been well established, less is known regarding the mechanisms by which early life trauma translates into self-destructive behavior in adulthood. Recent studies have begun to examine various dimensions of childhood adversity (eg, type of abuse/neglect, age of onset, severity, relationship of the abuser to the child, the gender of the child and of the perpetrator) and how they impact on the emergence of suicidality. Other studies have focused on personality traits that are known to contribute to suicidal behavior (eg, impulsivity and aggression) and how they may be developmentally linked to abusive experiences early in life. Diagnostic comorbidity has also been identified as a possible link between early abuse/neglect and suicidal behavior in adolescents and adults. In particular, diagnoses of Cluster B personality disorder (antisocial, borderline, narcissistic, and histrionic personality disorders) and PTSD–populations in which childhood abuse and neglect are highly prevalent–have been found to be risk factors for suicidal behavior. Earlier age of onset of major depressive disorder and panic disorder is also correlated with a history of childhood abuse/neglect and suicide. Neurobiologic studies are investigating biologic pathways and interactions between genetic and environmental (trauma) factors that lead to suicidal behavior. Protective factors such as social support, and religious or moral objections to suicide that mitigate the effect of childhood trauma on subsequent psychiatric illness and suicidality, have also been identified.

DIMENSIONS OF ADVERSE EXPERIENCE RELATED TO SUICIDAL BEHAVIOR

Type of Abuse

Although some studies have found a relationship between physical abuse and suicidal behavior, most studies show a much greater effect with a history of sexual abuse rather than physical abuse [22,41–43], with some studies reporting a greater risk for suicide attempts in those reporting more than one type of abuse [44]. Adult suicide attempters who report a history of physical or sexual abuse before the age of 15 years make their first attempt at an earlier age than attempters who do not report abuse [1,23]. In a review of the literature on childhood abuse and self-injury in adulthood, Santa Mina and Gallop [40] summarized that when trauma is sexual in nature and invasive, it is more likely to be correlated with suicidal behavior. More recently, Ystgaard and colleagues [43] found that physical abuse and sexual abuse are significantly and independently associated with repeated suicidal behavior. In a longitudinal study of childhood adversities and risk for suicidal ideation and attempts, Enns and colleagues [21] reported that childhood neglect, psychologic abuse, and physical abuse were strongly associated with new onset of suicidal ideation and suicide attempts. Two recent studies, however, found a differential effect of childhood sexual abuse versus physical abuse on adult behavior: sexual abuse in childhood is related to suicidal behavior in adulthood, whereas physical abuse in childhood is related to aggression and interpersonal violence [30,41].

Sexual abuse may be more specifically related to suicidal behavior because it is more closely associated with feelings of shame [45,46] or internal attributions of blame [47–50] that may increase vulnerability to internalizing behaviors such as self-harm and suicidality. For instance, female survivors of sexual abuse who reported abuse by an immediate family member before the age of 10 years recalled making internal attributions of blame when they were children that were predictive of a history of suicide attempts [51]. Less is known regarding the attributions related to physical abuse [52].

In addition, the familial dynamics surrounding sexual abuse, in contrast to physical abuse, may contribute to risk for suicide. For instance, emotional and psychologic abuse appear more closely related to sexual abuse than to physical abuse [53,54]. In addition, a history of childhood sexual and emotional abuse was highly correlated with intimate partner violence, PTSD, and suicide attempts among a community sample of women [53]. There is evidence that mothers who were sexually abused in childhood have higher rates of permissive parenting behaviors that may endanger their offspring in terms of sexual abuse (having difficulty establishing clear generational boundaries) [52,55] and use harsh physical discipline [54].

Gender of the Abuse Survivor

There is no evidence of a gender difference regarding the relationship between childhood abuse and suicidality. Although women report a higher incidence of childhood sexual abuse than men, Dube and colleagues [56] found that men also report significant levels of sexual abuse and that a history of suicide attempt was twice as likely among men and women who experienced childhood sexual abuse. A study by Roy and Janal [57] found no interaction between gender and childhood sexual abuse in determining attempter status, indicating that in terms of suicidal behavior, there is no gender difference in response to a history of sexual abuse.

Duration, Severity, and Perpetrator of Abuse

Very little is known regarding the relation of these dimensions of abuse with suicidal behavior. Zanarini and colleagues [58] found that the severity of reported childhood sexual abuse was significantly related to the severity of symptoms of borderline personality disorder (BPD), including impulsive and suicidal behaviors. A Swedish study found a significant relationship between age of onset of childhood sexual abuse and severity of psychiatric symptoms in general [59]. This study found that the most victims had not told anyone about the abuse for fear of not being believed [59].

IMPULSIVITY AND AGGRESSION ASSOCIATED WITH CHILDHOOD TRAUMA

Impulsivity [30,60] and aggression [61] may be personality traits that develop in response to early childhood experiences of trauma and loss. Earlier studies show a relationship between the presence of impulsive personality characteristics and suicidal behavior in individuals who have comorbid major depression and BPD [3,62,63]. The authors also found that depressed adults who report a history of physical abuse, sexual abuse, or both before age 15 years are more likely to have made a suicide attempt and also have higher levels of impulsivity and aggression [3,63]. Thus, the association between childhood trauma and self-destructive behavior in adulthood may be mediated in part by a relationship between the trauma and the development of the biologic and psychologic aspects of the traits of impulsivity and aggression. Alternatively, impulsivity and aggression could be mainly inherited traits that underlie the childhood abuse (perhaps at the hands of a first-degree relative who has trait impulsivity) in addition to the manifestation of adult-trait impulsivity. Twin [64,65], family [28,66,67], and adoption [68] studies have demonstrated the familial transmission of suicidal behavior. One set of causes of transmission of suicidal behavior is familial transmission of psychiatric illnesses such as mood disorder and substance use disorder [66,69–72]. Because increased suicidal risk persists even after controlling for familial transmission of major psychiatric disorders [73–75], however, other factors must also mediate the transmission of suicidal behavior from one generation to the next.

Twin studies find that genetic factors account for about half of the variance [65,74] and that environmental factors such as familial instability and childhood abuse contribute independently to the transmission of suicidal behavior [1,63,75–79].

Studies that control for other indices of familial instability [80,81] have identified sexual abuse of the individual as a factor that accounts for almost 20% of the population attributable risk for suicide attempt in young people. A number of the authors' studies of the familial transmission of abuse and suicidal behavior [30,66] have found that the familial transmission of suicidal behavior from proband to offspring is related to reported sexual abuse in the proband and to greater impulsive aggression and reported childhood sexual abuse in the offspring. In path analysis, offspring sexual abuse and offspring impulsivity were found to mediate the relationship between proband sexual abuse and off-spring suicide attempt. The relationship between the environment (sexual abuse) and the trait (impulsivity) variables is additive, not interactive. Thus, the path from proband sexual abuse to offspring sexual abuse and offspring suicide attempt is distinct from the path from proband sexual abuse and pro-band impulsivity to offspring impulsivity and offspring suicide attempt. This finding indicates that environmental and trait variables are familially transmit-ted and increase the risk for offspring suicidal behavior.

DIAGNOSTIC COMORBIDITY

Certain axis I and axis II disorders are known to be associated with a high prevalence of childhood physical and sexual abuse and neglect. These same diagnoses also increase the risk for suicidal behavior. PTSD is often seen in in-dividuals who have experienced adverse childhood experiences such as phys-ical abuse, sexual abuse, or both. The co-occurrence of PTSD with major depressive disorder enhances the risk for suicidal behavior, independently of other risk factors such as substance use or Cluster B personality disorders [35]. Further research [34], however, has found that this effect was attributable to co-occurring Cluster B personality disorders. Other studies support the role of Cluster B personality disorders, particularly BPD, as important in mediating the relationship between childhood abuse and suicidal behavior. Numerous studies [58,82–84] have documented high rates of reported abuse history in BPD, leading some theorists and researchers to conceptualize BPD as a form of PTSD. Although there are conflicting reports regarding the relationship of abuse to self-injury in BPD, self-injury has been associated with sequelae of abuse such as dissociation. Wagner and Linehan [39] found that BPD individ-uals who reported childhood sexual abuse did not self-mutilate more but made more lethal suicide attempts. An earlier study of the authors' [3] found that individuals who had BPD and reported a history of abuse were more likely to have made a suicide attempt than those who did not report abuse.

Although PTSD and Cluster B personality disorders are highly associated with adverse childhood experiences, they are also independently related to sui-cidal behavior [34]. Thus, an abuse-related diagnosis may be one of multiple mediators between abuse and suicidal behavior.

Childhood trauma has also been shown to be associated with an earlier age of onset of major depression [30,85]. In a study of the pathways from child-hood sexual abuse to deliberate self-harm, Gladstone and colleagues [85] found that among depressed women, a history of childhood sexual abuse was not associated with differences in level of depression, yet the abused women were more likely to have made a suicide attempt, engaged in deliberate self-harm, or both. The abused women also reported earlier age of onset of depres-sion and were more likely to have panic disorder. These conditions, however, did not seem to mediate the relationship between sexual abuse and self-harm behaviors; rather, in this study, there was a direct path between childhood sex-ual abuse and self-harm behaviors.

Substance use disorders are also risk factors for suicidal behavior. Makhija [86] reported that adolescents who were victims of childhood abuse show an even greater prevalence of suicidality and substance and alcohol misuse. Makhija [86] proposed that substance abuse may be a mediating link between childhood abuse and suicidal behavior in adolescents. A history of childhood abuse is also correlated with higher rates of substance and alcohol use in adults, which in turn exacerbates suicidal behavior in adults [87].

PROTECTIVE FACTORS

A number of studies have also investigated the factors that protect an individual from engaging in self-destructive behavior despite a history of childhood abuse/neglect. The presence of a caring adult, high quality of adult relationships, less affiliation with delinquent peer groups, family connectedness [88], and involvement in sports throughout childhood and adolescence [89] have been found to mitigate the association between abuse history and adult psychopathology. Reasons for living, moral objections to suicide, and religious affiliation [90] are also protective factors against suicidal behavior in adults who have major depression and a history of abuse.

NEUROBIOLOGIC CORRELATES OF TRAUMA AND SUICIDAL BEHAVIOR

A consistent finding of neurobiologic studies is that low serotonergic functioning is associated with increased impulsivity, self-destructive behavior, and aggressive behavior in adults [91,92]. Early childhood environmental factors might contribute to lower serotonergic functioning or to the development of personality traits of impulsivity and aggression. There is evidence from nonhuman primate studies that genetic transmission and environmental factors such as maternal deprivation contribute to the presence of biologic correlates of impulsivity. Peer-raised monkeys reset their cerebral spinal fluid 5-hydroxyindoleacetic acid levels at a lower level compared with maternally raised monkeys, and this effect endures for years and is associated with impulsive and aggressive behaviors [93]. In a separation paradigm study with rhesus macaques, those raised by peers only and that had the short allele of the human serotonin transporter–linked promoter region polymorphism exhibited more pathologic behaviors (ie, despair, agitation, and behavioral pathology) [94]. Similar findings of the relationship among maternal separation, decreased expression of serotonin, and depressive symptomatology have been found in rodents [95–98].

Human genetic studies are providing preliminary evidence that certain gene polymorphisms related to serotonergic functioning moderate the relationship between childhood trauma and depression/suicidal behavior. Roy and colleagues [33] reported that childhood trauma interacts with low expressing 5-HTTLPR genotypes to increase the risk of suicidal behavior among patients who have substance dependence. Gibb and colleagues [31] found that 5-HTTLPR genotype moderated the link between adult inpatients' histories of suicide attempts and childhood physical and sexual abuse, but not emotional abuse. In a study of a functional polymorphism in the Monoamine Oxidase A (MAO A) gene promoter, found to be altered in mood disorders and associated with aggressive behavior, Huang and colleagues [32] found that lower expression of this polymorphism favored more pronounced impulsiveness in adulthood in men (but not in women) reporting a history of early abuse. They also suggested that this polymorphism may be a marker for impulsivity that in turn may contribute to the risk for abuse and could be further aggravated by abuse.

Parental neglect and disrupted attachment behaviors may also have biologic underpinnings. The peptide hormone oxytocin is known from animal studies [99] to play an important role in regulating affiliative behaviors such as maternal and parenting behaviors. Bartz and Hollander [99] reviewed the current state of thought regarding the relationship between oxytocin and psychiatric disorders related to disrupted attachment—specifically autism, social phobia, obsessive-compulsive disorder, BPD, and schizophrenia. Researchers speculate that oxytocin supports affiliation through its role in stress reduction, and vasopressin, although the mechanisms are not clear. They suggest that adverse experiences in early childhood can alter brain development through its effects on the oxytocin-vasopressin stress response system.

MODELS OF ADVERSE EXPERIENCE AND SUICIDAL BEHAVIOR
A number of theoretic models provide useful frameworks within which to further understand and study the mechanisms by which early childhood trauma can contribute to suicidal behavior. Cole and Putnam [100] outlined a model of the effect of incest on self and social functioning. They observed that suicidal behavior may be a manifestation of self-dysregulation due to incest. They recommended comprehensive measures of self and social functioning when doing research on the consequences of incest on adult psychopathology.

According to Linehan [101], the chronic suicidal behavior characteristic of individuals who have BPD is a result of emotional, behavioral, cognitive, and interpersonal dysregulation. This theory attributes this dysregulation to a transaction between an inborn emotional vulnerability and an invalidating environment. Linehan [101] also applies learning theory to explain how the emotionally vulnerable individual develops self-destructive behaviors to get a nurturing response from the invalidating environment. As the behaviors escalate, they are intermittently reinforced, making them very difficult to unlearn. The most egregious example of an invalidating environment would be one in which sexual abuse, physical abuse, or neglect was present. In addition to being a clear example of invalidation of the child's needs, the experience of childhood abuse and neglect is often characterized by much inconsistency and conflict because the child experiences nurturing and abuse/neglect from the same caretaker. This theory has implications for further understanding the interaction of biologic and environmental risk factors for suicidal behavior.

Although childhood abuse and neglect are examples of an invalidating environment within this model, further research is needed to more fully understand the similarities and the differences related to childhood physical/sexual abuse and experiences of physical and emotional neglect. Because abuse and neglect often co-occur within the same family environment, it is difficult to tease apart the differential effects of these experiences on subsequent development.

A comprehensive diathesis-stress model of suicidal behavior has been described by Mann and colleagues [13]. In this model, early childhood abuse constitutes an environmental factor that might contribute to the diathesis (the vulnerability or propensity to act on suicidal ideation), possibly by altering stress responsivity, and to the stressor, which might be events that trigger memories of the abuse.

SUMMARY

A history of childhood abuse, particularly sexual abuse, creates a vulnerability to suicidal behavior in adulthood. Neglect also appears to convey a similar liability. Other childhood adverse experiences such as parental loss and other forms of trauma have not received as much research attention.

References

[1] Boudewyn AC, Liem JH. Childhood sexual abuse as a precursor to depression and self-destructive behavior in adulthood. J Trauma Stress 1995;8:445–59.

[2] Briere J, Runtz M. Differential adult symptomatology associated with three types of child abuse histories. Child Abuse Negl 1990;14:357–64.

[3] Brodsky B, Malone K, Ellis S, et al. Characteristics of borderline personality disorder associated with suicidal behavior. Am J Psychiatry 1997;154:1715–9.

[4] Brown GR, Anderson B. Psychiatric morbidity in adult inpatients with childhood histories of sexual and physical abuse. Am J Psychiatry 1991;148:55–61.

[5] Bryant SL, Range LM. Type and severity of child abuse and college students' lifetime suicidality. Child Abuse Negl 1997;21(12):1169–76.

[6] Davidson JR, Hughes DC, Gerge LK, et al. The association of sexual assault and attempted suicide within the community. Arch Gen Psychiatry 1996;53(6):550–5.

[7] Dubo ED, Zanarini MC, Lewis RE, et al. Childhood antecedents of self-destructiveness in borderline personality disorder. Can J Psychiatry 1997;42(1):63–9.

[8] Gould DA, Stevens NG, Ward NG, et al. Self-reported childhood abuse in an adult population in a primary care setting. Prevalence, correlates and associated suicide attempts. Arch Fam Med 1994;3(3):252–6.

[9] Grilo CM, Sanislow C, Fehon D, et al. Psychological and behavioral functioning in adolescent psychiatric inpatients who report histories of childhood abuse. Am J Psychiatry 1999;156:538–43.

[10] Kaplan ML, Asnis GM, Lipschitz DS, et al. Suicidal behavior and abuse in psychiatric outpatients. Compr Psychiatry 1995;36(3):229–35.

[11] Kaplan SJ, Pelcovitz D, Salzinger S, et al. Psychopathology of abused and neglected children and adolescents. J Am Acad Child Psychiatry 1983;22(3):238–44.

[12] Lipschitz DS, Winegar RK, Nicolaou AL, et al. Perceived abuse and neglect as risk factors for suicidal behavior in adolescent inpatients. J Nerv Ment Dis 1999;187(1):32–9.

[13] Mann JJ, Waternaux C, Haas GL, et al. Toward a model of suicidal behavior in psychiatric patients. Am J Psychiatry 1999;156(2):181–9.

[14] Mullen PE, Martin JL, Anderson JC, et al. Childhood sexual abuse and mental health in adult life. Br J Psychiatry 1993;163:721–32.

[15] Roberts J, Hawton K. Child abuse and attempted suicide. Br J Psychiatry 1980;137:319–23.

[16] Romans SE, Martin JL, Anderson JC, et al. Sexual abuse in childhood and deliberate self-harm. Am J Psychiatry 1995;153(9):1336–42.

[17] Shaunesey K, Cohen JL, Plummer B, et al. Suicidality in hospitalized adolescents; relationship to prior abuse. Am J Orthopsychiatry 1993;63:113–9.

[18] Stepakoff S. Effects of sexual victimization on suicidal ideation and behavior in US college women. Suicide Life Threat Behav 1998;28(1):107–26.

[19] Van der Kolk BA, Perry JC, Herman JL. Childhood origins of self-destructive behavior. Am J Psychiatry 1991;148:1665–71.

[20] Windle M, Windle RC, Scheidt DM, et al. Physical and sexual abuse and associated mental disorders among alcoholic inpatients. Am J Psychiatry 1995;12:1322–8.

[21] Enns MW, Cox BJ, Afifi TO, et al. Childhood adversities and risk for suicidal ideation and attempts: a longitudinal population-based study. Psychol Med 2006;36(12):1269–78.

[22] Molnar BE, Berkman LF, Buka SL. Psychopathology, childhood sexual abuse and other childhood adversities: relative links to subsequent suicidal behavior in the US. Psychol Med 2001;31(6):965–77.

[23] Fergusson DM, Horwood LJ, Woodward LJ. The stability of child abuse reports: a longitudinal study of the reporting behaviour of young adults. Psychol Med 2000;30:529–44.

[24] Maughan B, Rutter M. Retrospective reporting of childhood adversity: issues in assessing long-term recall. J Personal Disord 1997;11(1):19–33.

[25] Bernstein DP, Fink L, Handelsman L, et al. Initial reliability and validity of a new retrospective measure of child abuse and neglect. Am J Psychiatry 1994;151(8):1132–6.

[26] Posner K, Oquendo M, Gould M, et al. Columbia classification algorithm of suicide assessment (C-CASA): classification of suicidal events in the FDA's pediatric suicidal risk analysis of antidepressants. Am J Psychiatry 2007;164(7):1035–43.

[27] Silverman MM, Berman AL, Sanddal ND, et al. Rebuilding the tower of Babel: a revised nomenclature for the study of suicide and suicidal behaviors. Part 1: background, rationale, and methodology. Suicide Life Threat Behav 2007;37(3):248–63.

[28] Brent DA, Oquendo M, Birmaher B, et al. Familial transmission of mood disorders: convergence and divergence with transmission of suicidal behavior. J Am Acad Child Adolesc Psychiatry 2004;43(10):1259–66.

[29] Brent DA, Perper JA, Moritz G, et al. Familial risk factors for adolescent suicide: a case-control study. Acta Psychiatr Scand 1994;89:52–8.

[30] Brodsky B, Mann J, Stanley B. Familial transmission of suicidal behavior: factors mediating the relationship between childhood abuse and offspring suicide attempts. J Clin Psychiatry 2008 Mar 25;e1–e13 [Epub ahead of print].

[31] Gibb BE, McGeary JE, Beevers CG. Serotonin transporter (5-HTTLPR) genotype, childhood abuse, and suicide attempts in adult psychiatric inpatients. Suicide Life Threat Behav 2006;36(6):687–93.

[32] Huang YY, Cate SP, Battistuzzi C, et al. An association between a functional polymorphism in the monoamine oxidase A gene promoter, impulsive traits and early abuse experiences. Neuropsychopharmacology 2004;29(8):1498–505.

[33] Roy A, Hu XZ, Janal MN, et al. Interaction between childhood trauma and serotonin transporter gene variation in suicide. Neuropsychopharmacology 2007;32(9):2046–52 [Epub Mar 14, 2007].

[34] Oquendo M, Brent DA, Birmaher B, et al. Posttraumatic stress disorder comorbid with major depression: factors mediating the association with suicidal behavior. Am J Psychiatry 2005;162(3):560–6.

[35] Oquendo MA, Friend JM, Halberstam B, et al. Association of comorbid posttraumatic stress disorder and major depression with greater risk for suicidal behavior. Am J Psychiatry 2003;160(3):580–2.

[36] DeBellis M. The psychobiology of neglect. Child Maltreat 2005;10(2):150–72.

[37] Yehuda R. Biology of posttraumatic stress disorder. J Clin Psychiatry 2001;62(Suppl 17):41–6.

[38] Chaffin M, Wherry J, Newlin C, et al. The abuse dimensions inventory: initial data on a research measure of abuse severity. J Interpers Violence 1999;12(4):569–89.

[39] Wagner AW, Linehan MM. Relationship between childhood sexual abuse and topography of parasuicide among women with borderline personality disorder. J Personal Disord 1994;8:1–9.

[40] Santa Mina EE, Gallop RM. Childhood sexual and physical abuse and self-harm and adult suicidal behaviour: a literature review. Can J Psychiatry 1998;43(8):793–800.

[41] McHolm AE, MacMillan HL, Jamieson E. The relationship between childhood physical abuse and suicidality among depressed women: results from a community sample. Am J Psychiatry 2003;160(5):933–8.

[42] Ogata SN, Silk KR, Goodrich S, et al. Childhood sexual and physical abuse in adult patients with borderline personality disorder. Am J Psychiatry 1990;147:1008–13.

[43] Ystgaard M, Nestetun I, Loeb M, et al. Is there a specific relationship between childhood sexual and physical abuse and repeated suicidal behavior? Child Abuse Negl 2004;28(8):863–75.

[44] Anderson PL, Tiro JA, Price AW, et al. Additive impact of childhood emotional, physical and sexual abuse on suicide attempts among low-income African American women. Suicide Life Threat Behav 2002;32(2):131–8.

[45] Feiring C, Taska LS. The persistence of shame following sexual abuse: a longitudinal look at risk and recovery. Child Maltreat 2005;10(4):337–49.

[46] Feiring C, Taska L, Lewis M. A process model for understanding adaptation to sexual abuse: the role of shame in defining stigmatization. Child Abuse Negl 1996;20(8): 767–82.

[47] Barker-Collo SL. Adult reports of child and adult attributions of blame for childhood sexual abuse: predicting adult adjustment and suicidal behaviors in females. Child Abuse Negl 2001;25(10):1329–41.

[48] Feiring C, Taska L, Chen K. Trying to understand why horrible things happen: attribution shame, and symptom development following sexual abuse. Child Maltreat 2002;7: 26–41.

[49] Feiring C, Taska L, Lewis M. Adjustment following sexual abuse discovery: the role of shame and attributional style. Dev Psychol 2002;38(1):79–92.

[50] Quas JA, Goodman GS, Jones D. Predictors of attributions of self-blame and internalizing behavior problems in sexually abused children. J Child Psychol Psychiatry 2003;44(5): 723–36.

[51] Valle LA, Silovsky JF. Attributions and adjustment following child sexual and physical abuse. Child Maltreat 2002;7(1):9–24.

[52] Seedat S, Stein MB, Forde DR. Association between physical partner violence, posttraumatic stress, childhood trauma, and suicide attempts in a community sample of women. Violence Vict 2005;20(1):87–9.

[53] Bifulco A, Moran PM, Baines R, et al. Exploring psychological abuse in childhood: II. Association with other abuse and adult clinical depression. Bull Menninger Clin 2002;66(3): 241–58.

[54] DiLillo D, Damashek A. Parenting characteristics of women reporting a history of childhood sexual abuse. Child Maltreat 2003;8(4):319–33.

[55] Ruscio AM. Predicting the child-rearing practices of mothers sexually abused in childhood. Child Abuse Negl 2001;25(3):369–87.

[56] Dube SR, Anda RF, Whitefield CL, et al. Long-term consequences of childhood sexual abuse by gender of victim. Am J Prev Med 2005;28(5):430–8.

[57] Roy A, Janal M. Gender in suicide attempt rates and childhood sexual abuse rates: is there an interaction? Suicide Life Threat Behav 2006;36(3):329–35.

[58] Zanarini MC, Yong L, Frankenburg FR, et al. Severity of reported childhood sexual abuse and its relationship to severity of borderline psychopathology and psychosocial impairment among borderline inpatients. J Nerv Ment Dis 2002;190(6):381–7.

[59] Lundqvist G, Hansson K, Svedin CG. The influence of childhood sexual abuse factors on women's health. Nord J Psychiatry 2004;58(5):395–401.

[60] Roy A. Childhood trauma and impulsivity. Possible relevance to suicidal behavior. Arch Suicide Res 2005;9(2):147–51.

[61] Keilp JG, Gorlyn M, Oquendo MA, et al. Aggressiveness, not impulsiveness or hostility, distinguishes suicide attempters with major depression. Psychol Med 2006;7:1–10.

[62] Black DW, Blum N, Pfohl B, et al. Suicidal behavior in borderline personality disorder: prevalence, risk factors, prediction and prevention. J Personal Disord 2004;18(3): 226–39.

[63] Brodsky BS, Oquendo MA, Ellis SP, et al. The relationship of childhood abuse to impulsivity and suicidal behavior in adults with major depression. Am J Psychiatry 2001;158:1871–7.

[64] Roy A, Segal NL, Centerwall BS, et al. Suicide in twins. Arch Gen Psychiatry 1991;48: 29–32.

[65] Statham DJ, Heath AC, Madden PA, et al. Suicidal behaviour: an epidemiological and genetic study. Psychol Med 1998;28:839–55.

[66] Brent DA, Oquendo MA, Birmaher B, et al. Familial pathways to early-onset suicide attempt: a high-risk study. Arch Gen Psychiatry 2002;59:801–7.

[67] Schulsinger F, Kety SS, Rosenthal D, et al. A family study of suicide. In: Schou M, Stromgren E, editors. Origin, prevention and treatment of affective disorders. New York: Academic Press; 1979. p. 277–87.

[68] Wender PH, Kety SS, Rosenthal D, et al. Psychiatric disorders in the biological and adoptive families of adopted individuals with affective disorders. Arch Gen Psychiatry 1986;43:923–9.

[69] Egeland JA, Sussex JN. Suicide and family loading for affective disorders. JAMA 1985;254(7):915–91.

[70] Johnson BA, Brent DA, Bridge J, et al. The familial aggregation of adolescent suicide attempts. Acta Psychiatr Scand 1998;97:18–24.

[71] Kaufman J, Birmaher B, Brent DA, et al. Psychopathology in the relatives of depressed-abused children. Child Abuse Negl 1998;22:171–81.

[72] Mann JJ, Bortinger J, Oquendo MA, et al. Family history of suicidal behavior and mood disorders in probands with mood disorders. Am J Psychiatry 2005;162(9):1672–9.

[73] Brent DA, Bridge J, Johnson BA, et al. Suicidal behavior runs in families. A controlled family study of adolescent suicide victims. Arch Gen Psychiatry 1996;53:1145–52.

[74] Brent DA, Mann JJ. Family genetic studies, suicide, and suicidal behavior. Am J Med Genet C Semin Med Genet 2005;133(1):13–24.

[75] Gould MS, Fisher P, Parides M, et al. Psychosocial risk factors of child and adolescent completed suicide. Arch Gen Psychiatry 1996;53:1155–62.

[76] Adams KS, Bouckoms A, Streiner D. Parental loss and family stability in attempted suicide. Arch Gen Psychiatry 1982;39:1081–5.

[77] Brand EF, King CA, Olson E, et al. Depressed adolescents with a history of sexual abuse: diagnostic comorbidity and suicidality. J Am Acad Child Adolesc Psychiatry 1996;35: 34–41.

[78] Bryer JB, Nelson B, Miller JB, et al. Childhood sexual and physical abuse as factors in adult psychiatric illness. Am J Psychiatry 1987;144:1426–30.

[79] Munro A. Parent-child separation: is it really a cause of psychiatric illness in adult life? Arch Gen Psychiatry 1969;20:598–604.

[80] Dinwiddie S, Heath AC, Dunne MP, et al. Early sexual abuse and lifetime psychopathology: a co-twin control study. Psychol Med 2000;30:41–52.

[81] Nelson EC, Heath AC, Madden PAF, et al. Association between self-reported childhood sexual abuse and adverse psychosocial outcomes: results from a twin study. Arch Gen Psychiatry 2002;59:139.

[82] Brodsky B, Stanley B. Developmental effects on suicidal behavior: the role of abuse in childhood. Clin Neurosci Res 2001;1:331–6.

[83] Herman JL, Perry JC, Van der Kolk BA. Childhood trauma in borderline personality disorder. Am J Psychiatry 1989;146(4):490–5.

[84] Stanley B, Brodsky B. Risk factors and treatment of suicidality in borderline personality disorder. Clin Neurosci Res 2001;1:351–61.

[85] Gladstone GL, Parker GB, Mitchell PB, et al. Implications of childhood trauma for depressed women: an analysis of pathways from childhood sexual abuse to deliberate self-harm and revictimization. Am J Psychiatry 2004;161(8):1417–25.

[86] Makhija N. Childhood abuse and adolescent suicidality: a direct link and an indirect link through alcohol and substance misuse. Int J Adolesc Med Health 2007;19(1):45–51.

[87] Makhija N, Sher L. Childhood abuse, adult alcohol use disorders and suicidal behaviour. QJM 2007;100(5):305–9 [Epub April 21, 2007].

[88] Eisenberg ME, Ackard DM, Resnick MD. Protective factors and suicide risk in adolescents with a history of sexual abuse. J Pediatr 2007;151(5):482–7 [Epub Sep 17, 2007].

[89] Fergusson DM, Beautrais AL, Horwood LJ. Vulnerability and resiliency to suicidal behaviours in young people. Psychol Med 2003;33(1):61–73.

[90] Dervic K, Grunebaum M, Burke AK, et al. Protective factors against suicidal behavior in depressed adults reporting childhood abuse. J Nerv Ment Dis 2006;194(12):971–4.

[91] Mann JJ, Brent DA, Arango V. The neurobiology and genetics of suicide and attempted suicide: a focus on the serotonergic system. Neuropsychopharmacology 2001;23(5):467–77.

[92] Stanley M, Mann JJ. Increased serotonin-2 binding sites in frontal cortex of suicide victims. Lancet 1983;1(8318):214–6.

[93] Higley JD, Suomi SJ, Linnoila M. A longitudinal assessment of CSF monoamine metabolite and plasma cortisol concentrations in young rhesus monkeys. Biol Psychiatry 1992;32(2):127–45.

[94] Spinelli S, Schwandt ML, Lindell SG, et al. Association between the recombinant human serotonin transporter linked promoter region polymorphism and behavior in rhesus macaques during a separation paradigm. Dev Psychopathol 2007;19(4):977–87.

[95] Bhansali P, Dunning J, Singer SE, et al. Early life stress alters adult serotonin 2C receptor pre-mRNA editing and expression of the alpha subunit of the heterotrimeric G-protein G q. J Neurosci 2007;27(6):1467–73.

[96] Lee JH, Kim HJ, Kim JG, et al. Depressive behaviors and decreased expression of serotonin reuptake transporter in rats that experienced neonatal maternal separation. Neurosci Res 2007;58(1):32–9.

[97] Lim MM, Young L. Neuropeptidergic regulation of affiliative behavior and social bonding in animals. Horm Behav 2006;50(4):518–28.

[98] Vicentic A, Francis D, Moffett M, et al. Maternal separation alters sertonergic transporter densities and serotonergic 1A receptors in rat brain. Neuroscience 2006;140(1):355–65.

[99] Bartz JA, Hollander E. The neuroscience of affiliation: forging links between basic and clinical research on neuropeptides and social behavior. Horm Behav 2006;50(4):518–28.

[100] Cole PM, Putnam FW. Effect of incest on self and social functioning: a developmental psychopathology perspective. J Consult Clin Psychol 1992;60(2):174–84.

[101] Linehan M. Cognitive behavior therapy of borderline personality disorder. New York: Guilford Press; 1993.

Psychiatr Clin N Am 31 (2008) 237–246

PSYCHIATRIC CLINICS
OF NORTH AMERICA

Interaction of Child and Family Psychopathology Leading to Suicidal Behavior

Gil Zalsman, MD[a,b,c,*], Tomer Levy, MD[a,d], Gal Shoval, MD[a,b]

[a]Sackler School of Medicine, Tel Aviv University, Tel Aviv, Israel
[b]Child and Adolescent Department, Geha Mental Health Center,
Tel Aviv University, 1 Helsinki Street, P.O. Box 102, Petach Tiqwa 49100, Israel
[c]Neuroscience Division, Columbia University, New York, NY, USA
[d]Geha Mental Health Center, Tel Aviv University, 1 Helsinki Street,
P.O.Box 102, Petach Tiqwa 49100, Israel

SUICIDAL BEHAVIOR AMONG CHILDREN AND ADOLESCENTS

According to the Centers for Disease Control and Prevention, suicide is the third leading cause of death in adolescents in the United States. Nonfatal forms of suicidal behavior are the most common reason for the psychiatric hospitalization of adolescents in many countries [1].

In 2001, approximately 1600 American youngsters aged 15 to 19 years committed suicide; 3.4 million youngsters in this age group seriously considered suicide; 1.7 million attempted suicide; and 590,000 made a suicide attempt that required medical attention [2].

Not all suicidal ideation or behavior in pediatric populations is directly attributable to depression [3]. One major survey, the Biannual Youth Risk Behavior survey [4], found that during the preceding 12 months, 28.6% of high school students nationwide felt sad or hopeless almost every day for at least 2 weeks in a row and stopped performing some of their usual activities; 16.9% seriously considered attempting suicide; 16.5% made a plan to attempt suicide; 8.5% actually attempted suicide one or more times; and 2.9% made a suicide attempt requiring medical care [4].

RISK FACTORS FOR SUICIDE AMONG CHILDREN AND ADOLESCENTS

Risk factors for suicidality are discussed elsewhere in this issue and are not specific for children and adolescents. Suicidal behavior in adolescents is linked to a wide variety of psychiatric disorders, including affective illness, alcohol and

*Corresponding author. Child and Adolescent Department, Geha Mental Health Center, Tel Aviv University, 1 Helsinki Street, P.O.Box 102, Petach Tiqwa 49100, Israel. *E-mail address*: zalsman@post.tau.ac.il (G. Zalsman).

0193-953X/08/$ – see front matter
doi:10.1016/j.psc.2008.01.009

substance abuse, conduct disorder, and schizophrenia [5]. More than 90% of adolescent and adult suicide victims appear to have at least one Axis I disorder [6].

Because most psychiatric patients do not attempt or commit suicide, psychiatric disorder may be a necessary, although insufficient, precursor for suicide. Similar to other investigators [7,8], the authors found evidence suggesting that certain psychopathologic dimensions, namely a tendency to impulsive aggression and anxiety, may predispose to suicidal behavior and completed suicide in this age group [1,9–11]. The risk for suicide is substantially increased when psychiatric disorders and certain personality traits occur concurrently.

Currently, the most common biologically correlated system related to suicidality, impulsive violence, and anxiety is the serotonergic system [8,11,12]. Platelet $5HT_2$ receptors have been shown to have lower responsiveness and sensitivity in suicide attempters compared with nonattempters. A strong correlation seems to exist between the medical damage resulting from a suicide attempt and the number of 5HT receptors [8,11]. After the finding of higher affinity (B_{MAx}) in the $5HT_{2A}$ receptors in suicidal patients, independent of diagnosis [13–15], postmortem studies have shown higher $5HT_{2A}$ receptor binding capacity in postmortem brains of adolescent suicide victims [14], hence replicating the abnormalities observed in adults.

Low platelets, low serum, and low cerebrospinal fluid 5-hydroxyindolacetic acid (5-HIAA) levels were found to be related to suicidal behavior, especially more lethal suicide attempts, regardless of psychiatric diagnosis [12,16,17].

FAMILIAL TRANSMISSION OF SUICIDAL BEHAVIOR

Suicidal behavior runs in families [18,19]. Despite much variability in the methodology of the studies, results consistently show familial aggregation of suicidal behavior. Longitudinal community studies show that family history of suicidal behavior is one of the precursors of youthful suicidal behavior, such as depression, suicidal ideation, behavioral problems, and child maltreatment [20].

The transmission of suicidal behavior may occur through pure genetic transmission (specific genes and loci), pure environmental transmission (eg, modeling, abuse), or interaction of these two factors (gene–environment interaction) [12,18,21–24].

THE GENETICS AND INHERITANCE OF SUICIDE

Twin and Adoption Studies

In a review of all published twin case reports for suicide, Roy and Segal [25] found higher rates of concordance for suicide and suicidal behavior in monozygotic (MZ) versus dizygotic (DZ) twins (14.9% versus 0.7%, and 23.0% versus 0.7% respectively). Among twin suicide victims, Roy and colleagues [26] found an even higher concordance rate for suicide attempts in surviving MZ than DZ twins (38% versus 0%), supporting the view that the clinical phenotype for concordance included both completed suicide and suicide attempts. Because these meta-analyses used reported case series, they are not necessarily representative of all twins among whom suicide occurred. The differential concordance rate for suicide for MZ versus DZ twins does not seem to be caused by greater bereavement reactions in MZ twins, because the risk for a suicide attempt after the nonsuicide death of a co-twin is similar in MZ versus DZ twins (1.4% versus 3.3%) [25].

Fu and colleagues [27] examined the relationship of suicidal ideation and behavior in 3372 male twin pairs in the Vietnam Era Twin registry. MZ twins were more likely to be concordant for suicide attempts than were DZ twins, even after adjusting for other risk factors of suicidal behavior (area of responsibility [AOR], 12.06 versus 7.41, respectively); this was also the case for suicidal ideation (AOR, 2.95 versus 1.55, respectively). The unadjusted heritabilities for suicidal ideation and attempt were 43% and 30%, respectively.

This twin study is unique in that the estimates of the genetic component of risk for suicide ideation and attempt were estimated, after adjustment for psychiatric disorder, combat history, and sociodemographic variables, and were 36.0% and 17.4%, respectively [27].

Schulsinger [28] performed the classic adoption study on suicide in Denmark, comparing the rates of suicide among the biological and adoptive relatives of adoptees who committed suicide with a matched living adoptee control group. The sixfold higher rate of suicide in the biological relatives of the suicide adoptees, and the absence of suicide among the adopted relatives of the suicide versus control adoptees, support a genetic rather than environmental effect. The rate of suicide was higher in the biological relatives of suicide adoptees regardless of whether the adoptees were psychiatric patients. However, whether the genetic liability to suicide was attributable to the transmission of major psychiatric disorder was impossible to determine [28].

Suicide and Serotonin

In adults, many significant abnormalities have been found in the serotonergic system in both suicide attempters and completers [29]. Although studies of candidate genes are still in an early phase, some emerging results suggest that genetic factors influencing suicide risk may operate, at least partially, through the serotonergic neurotransmitter system [21,22]. The abnormalities can be transmitted either genetically or through in utero exposure. Further studies are needed to establish the mode of the biological vulnerability transmission.

ENVIRONMENTAL FACTORS

Studies link suicidal behavior among children and adolescents to specific family stressors, such as family discord, parenting problems, a history of insulting behavior, and sexual abuse. One study of children aged 15 years or younger compared 481 subjects who exhibited symptomatic depression with 147 who had this symptom and also had suicidal ideation [30]. Suicidal ideation was associated with disturbed, hostile intrafamilial relationships. No specific psychiatric, emotional, or conduct disorder symptoms were found to differentiate the groups. Similarly, no extrafamilial and social characteristics were found to differentiate the groups. The children who had suicidal ideation had no more disturbance of peer relationships or social withdrawal than did the nonsuicidal, depressed subjects. Another study compared adolescent suicide attempters with depressed and nondepressed adolescents, who never attempted suicide, regarding life events that occurred in childhood and adolescence [31]. Life event data about childhood and adolescence were gathered from three groups of adolescents: 48 suicide attempters, 66 depressed nonattempting adolescents, and 43 nondepressed nonattempting adolescents. The group of adolescents who attempted suicide differed from both other groups in that they had experienced more turmoil in their families, beginning in childhood and not stabilizing during adolescence. Brent and colleagues [32] compared 67 adolescent suicide victims and 67 demographically matched living controls regarding family constellation, familial stressors, and familial loading for psychopathology. One of this study's conclusions was that lifetime history of parent–child discord was one of the factors most closely associated with adolescent suicide.

A different study [33] based on a previous community survey study of 1050 adolescents [34] showed an association between poor parent–child communication and suicide, especially between fathers and suicide victims. However, family history of suicidal behavior persisted as a risk factor even after adjusting for poor parent–child communication, indicating multifactorial origins. In the birth cohort of New Zealand children (aged ≤16 years), the extent to which young people expressed suicidal tendencies was correlated with the extent to which the young person had been exposed to adverse family circumstances, such as low maternal emotional response and family conflict [35].

Compared with first-degree relatives of normal children, those of child suicide attempters had more antisocial personality disorder, assaultive behavior, and substance abuse [36]. Another factor identified as a potential precursor of suicidal behavior among children is parental history of child sexual abuse. In a prospective study of offspring of parents who had mood disorders, Melhem and colleagues [20] followed up 365 offspring of 203 parents for up to 6 years, showing that one of the two most significant predictors of suicide incidents was a history of sexual abuse. The authors suggest that because parental sexual abuse is related to various factors that might affect suicidal risk in children, such as parental aggression, mood disorder, posttraumatic stress disorder, borderline personality disorder, and substance abuse, the salience of parental history of abuse in predicting child-onset suicidal behavior requires clarification from further longitudinal studies [31,32,37]. Relationships between the extent of childhood sexual abuse and risk for suicidal behavior are consistent, with patients reporting sexual abuse involving intercourse having the highest risk for disorder [38].

The literature provides clues about the possible mechanisms of transmission of suicidal behavior in the setting of insulting treatment and physical abuse. Cross-sectional studies have shown that the familial aggregation for suicidal behavior is related to the trait of impulsive aggression. Higher levels of impulsive aggression in those who attempt or complete suicide are associated with higher levels of impulsive aggression in parents and are associated with child suicidal behavior [37]. In one cross-sectional study, the familial transmission of suicidal behavior seemed to be mediated by the transmission of impulsive aggression from parent to child [39]. The results of the prospective study by Melhem and colleagues [20] indicate that impulsive aggression among offspring serves as a precursor to early-onset suicidal behavior. Familial transmission of impulsive aggression may also be under genetic control [24].

PSYCHOPATHOLOGY AND SUICIDAL TRANSMISSION

Abundant literature documents impairment in multiple areas of functioning in the adolescent offspring of depressed parents. Maternal depression has been associated with offspring delinquency, alcohol problems, academic difficulties, and interpersonal conflicts. Paternal depressive symptoms are associated with lower cognitive competence and greater father–child conflict [40]. Recent evidence shows that treatment of maternal depression results in improved psychiatric and functional outcomes for children [41].

Tsuang [42] compared the risk for suicide among first-degree relatives of 195 patients who had schizophrenia and 315 patients who were manic–depressive, of whom 29 had committed suicide. Results show a 7.9% risk among relatives of patients who died of suicide, 2.1% in relatives of the nonsuicide patients, and 0.3% in the relatives of nonpatient surgical control group. These findings suggest that psychiatric disorders and suicide attempts in the family are precursors for suicide attempt in relatives, and that psychopathology in the family does not account exclusively for the transmission of suicide.

Studies comparing the risk for suicidal behavior in relatives of suicide probands while controlling for differences in family psychopathology show congruent results. In a population-based study in Denmark, Qin and colleagues [43] found that family history of completed suicide was a risk factor for suicide, independent of the effect of family history of mental disorders [44]. Similarly, Runeson and Asberg [45] found evidence of familial clustering of suicide in the general population in Sweden, even after adjusting for the presence of psychiatric disorders in the proband and family [45]. In a study drawing data from a representative sample (n = 8098) of household adults in the United States [46], results showed that parental suicide attempt was associated with increased odds of suicidal ideation (odds ratio [OR], 3.5) and suicide attempt (OR, 4.6) among offspring. This finding was still significant after adjustment for comorbid mental disorders (OR, 2.0 and 2.2, respectively). However, control for mental disorders somewhat reduced the association, suggesting that some component of parent–offspring resemblance in suicidality may be mediated by intervening mental health factors [46]. Roy [47], comparing 243 patients who had a family history of suicide and 5602 patients who did not, found that family history of suicide significantly increased the risk for a suicide attempt in patients who had a wide variety of diagnoses, including schizophrenia, unipolar and bipolar affective disorders, depression, and personality disorders. These findings support the view that the tendency to suicidal behavior is transmitted independently of the type of psychiatric disorder [47]. In a family study of 58 adolescent suicide victims compared with 55 community controls, Brent and colleagues [18] showed that after controlling for differences in rates of psychopathology between the group of first-degree relatives who had suicidal ideation and the group of first-degree relatives who had suicidal behavior, the difference in OR between these groups was no longer significant. This finding suggests that suicidal ideation is related to psychopathology, but that the tendency to act on suicidal ideation is familially transmitted [18].

Thus, current data suggest that familial transmission of suicidal ideation and behavior is based on diathesis that was transmitted either additively to the psychopathology or independently, leaving the magnitude and mechanisms of interaction between these parameters requiring further investigation.

GENE–ENVIRONMENT INTERACTIONS

Childhood adversity may produce a biological and clinical diathesis for mood disorder that endures into adulthood. Childhood separation from parents, sexual and physical abuse, and adult losses may precede the onset of major depression. Current stressful life events have a relationship with the onset of major depression, modulated at least in part through an interaction with genetic predisposition [48–50]. Life events predict depression and suicidal ideation or a suicide attempt in children, adolescent and young adult carriers of the S allele of the 5-HTTLPR polymorphism [48–50].

After Caspi and colleagues [51] showed the interaction between stressful life events and the serotonin transporter promoter polymorphism (5-HTTLPR), many researchers attempted to replicate this finding. It is well known that early childhood abuse and neglect seem to contribute to the familial transmission of suicidal behavior through compounding genetic vulnerability. Studies in nonhuman primates show that early neglect by parents results in alterations in serotonin function in the brain, with attendant increases in impulsivity and aggression, especially in those who are genetically vulnerable [52]. Parents who attempt suicide often have risk factors, such as impulsive aggression, that not only may be passed on to their children but also may affect the parent's ability to provide an optimal environment for child rearing [24,39,53].

The gene for the serotonin transporter promoter, especially the polymorphism 5-HTTLPR, became a major candidate gene in the study of suicidal behavior. The polymorphism used by Caspi and colleagues [51] seems to have some other variants, particularly in Japanese individuals, that are rare in Caucasians. A third functional allele is described, L_G with an $A \rightarrow G$ polymorphism at position 6 of the first of two 22 base-pair–imperfect repeats that define the 16-repeat L allele. Originally described by Nakamura and colleagues [54], L_G is equivalent in expression to the S allele. The allelic frequency of L_G is 0.09 to 0.14 in Caucasians and 0.24 in African Americans, and the three alleles, S, L_A, and L_G, seem to act codominantly, possibly explaining some discordant published findings. Some studies using biallelic S/L genotyping show a higher frequency of the low activity allele (S) in mood disorders and in suicidal behavior. The authors' group has replicated Caspi and colleagues' [51] finding, with some methodological variations using the three alleles of the 5-HTTLPR [55].

Other replications in children and adolescents followed Caspi and colleagues' study. In a study of gene–environment interaction in adolescent depression, Eley and colleagues [56] found a significant genotype–environmental risk interaction for 5-HTTLPR in women only, with the effect occurring in the same direction as Caspi and colleagues', reaffirming that an important source of genetic heterogeneity is exposure to environmental risk. The sample was selected from 1990 adolescents aged 10 to 20 years. Those who had depression symptoms in the top or bottom 15% were identified and divided into high or low environmental risk groups. DNA was obtained from four quadrants of high or low depression and high or low environmental risk. Markers within, or close to, each of the serotonergic genes were genotyped. Environmental risk group was a nonsignificant predictor while gender was a significant predictor of the depression group. HTR2A and tryptophan hydroxylase significantly predicted the depression group independent of the effects of gender, environmental risk group, and their interaction. A trend was also seen for an effect of 5-HTTLPR, which was significant in female subjects [56].

Kaufman and colleagues [57] replicated the study by Caspi and colleagues using a different angle. Quality and availability of social supports were found to moderate risk for depression associated with a history of maltreatment and the presence of the short allele of the 5-HTTLPR. Maltreated children with the s/s genotype and no positive supports had the highest depression ratings, showing scores twice as high as the nonmaltreated comparison children who had the same genotype. However, the presence of positive supports reduced risk associated with maltreatment and the s/s genotype, so that maltreated children who had this profile showed only minimal increases in their depression scores [57].

SUMMARY

Although the existing evidence cumulatively suggest that suicidal behavior has a strong familial risk and may be partly genetically transmitted, several questions remain about the applicability of these findings. First, whether the relationship between family history of suicidal ideation and suicide attempt and increased risk for suicide behavior can be generalized from youth to adults is unclear. Secondly, previous studies suggest that family history of suicide attempts and suicide completion is associated with an increased familial risk for suicidal behavior. However, these studies did not examine the relationship between family history of suicidal ideation and the risk for suicidal ideation in the community. Finally, the extent to which parent–offspring resemblance in suicidal behavior reflects a specific association in suicide response or a more pervasive association involving mental health problems in general must be clarified.

As this article shows, the risk for suicide attempt among offspring of suicide completers is multifactorial, challenging experts to develop a strategy that includes assessment and management that consider these factors. Although treatment of depression is necessary, antisuicide treatment strategies that solely target depression may not be sufficient to reduce suicidal risk. Other factors, such as impulsive aggression and parental history of sexual abuse, also contribute to suicidal risk. As emphasized by previous studies of adults and the studies by Brent and colleagues of familial pathways, assessment and management of impulsive aggression is likely critical to preventing onset or recurrence of suicidal behavior.

In adult attempters, psychosocial and pharmacologic interventions that increase emotional regulation and decrease impulsive aggression are among the few interventions proven to diminish the risk for further attempts. Further studies are needed to assess if this is also true in children and adolescents.

References

[1] Apter A, Gothelf D, Orbach I, et al. Correlation of suicidal and violent behavior in different diagnostic categories in hospitalized adolescent patients. J Am Acad Child Adolesc Psychiatry 1995;34(7):912–8.

[2] Shaffer D, Waslick B. The many faces of depression in children and adolescents. 1st edition. Washington, DC: American Psychiatric Association; 2002.

[3] Zalsman G, Brent DA, Weersing VR. Depressive disorders in childhood and adolescence: an overview: epidemiology, clinical manifestation and risk factors. Child Adolesc Psychiatr Clin N Am 2006;15(4):827–41, vii.

[4] Grunbaum JA, Kann L, Kinchen S, et al. Youth risk behavior surveillance—United States, 2003 (Abridged). J Sch Health 2004;74(8):307–24.

[5] Shaffer D. Epidemiological aspects of some problems in child and adolescent psychiatry. Epidemiol Psichiatr Soc 1998;7(3):151–5.

[6] Brent DA. Risk factors for adolescent suicide and suicidal behavior: mental and substance abuse disorders, family environmental factors, and life stress. Suicide Life Threat Behav 1995;25 Suppl:52–63.

[7] Mann JJ. A current perspective of suicide and attempted suicide. Ann Intern Med 2002;136(4):302–11.

[8] Mann JJ. Neurobiology of suicidal behaviour. Nat Rev Neurosci 2003;4(10):819–28.

[9] Apter A, Kotler M, Sevy S, et al. Correlates of risk of suicide in violent and nonviolent psychiatric patients. Am J Psychiatry 1991;148(7):883–7.

[10] Apter A, Bleich A, King RA, et al. Death without warning? A clinical postmortem study of suicide in 43 Israeli adolescent males. Arch Gen Psychiatry 1993;50(2):138–42.

[11] Apter A, Plutchik R, van Praag HM. Anxiety, impulsivity and depressed mood in relation to suicidal and violent behavior. Acta Psychiatr Scand 1993;87(1):1–5.

[12] Zalsman G, Oquendo MA, Greenhill L, et al. Neurobiology of depression in children and adolescents. Child Adolesc Psychiatr Clin N Am 2006;15(4):843–68, viii.

[13] Pandey GN, Pandey SC, Dwivedi Y, et al. Platelet serotonin-2A receptors: a potential biological marker for suicidal behavior. Am J Psychiatry 1995;152(6):850–5.

[14] Pandey GN, Dwivedi Y, Rizavi HS, et al. Higher expression of serotonin 5-HT(2A) receptors in the postmortem brains of teenage suicide victims. Am J Psychiatry 2002;159(3):419–29.

[15] Pandey GN, Dwivedi Y, Rizavi HS, et al. Decreased catalytic activity and expression of protein kinase C isozymes in teenage suicide victims: a postmortem brain study. Arch Gen Psychiatry 2004;61(7):685–93.

[16] Tyano S, Zalsman G, Ofek H, et al. Plasma serotonin levels and suicidal behavior in adolescents. Eur Neuropsychopharmacol 2006;16(1):49–57.

[17] Zalsman G, Anderson GM, Peskin M, et al. Relationships between serotonin transporter promoter polymorphism, platelet serotonin transporter binding and clinical phenotype in suicidal and non-suicidal adolescent inpatients. J Neural Transm 2005;112(2):309–15.

[18] Brent DA, Bridge J, Johnson BA, et al. Suicidal behavior runs in families. A controlled family study of adolescent suicide victims. Arch Gen Psychiatry 1996;53(12):1145–52.

[19] Egeland JA, Sussex JN. Suicide and family loading for affective disorders. JAMA 1985;254(7):915–8.

[20] Melhem NM, Brent DA, Ziegler M, et al. Familial pathways to early-onset suicidal behavior: familial and individual antecedents of suicidal behavior. Am J Psychiatry 2007;164(9): 1364–70.

[21] Mann JJ, Brent DA, Arango V. The neurobiology and genetics of suicide and attempted suicide: a focus on the serotonergic system. Neuropsychopharmacology 2001;24(5):467–77.

[22] Zalsman G, Frisch A, Apter A, et al. Genetics of suicidal behavior: candidate association genetic approach. Isr J Psychiatry Relat Sci 2002;39(4):252–61.

[23] Zalsman G, Posmanik S, Fischel T, et al. Psychosocial situations, quality of depression and schizophrenia in adolescents. Psychiatry Res 2004;129(2):149–57.

[24] Brent DA, Mann JJ. Family genetic studies, suicide, and suicidal behavior. Am J Med Genet C Semin Med Genet 2005;133(1):13–24.

[25] Roy A, Segal NL, Centerwall BS, et al. Suicide in twins. Arch Gen Psychiatry 1991;48(1): 29–32.

[26] Roy A, Segal NL, Sarchiapone M. Attempted suicide among living co-twins of twin suicide victims. Am J Psychiatry 1995;152(7):1075–6.

[27] Fu Q, Heath AC, Bucholz KK, et al. A twin study of genetic and environmental influences on suicidality in men. Psychol Med 2002;32(1):11–24.

[28] Schulsinger F. The experience from the adoption method in genetic research. Prog Clin Biol Res 1985;177:461–78.

[29] Mann JJ, Arango V, Underwood MD. Serotonin and suicidal behavior. Ann N Y Acad Sci 1990;600:476–84.

[30] Kosky R, Silburn S, Zubrick S. Symptomatic depression and suicidal ideation—a comparative-study with 628 children. J Nerv Ment Dis 1986;174(9):523–8.

[31] Kienhorst CWM, Dewilde EJ, Diekstra RFW, et al. Differences between adolescent suicide attempters and depressed adolescents. Acta Psychiatr Scand 1992;85(3):222–8.

[32] Brent DA, Johnson BA, Perper J, et al. Personality disorder, personality traits, impulsive violence, and completed suicide in adolescents. J Am Acad Child Adolesc Psychiatry 1994;33(8):1080–6.

[33] Gould MS, Fisher P, Parides M, et al. Psychosocial risk factors of child and adolescent completed suicide. Arch Gen Psychiatry 1996;53(12):1155–62.

[34] Wagner BM, Cole RE, Schwartzman P. Psychosocial correlates of suicide attempts among junior and senior high-school youth. Suicide Life Threat Behav 1995;25(3):358–72.

[35] Fergusson DM, Lynskey MT. Childhood circumstances, adolescent adjustment, and suicide attempts in a New-Zealand birth cohort. J Am Acad Child Adolesc Psychiatry 1995;34(5): 612–22.

[36] Pfeffer CR, Normandin L, Kakuma T. Suicidal children grow up: suicidal-behavior and psychiatric disorders among relatives. J Am Acad Child Adolesc Psychiatry 1994;33(8): 1087–97.

[37] Brent DA, Birmaher B. Clinical practice. Adolescent depression. N Engl J Med 2002; 347(9):667–71.

[38] Beautrais AL, Joyce PR, Mulder RT, et al. Prevalence and comorbidity of mental disorders in persons making serious suicide attempts: a case-control study. Am J Psychiatry 1996; 153(8):1009–14.

[39] Brent DA, Oquendo M, Birmaher B, et al. Peripubertal suicide attempts in offspring of suicide attempters with siblings concordant for suicidal behavior. Am J Psychiatry 2003; 160(8):1486–93.

[40] Lewinsohn PM, Olino TM, Klein DN. Psychosocial impairment in offspring of depressed parents. Psychol Med 2005;35(10):1493–503.

[41] Pilowsky DJ, Wickramaratne PJ, Rush AJ, et al. Children of currently depressed mothers: a STAR*D ancillary study. J Clin Psychiatry 2006;67(1):126–36.

[42] Tsuang MT. Risk of suicide in the relatives of schizophrenics, manics, depressives, and controls. J Clin Psychiatry 1983;44(11):396–400.

[43] Qin P, Agerbo E, Mortensen PB. Suicide risk in relation to family history of completed suicide and psychiatric disorders: a nested case-control study based on longitudinal registers. Lancet 2002;360(9340):1126–30.

[44] Qin P, Agerbo E, Mortensen RB. Suicide risk in relation to family history of completed suicide and hospitalized psychiatric disorders. Acta Psychiatr Scand 2002;105:44.

[45] Runeson B, Asberg M. Family history of suicide among suicide victims. Am J Psychiatry 2003;160(8):1525–6.

[46] Goodwin RD, Beautrais AL, Fergusson DM. Familial transmission of suicidal ideation and suicide attempts: evidence from a general population sample. Psychiatry Res 2004; 126(2):159–65.

[47] Roy A. Family history of suicide. Arch Gen Psychiatry 1983;40(9):971–4.

[48] Caspi A, Moffitt TE. Gene-environment interactions in psychiatry: joining forces with neuroscience. Nat Rev Neurosci 2006;7(7):583–90.

[49] Moffitt TE, Caspi A, Rutter M. Strategy for investigating interactions between measured genes and measured environment. Arch Gen Psychiatry 2005;62(5):473–81.

[50] Rutter M, Moffitt TE, Caspi A. Gene-environment interplay and psychopathology: multiple varieties but real effects. J Child Psychol Psychiatry 2006;47(3–4):226–61.

[51] Caspi A, Sugden K, Moffitt TE, et al. Influence of life stress on depression: moderation by a polymorphism in the 5-HTT gene. Science 2003;301(5631):386–9.

[52] Suomi SJ. Gene-environment interactions and the neurobiology of social conflict. Ann N Y Acad Sci 2003;1008:132–9.

[53] Brent DA, Oquendo M, Birmaher B, et al. Familial transmission of mood disorders: convergence and divergence with transmission of suicidal behavior. J Am Acad Child Adolesc Psychiatry 2004;43(10):1259–66.

[54] Nakamura M, Ueno S, Sano A, et al. The human serotonin transporter gene linked polymorphism (5-HTTLPR) shows ten novel allelic variants. Mol Psychiatry 2000;5(1):32–8.

[55] Zalsman G, Huang YY, Oquendo MA, et al. Association of a triallelic serotonin transporter gene promoter region (5-HTTLPR) polymorphism with stressful life events and severity of depression. Am J Psychiatry 2006;163(9):1588–93.

[56] Eley TC, Sugden K, Corsico A, et al. Gene-environment interaction analysis of serotonin system markers with adolescent depression. Mol Psychiatry 2004;9:908–15.

[57] Kaufman J, Yang BZ, Douglas-Palumberi H, et al. Social supports and serotonin transporter gene moderate depression in maltreated children. Proc Natl Acad Sci U S A 2004;101(49): 17316–21.

Psychiatr Clin N Am 31 (2008) 247–269

PSYCHIATRIC CLINICS
OF NORTH AMERICA

ELSEVIER
SAUNDERS

Stress, Genes and the Biology of Suicidal Behavior

Dianne Currier, PhD*, J. John Mann, MD

Division of Molecular Imaging and Neuropathology, Department of Psychiatry, Columbia University, 1051 Riverside Drive, NYSPI Unit #42, New York, NY 10032, USA

SUICIDAL BEHAVIOR AND GENETICS

Family, twin, and adoption studies provide evidence of the heritability of suicide and attempted suicide, partly independent of the familial transmission of major psychiatric disorders [1]. Based on case reports and register-based studies, estimates of heritability for suicide among twins range from 21% to 50%. General population studies show heritability contributes between 30% and 55% to the broader phenotype of suicidal behavior (attempts, thoughts, plans) [2]. Identifying the relevant genes and the neurobiologic pathways through which they contribute to the origin of suicidal behavior is important for designing and implementing preventative strategies. The first wave of genetic studies sought to identify genes involved in suicide or attempted suicide through linkage studies or specific single nucleotide polymorphisms (SNPs) in association studies. Emerging approaches have the goal of investigating functional genomics using microarray technologies to profile expression of thousands of genes simultaneously [3] or performing a genome-wide array for hundreds of thousands of SNPs.

Candidate genes for association studies have been generally selected based on evidence from neurobiologic studies in suicide. Consequently, the serotonergic system has been most extensively investigated, along with other target systems, including the dopaminergic and noradrenergic systems; neurotrophins, such as brain-derived neurotrophic factor; and, more recently, genes related to the hypothalamic-pituitary-adrenal (HPA) axis. Although association studies have been the most common design, replication of findings has proven difficult for individual SNP association studies for several reasons, including differences in study sample size and composition with respect to diagnosis; different definitions of suicidality, including suicide, nonfatal attempts, or suicidal ideation; the effects of ethnicity/race-related stratification; and the effect of or interactions with environmental factors.

Environment, particularly during childhood developmental periods, can influence the effect of genetic variants on neurobiologic function. Another factor

*Corresponding author. *E-mail address*: dmc2111@columbia.edu (D. Currier).

0193-953X/08/$ – see front matter
doi:10.1016/j.psc.2008.01.005

contributing to the disparity in results may be the complexity of the suicidal behavior phenotype, although this may be less of a problem because suicide, nonfatal suicide attempts and suicidal ideation are all partly heritable and perhaps involve many of the same genes. Nevertheless, many genes and epigenetic factors are probably involved in the diathesis for suicidal behavior. Moreover, the rarity of completed suicide means that studies may be underpowered to detect the effect of a single SNP or gene. To address the matter of a low base rate of suicide, one approach is to focus on endophenotypes for suicidal behavior that are more prevalent and can often be more narrowly and specifically defined and measured. These may include clinical traits, such as impulsive aggression; cognitive function; or neurobiologic functioning, such as amygdala responsivity.

Much remains unknown regarding which genes have the most influence in suicidal behavior and the neurobiologic mechanisms through which genetic variants affect the risk for suicidal behavior. This article reviews published findings that together begin to form a picture of the genes, their functional effects, and their involvement in endophenotypes that are putative pathways to suicidal acts.

SEROTONERGIC SYSTEM

Approximately 30 years of research documents abnormalities in the serotonergic system in suicide and nonfatal suicidal behavior [4]. Therefore, the serotonergic system has been most scrutinized for genetic variants potentially contributing to serotonergic system dysfunction and thereby to suicidal behavior. Candidate genes from the serotonergic system that have been examined with respect to suicidal behavior include SNPs in genes for the serotonin transporter; serotonin receptors, including $5\text{-}HT_{2A}$, $5\text{-}HT_{1A}$, and $5\text{-}HT_{1B}$; tryptophan hydroxylases I and II (the rate-limiting enzymes in serotonin synthesis); and monoamine oxidase A, which is involved in the breakdown of monoamines, including serotonin.

Serotonin Transporter

Postmortem studies of depressed suicides report fewer serotonin transporters in prefrontal cortex (suicide or major depression), hypothalamus (suicide), occipital cortex (major depression), and brainstem (suicide and major depression) [5]. Of relevance in identifying the responsible brain circuitry in suicide, this prefrontal cortex deficit seems localized to the ventromedial prefrontal cortex (a brain region involved in willed action and decision making), whereas major depression is associated with lower binding throughout the prefrontal cortex [6].

The cause of lower transporter binding has been the target of inquiry. The serotonin transporter gene is located on chromosome 17 and has a common, functional promoter polymorphism (5-HTTLPR). Initially a short variant (S allele) of the polymorphism was found to have lower transcriptional efficiency and less transporter expression, binding, and 5-HT uptake in lymphoblasts [7]. The so-called "long" or "L" variant was subsequently found to comprise low-expressing (L_G) and higher-expressing (L_A) variants [8,9]. In healthy volunteers, two positron emission tomography (PET) studies using the high-affinity ligand [^{11}C]DASB reported altered serotonin transporter binding in midbrain [10] and putamen [11] associated with 5-HTTLPR genotype; however, these and other imaging studies find no evidence of genotype effect on serotonin transporter binding in the amygdala, thalamus, prefrontal cortex, or anterior cingulate [6,12–14].

Multiple studies in healthy adults have reported that individuals who have the lower-expressing s/s genotype show increased amygdala activity when exposed to angry or fearful faces, negative words, or aversive pictures [15]. Two recent studies examine whether genotype affects resting amygdalar activity (ie, when exposed to neutral rather than negative stimuli) [16,17]. These studies use spin labeled perfusion functional MRI (fMRI) methods, which quantify absolute cerebral blood flow, rather than the blood-oxygen–level dependent (BOLD) method, which is only informative in comparing changes in state. Both report that, compared with the l/l group, the s/s group or s/s and s/l combined group had significantly higher resting cerebral blood flow in the amygdala [16,17]. These findings suggest that the presence of the low-expressing allele may contribute to a more generalized alteration in amygdala function that may underlie the observed increased sensitivity to emotional stimuli. Canli and colleagues [16] also noted that life stress interacted with genotype with respect to amygdala function, whereby amygdala activation at rest correlated positively with life stress in short variant carriers, but correlated negatively with life stress in noncarriers. A similar effect was noted in the hippocampus. The amygdala is densely innervated by serotonergic neurons and 5-HT receptors are abundant [18–20], and thus the serotonergic abnormalities seen in suicides may indicate altered amygdala function.

5-HTTLPR and Suicidal Behavior

More than 20 studies have examined the 5-HTTLPR polymorphism with respect to suicidal behavior, with both negative and positive findings. Meta-analyses of 12 studies comprising 1599 subjects found a significant association between the 5-HTTLPR low-expressing S allele and suicidal behavior [21]. Another meta-analysis found that the S allele was more frequent in suicide attempters within individual diagnostic categories and was associated with violent rather than nonviolent suicide attempts [22].

The 5-HTTLPR lower-expressing alleles have been associated with violent behavior [23–25]. The relationship between impaired serotonergic function and aggression is well established [26]. The 5-HTTLPR gene may be related to impulsivity and aggression through observed alterations in amygdala function, because the amygdala, along with the prefrontal cortex and orbital cortex, is believed to play a role in the emergence of violent behavior by way of faulty regulation of negative emotion [27].

SEROTONIN RECEPTORS

Greater postmortem 5-HT_{2A} receptor binding was observed in the prefrontal cortex of suicide victims compared with nonsuicides in some studies [28–32]. Youths who died by suicide had increased protein levels and gene expression, which may partially explain observed higher binding [32]. Higher 5-HT_{2A} binding has also been reported in the amygdala in depressed suicides [33], and suicide victims with and without depressive diagnoses show evidence that 5-HT_{2A} receptors are up-regulated in the dorsal prefrontal cortex (areas 8 and 9) but unchanged in the rostral pole of the prefrontal cortex (area 10) [34]. Not all studies concur, and several observe no difference in 5-HT_{2A} receptors in the prefrontal cortex in depressed suicides compared with controls [35–42].

In nonfatal suicide attempts, multiple platelet studies of 5-HT_{2A} receptors, serotonin reuptake sites, and serotonin second messenger systems have reported higher platelet 5-HT_{2A} receptor numbers in suicide attempters compared with nonattempters and healthy controls [43]. These findings indicate impaired 5-HT_{2A} receptor–mediated signal transduction in the prefrontal cortex of suicides [44], and blunted 5-HT_{2A} receptor in patients who had major depression and made a high-lethality suicide attempt compared with those who made a low-lethality suicide attempt [45]. This defect in signal transduction, if present in the brain, would suggest that although a greater density of 5-HT_{2A} receptors may be present, the signal that is transduced by 5-HT_{2A} receptor activation may be blunted, which would compound deficient serotonergic activity as seen in the lower levels of brainstem serotonin or 5-HIAA in suicide victims [35,36,46–50].

5-HT Receptor Genes and Suicidal Behavior

Studies of 5-HT_{2A} receptor gene and suicidal behavior have largely focused on the T102C SNP. The T102C SNP was not associated with suicide in postmortem studies, but sample sizes are small [51–54]. Positive associations have been reported with suicide attempt in depressed individuals [55] and with suicidal ideation [56]; however, multiple studies have shown negative results in varied populations and diagnostic groups for both ideation and attempt [57–61]. Meta-analysis of 9 studies found no association between the T102C polymorphism and suicide attempt or suicide [21], and a recent expanded meta-analysis of 25 studies confirmed this lack of association [62].

Huang and colleagues [63] reported decreased 5-HT_{1B} binding in the prefrontal cortex of suicides and nonsuicides associated with the C allele of C129T and G allele of G861C SNPs. Multiple studies of the common G861C SNP in the 5-HT_{1B} receptor gene coding region report no association of genotype and suicide [63–65] or suicide attempt [66–68]. The observation that 5-HT_{1B} knockout mice exhibit aggressive behavior [69], suggested that this gene may be involved in the aggressive/impulsive endophenotype of suicidal behavior. Investigations of the two common SNPs in this gene have examined association with aggression or impulsive traits and suicide directly. The G861C SNP was shown to be involved in aggression and impulsivity, with increased C allele frequency in antisocial alcoholics [70], although a German study of alcoholics found lower C allele frequency in those who had antisocial and conduct disorders [71].

Other serotonin receptors have been less studied with respect to genetic involvement in suicidal behavior. An overrepresentation of $5\text{-}HT_{1A}$ 1018G allele in suicides compared with controls has been reported by some [72], but others find no association [73–75]. Studies of the $5\text{-}HT_{2C}$ [76] and $5\text{-}HT_6$ receptor [77] and a study of seven other serotonin receptor genes [78] indicate no association with suicidality.

Aside from the $5\text{-}HT_{1B}$ receptor gene and aggression, few other studies of 5-HT receptor polymorphisms have investigated associations with endophenotypes. Giegling and colleagues [79] examined multiple $5\text{-}HT_{2A}$ SNPs, and found that CC-homozygotes for the functional SNP rs6311 reported more anger- and aggression-related behavior, and that the C allele and the G–C haplotype combination of rs594242–rs6311 were related to nonviolent and impulsive suicidal acts. A study of multiple SNPs in the $5\text{-}HT_{2C}$ and $5\text{-}HT_{1A}$ genes found no effect of measures of state and trait anger or aggression in Caucasian suicides or in suicide attempters with various psychiatric diagnosis or in healthy volunteers [80].

TRYPTOPHAN HYDROXYLASE

Tryptophan hydroxylase (TPH) is the rate-limiting enzyme in the synthesis of serotonin. Two isoforms of TPH have been identified, TPH1 and TPH2, with the latter expressed primarily in the brain, and their genes are on different chromosomes. Postmortem studies comparing depressed suicides with controls report greater density and number of TPH-immunoreactive neurons in the dorsal raphe nucleus (DRN) [81] and higher TPH immunoreactivity in the DRN but not the median raphe nucleus in depressed suicides [82], although others find less TPH immunoreactivity in the DRN of depressed alcoholics, suggesting a common mechanism in major depression [83]. Compared with controls, depressed alcoholic suicides had 46% higher TPH immunoreactivity in the dorsal subnucleus but no other dorsal raphe subregion [84]. Higher levels of TPH2 mRNA and protein were found in the DRN of drug-free suicides [85]. This over-expression may be caused by a stress response, because it has been reported to occur in animal models of stress.

Two common polymorphisms in intron 7 of TPH1 are in very high linkage disequilibrium: A218C and A779C (originally classified as U and L for upper and lower band, respectively). A218C has been linked to altered 5-HT function. In a postmortem study, the AA genotype was associated with higher TPH immunoreactivity and lower 5-HT2A binding in the prefrontal cortex compared with other genotypes in suicides and nonsuicides, whereas another TPH1 polymorphism, A-1438, had no effect on either serotonergic marker [86]. Manuck and colleagues [87] found an attenuated prolactin response to fenfluramine in C allele of A779C relative to LL homozygotes in healthy volunteers, but New and colleagues [88] observed no relationship with respect to this polymorphism between genotypes and prolactin response to fenfluramine in male patients who had personality disorder. Jönsson and colleagues [89] reported a relationship to cerebrospinal fluid 5-HIAA in male healthy volunteers but not females; however, we did not find such a relationship in subjects who had mood disorder [90]. The differences in study population may account for the lack of replication.

Tryptophan Hydroxylase Genes and Suicidal Behavior

Multiple reports exist of both positive and negative associations with suicide and suicide attempt and the intron 7 A128C SNP. Initially, meta-analysis found no association with suicide or suicide attempt [91]; however, subsequent expanded meta-analyses found an association of this polymorphism with suicidal behavior in Caucasian [92,93] and mixed populations [94]. Positive associations have been reported for the A779C SNP C allele and suicidal behavior in alcoholic offenders [95] and surviving monozygotic twins of suicides [96]; however, another study reported an opposite result, with the A allele more frequent in depressed suicide attempters than in nonattempters [97].

The A allele of the TPH1 A779C polymorphism has been associated with higher scores for state anger, trait anger, and angry temperament in suicide attempters and controls [98], with higher aggressive hostility [99] and aggression and outwardly expressed anger in healthy volunteers [87] compared with CC homozygotes. Another study in men who had schizophrenia failed to replicate this finding [100]. Rujescu and colleagues [98] also found the TPH1 A allele of the 218C SNP to be associated with higher anger scores in a combined sample of suicide attempters and controls, which is not surprising, because the two SNPs are in strong linkage disequilibrium. A study of nonpsychotic inpatients and nonimpulsive controls found no difference in A218C genotype between the groups, although the patient group had several behavioral tendencies associated with the C allele [101].

Haplotype and association studies of different SNPs suggest involvement of the *TPH2* gene with suicide [102] and suicide attempt [103,104]; however, not all studies agree [105–107]. Almost no reports exist of functional consequences of *TPH2* gene variation. One recent study in healthy volunteers found evidence of a frequent functional *cis*-acting polymorphism in the *TPH2* gene that affected mRNA expression. In that study, low levels of TPH2 mRNA expression in the pons were associated with the CTGTG combination of alleles and high levels of expression with the TAAGA combination of alleles for the SNPs rs2171363, rs4760815, rs7305115, rs6582076, and rs9325202 [108]. This specific haplotype has not been investigated with respect to suicidal behavior.

TPH2 has been little studied with respect to endophenotypes of suicidal behavior. However, studies in healthy volunteers found an effect of the TPH2 −703 G/T SNP on amygdala responses to emotional stimuli [109], and the TT genotype of this SNP was associated with more errors in the attention network test, a possible indicator of impaired impulse control, and decreased performance in executive control, explaining more than 10% of the variance in these two indicators of attention [110].

MONOAMINE OXIDASE A

Monoamine oxidase (MAO) A plays a key role in metabolism of amines. Low MAO A activity (approximately 80% reduced in activity is required to get a detectable effect) results in elevated levels of serotonin, norepinephrine, and dopamine in the brain. The MAO A gene has a 13 to 30 bp uVNTR (variable number tandem repeat) in the promoter region, in which alleles with 3.5 or 4 repeats (referred to alleles 2 and 3) transcribed 2 to 10 times more efficiently than those with 3 or 5 repeats (referred to alleles 1 and 4) [111]. The 2 and 3 alleles were associated lower prolactin responses to fenfluramine challenge in men [112] and higher levels of CSF 5-HIAA in healthy women [113] and men [114]. In an fMRI study in healthy volunteers, Meyer-Lindenberg and colleagues [115] showed that the low expression variant was associated with limbic volume reductions and amygdalar hyper-responsivity during emotional arousal, and diminished reactivity of the regulatory prefrontal regions compared with the higher expressing alleles. Thus, a potential pathway for genetic involvement in suicidal behavior is through altered affect and behavioral regulation, partly resulting from partially genetically related alterations in serotonergic system function.

Monoamine Oxidase Genes and Suicidal Behavior

MAO A uVNTR is mostly found to be unassociated with suicide or suicide attempt [116–119]. One study found an association with history of suicide attempt, particularly in women who had bipolar disorder [120], but not in major depressive disorder. Courtet and colleagues [121], in a sample of European Caucasian suicide attempters who had mixed psychiatric diagnoses and controls, found no association with suicidality, although they did observe a higher frequency of higher-expressing alleles in men who made a violent suicide attempt compared with men who made a nonviolent attempt.

Human and rodent studies provide evidence of the involvement of MAO A in aggression [122,123]. The MAO A uVNTR has been examined for associations with aggression and violence. In a study of multiple domains of aggressive and disruptive behavior in patients who had personality disorder, aggression and other domains of disruptive outward-bound behavior traits were associated with MAO A uVNTR [124]. Meyer-Lindenberg and colleagues [115] used fMRI and found the low-expressing alleles to be associated with increased risk for violent behavior, as well as alterations in the corticolimbic circuitry involved in affect regulation, emotional memory, and impulsivity, and believed to be involved in the emergence of aggressive behavior [27]. Moreover, two fMRI studies observed an effect of MAO A genotype during response tasks indicative of impulsivity [125,126].

STRESS, GENES, AND SEROTONIN

Caspi and colleagues [127] observed that life events predicted onset of depressive episode only in individuals with the low expressing 5-HTTLPR S allele. This finding has been replicated multiple times, although not in every case [128]. Moreover, Caspi and colleagues [127] found that childhood maltreatment predicted adult depression that seemed to be triggered by stress but more so in individuals who had the S allele, a finding that has also been replicated in some and not others [128]. Regarding suicidal behavior, Caspi and colleagues [127] found the same relationship among life events, the S allele, and suicide attempt and ideation, but did not report on suicidality with respect to childhood maltreatment/genotype interaction. Childhood adversity–genotype interactions and suicidal behavior are reported in mixed-diagnosis inpatients [129] and abstinent African-American substance dependence patients [130].

Gene–environment interactions for the 5-HTTLPR have been investigated with respect to behavioral and putative biologic endophenotypes for suicidal behavior, including aggression and amygdala responsivity. Reif and colleagues [131] found an interaction effect of childhood environment and 5-HTTLPR genotype on violent behavior, whereby high adversity in childhood was associated with later-life violence if the short promoter alleles were present. Gene and early-life environment effects on later-life aggressive or violent traits have also been sought for the MAO A uVNTR. Adverse child-rearing in combination with a lower-expressing variant of the MAO A gene was also found to contribute, in men only, to the development of antisocial behavior and more impulsivity, both of which may contribute to suicidal behavior [116,132]. In other studies of the MAO A uVNTR, Foley and colleagues [133] found the low-expressing alleles more frequent in conduct disorder in the presence of an adverse childhood environment, and Nilsson and colleagues [134] found that the short allele interacted with adverse psychosocial risk factors, including adverse living environment and violent victimization, in adolescent boys to increase violent behaviors. Another study reported that in women who had a history of childhood sexual abuse, the low-expressing allele was associated with alcoholism and particularly antisocial alcoholism, whereas nonabused women showed no relationship between genotype and antisocial personality disorder or alcoholism [135]. Not all studies observed a moderating effect of MAO A genotype on childhood/adolescent maltreatment and antisocial or violent behavior [136,137].

Elucidating the neurobiologic underpinnings of this type of gene–early-life environment interaction is a complex task. Animal and human studies show that early-life stress has an effect on the development and functioning of the serotonergic system in adulthood. Adult rats exposed to maternal separation in early life show evidence of autoreceptor supersensitivity indicative of enduring alteration in 5-HT transporter and $5-HT_{1A}$ autoreceptors [138]. In humans, a history of childhood abuse has been associated with blunted prolactin response to different serotonergic agonists in children who have depression [139], boys in juvenile detention [140], and adult women who have borderline personality disorder [141]. Prolactin release is mediated by way of 5-HT$_{1A}$ and 5-HT$_{2A}$ receptors, and these findings suggest sensitization of these receptors from early-life stress.

The detrimental effect of early-life stress on the development and function of the serotonergic system may in and of itself confer increased risk for suicidal behavior, for example through increased aggression and impulsivity. Moreover, given that there may be underlying genetic differences in level of serotonergic system function, those who have low-function genotypes may be more vulnerable to the detrimental effects of early-life stress on 5-HT function. Animal studies have observed such effects. Monkeys exposed to maternal deprivation in infancy and having the 5-HTTLPR lower expressing S allele manifest a lowering of cerebrospinal fluid 5-HIAA that persists into adulthood, whereas monkeys with the higher expressing alleles exposed to maternal deprivation in infancy do not show these alterations [142]. Similar studies in human samples would be instructive.

Another pathway among genes, stress, and suicidal behaviors may be through the effects of impaired serotonergic function on stress-response regulation later in life. Studies in animals and humans show that the serotonergic system is involved in the regulation of stress response by way of the HPA axis, and that impairments in the serotonergic system may deteriorate HPA function [143]. Therefore, individuals who have lower 5-HT function because of genes or early environment effects would show altered HPA axis function. A recent study reports that the low-expressing S allele was associated with higher levels of waking cortisol in nondepressed older adults [144]; however, others found no association of 5-HTTLPR genotype and plasma cortisol [145,146]. Early life experience is likely to mediate this relationship, and animal studies have examined this. In 6-month-old macaque monkeys exposed to social stress, peer-reared animals with the S allele had a higher adrenocorticotrophic hormone response, an HPA axis hormone related to stress response, compared with peer-reared animals without that allele and animals with the allele who were maternally reared [147]. Therefore, studies of the serotonergic system suggest that elucidating the genetics of suicidal behavior involves examining not only genes but also early-life environment, biologic and behavioral endophenotypes, and interactions among biologic systems.

OTHER SYSTEMS
Noradrenergic System
The noradrenergic system has been investigated with respect to suicidal behavior as it is involved in the regulation of stress response. Postmortem studies of suicides have reported fewer noradrenergic neurons in the locus coeruleus of suicide victims who have major depression [148] and increased brainstem levels of tyrosine hydroxylase [149]. Binding to α_2-adrenergic receptors in brains of suicides have been reported variously as increased, decreased, or unchanged [150].

Few studies have been conducted of genes related to the noradrenergic system. $\alpha2_A$-adrenoceptors located in the locus coeruleus exert a tonic inhibitory modulation on the firing activity of noradrenergic cells and the release of norepinephrine in projecting areas [151]. Sequiera and colleagues [152], examining the α_2-adrenergic receptor gene in Canadian suicides, found the rare allele of N251K functional SNP that results in an asparagine to lysine amino acid change was present only in suicide victims, but only in three cases. A subsequent study could not replicate this finding, failing to detect the polymorphism in a large sample of 214 suicides and 176 controls [153].

Tyrosine hydroxylase (TH) is the rate-limiting step for catecholamine synthesis, and Persson and colleagues [154] observed a nonsignificant tendency for the low-incidence TH-KI allele among suicides compared with controls, although a significant association of the K3 allele was seen in subgroup adjustment disorders and suicide attempt. Other studies report a trend for association [155] or no association [156].

Catechol-O-methyltransferase (COMT) is an enzyme that metabolizes the noradrenaline that diffuses in the synaptic cleft. COMT has a common functional polymorphism, Val158Met, that results in the substitution of valine with methionine. The Val allele has high COMT activity compared with the Met allele [157,158]. A recent meta-analysis of six studies with 519 cases and 933 controls found evidence suggesting an association between COMT Val158Met polymorphism and suicidal behavior, perhaps related to the lethality of suicide attempts [159]. Reports supporting this finding, showing association in schizophrenia between the low-functioning Met allele and impulsive aggression [160–162] and violent suicide attempts [163], and between the Met/Met genotype and outward-directed aggression in suicide attempters of varied psychiatric diagnosis [164]. Other studies find no relationship between aggression and the Met allele [165–168] or the opposite direction [169–171]. A postmortem study found the Val allele less prevalent and the heterozygote Val/Met more prevalent in male suicides than in controls [172].

No studies have shown the effect of early-life environment gene interaction on suicidal behavior with respect to genes related to the noradrenergic system. Given that early-life stress has been shown to modify noradrenergic system function in adulthood [173], examining possible genetic factors that contribute to this effect would be of interest.

Dopaminergic System

Abnormality of the dopaminergic systems has been reported in depressive disorders [174]; however, the role of the dopaminergic system in suicidal behavior is unclear. Reduced dopamine turnover was observed in the caudate, putamen, and nucleus accumbens in a postmortem study of depressed suicides [175]. However, no differences in number or affinity of the dopamine transporters was found in depressed suicides compared with controls [176]. Depressed suicide attempters had lower cerebrospinal fluid homovanillic acid (HVA), a dopamine metabolite [177], and lower urinary HVA, dihydroxyphenylacetic acid, and dopamine [178], but other studies find no evidence that cerebrospinal fluid HVA levels predict suicide or correlate with clinical factors related to suicide, such as aggression or impulsive traits [179–181]. In studies of violent offenders, significant correlations between cerebrospinal fluid HVA/5-HIAA ratio and psychopathic traits of aggression and violence are reported, suggesting that dysfunction in the relative activity of the two systems rather than the dopaminergic system alone may be important [182,183].

Few studies of dopaminergic system genes have been conducted with respect to suicidal behavior. In studies of dopamine receptor genes, the del allele of the of 141C Ins/Del polymorphism in the D2 receptor gene was not associated with suicide attempt but was found in excess in alcoholics who had suicidality [184]. An A-G polymorphism in the 3′utr of exon 8 of the D2 receptor gene was associated with increased number of suicide attempts in alcoholics [185]. No differences between Swedish suicide attempters of mixed psychiatric diagnoses [186] or Israeli adolescent suicide attempters and controls [187] were found in the dopamine receptor subtype 4 gene exon III 48 bp repeat polymorphism.

HYPOTHALAMIC-PITUITARY-ADRENAL AXIS

HPA axis function may be involved in suicidal behavior in the context of acute stress response to life events preceding a suicidal act in which impaired stress response mechanisms contribute to risk. It may also be involved in suicidal behavior if increased activity of stress response to adversity during development has deleterious effects on the development of other systems and brain structures implicated in suicidal behavior.

One measure of abnormal HPA axis function is nonsuppression of cortisol in response to dexamethasone administration (DST). Over a 15-year follow-up, individuals who were nonsuppressors of DST cortisol had an approximately 14-fold higher risk for suicide compared with suppressors [188], and the authors' recent meta-analysis found that DST nonsuppressors had a 4.5-fold risk for dying of suicide in individuals who had mood disorders [189]. Fewer neuroanatomic studies of HPA axis have been conducted with respect to suicide; however, reported anomalies include larger pituitary and larger adrenal gland volumes found postmortem and using MRI in vivo in depressed suicide victims [190–193], and fewer corticotropin-releasing hormone (CRH) binding sites in the prefrontal cortex of depressed suicide victims [194].

For nonfatal suicidal behavior, the DST results are inconclusive [195–201]; however, reports have shown that DST nonsuppression may be characteristic of more serious attempts that result in high medical damage [200,202] or the use of violent methods [199]. In other indices of HPA axis function, depressed adolescents who attempted suicide during a 10-year follow-up had elevated presleep cortisol compared with depressed nonattempters and healthy controls [203]. Depressed suicide attempters have attenuated plasma cortisol responses to fenfluramine [204–206], and cerebrospinal fluid CRH is lower in previous attempters compared with nonattempters [207,208], although not all studies agree [178].

Hypothalamic-Pituitary-Adrenal Axis Gene and Suicidal Behavior

Comparatively few genetic studies have been performed on the HPA axis function, and fewer still in relation to suicidal behavior. In studies of healthy volunteers, some evidence shows that genes play a role in basal HPA axis function, and limited and conflicting reports exist on the genetic role in HPA axis activity in response to various challenges or stressors [209]. Almost no studies of HPA axis genes have been performed regarding suicidal behavior. Recently, the CRH receptor was examined. One study reported linkage and association between SNP rs4792887 and suicide attempt among depressed men exposed to low lifetime levels of stress, but not those exposed to high-stress levels [210]. The authors suggest that this may indicate increased risk for suicidal behavior from an overactive stress response system. Another recent study found the I allele of the ACE I/D polymorphism to be more frequent in completed suicides than in controls [211].

Studies in animals [212–215] and humans [216–219] have shown that early-life stress results in abnormal HPA axis function in adulthood. No studies have been published examining early-life stress, genes, and suicidal behavior with respect to the HPA axis, although an early-life stress gene interaction of the CRH R1 gene and early-life stress on severity of depression has been reported [220]. Another study reported an interaction effect of a CRH R1 polymorphism and negative life stress on alcohol use behavior in adolescents [221]. Clearly studies investigating the genetic and gene/environment influences on basal HPA axis function and response to stressors are necessary for elucidating the genetic contributions to suicidal behavior.

SUMMARY

Regarding the genes and biology of suicidal behavior, stress can be considered from two perspectives. Firstly, exposure to stress in early life has lasting detrimental effects on the development and function of neurobiologic systems believed to be involved in suicide, including those that regulate behavior, affect, and cognitive function. Secondly, impairments in stress response systems may be directly involved in suicidal behavior. In both contexts, genes may contribute to altered neurobiologic function. Increasingly sophisticated association studies that include an examination of early-life stress, markers of biologic function, or intermediate phenotypes of suicidal behavior will further illuminate the complexities of the relationship between stress, genes, and suicidal behavior.

References

[1] Brent DA, Mann JJ. Family genetic studies, suicide, and suicidal behavior. Am J Med Genet C Semin Med Genet 2005;133:13–24.

[2] Voracek M, Loibl LM. Genetics of suicide: a systematic review of twin studies. Wien Klin Wochenschr 2007;119:463–75.

[3] Mirnics K, Levitt P, Lewis DA. Critical appraisal of DNA microarrays in psychiatric genomics. Biol Psychiatry 2006;60:163–76.

[4] Mann JJ. Neurobiology of suicidal behaviour. Nat Rev Neurosci 2003;4:819–28.

[5] Purselle DC, Nemeroff CB. Serotonin transporter: a potential substrate in the biology of suicide. Neuropsychopharmacology 2003;28:613–9.

[6] Mann JJ, Huang YY, Underwood MD, et al. A serotonin transporter gene promoter polymorphism (5-HTTLPR) and prefrontal cortical binding in major depression and suicide. Arch Gen Psychiatry 2000;57:729–38.

[7] Heils A, Teufel A, Petri S, et al. Allelic variation of human serotonin transporter gene expression. J Neurochem 1996;66:2621–4.

[8] Nakamura M, Ueno S, Sano A, et al. The human serotonin transporter gene linked polymorphism (5-HTTLPR) shows ten novel allelic variants. Mol Psychiatry 2000;5:32–8.

[9] Hu XZ, Lipsky RH, Zhu G, et al. Serotonin transporter promoter gain-of-function genotypes are linked to obsessive-compulsive disorder. Am J Hum Genet 2006;78:815–26.

[10] Reimold M, Smolka MN, Schumann G, et al. Midbrain serotonin transporter binding potential measured with [11C]DASB is affected by serotonin transporter genotype. J Neural Transm 2007;114:635–9.

[11] Praschak-Rieder N, Kennedy J, Wilson AA, et al. Novel 5-HTTLPR allele associates with higher serotonin transporter binding in putamen: a [(11)C] DASB positron emission tomography study. Biol Psychiatry 2007;62:327–31.

[12] Willeit M, Stastny J, Pirker W, et al. No evidence for in vivo regulation of midbrain serotonin transporter availability by serotonin transporter promoter gene polymorphism. Biol Psychiatry 2001;50:8–12.

[13] Shioe K, Ichimiya T, Suhara T, et al. No association between genotype of the promoter region of serotonin transporter gene and serotonin transporter binding in human brain measured by PET. Synapse 2003;48:184–8.

[14] Parsey RV, Hastings RS, Oquendo MA, et al. Effect of a triallelic functional polymorphism of the serotonin-transporter-linked promoter region on expression of serotonin transporter in the human brain. Am J Psychiatry 2006;163:48–51.

[15] Brown SM, Hariri AR. Neuroimaging studies of serotonin gene polymorphisms: exploring the interplay of genes, brain, and behavior. Cogn Affect Behav Neurosci 2006;6:44–52.

[16] Canli T, Qiu M, Omura K, et al. Neural correlates of epigenesis. Proc Natl Acad Sci U S A 2006;103:16033–8.

[17] Rao H, Gillihan SJ, Wang J, et al. Genetic variation in serotonin transporter alters resting brain function in healthy individuals. Biol Psychiatry 2007;62:600–6.

[18] Azmitia EC, Gannon PJ. The primate serotonergic system: a review of human and animal studies and a report on Macaca fascicularis. Adv Neurol 1986;43:407–68.

[19] Sadikot AF, Parent A. The monoaminergic innervation of the amygdala in the squirrel monkey: an immunohistochemical study. Neuroscience 1990;36:431–47.

[20] Smith HR, Daunais JB, Nader MA, et al. Distribution of [3H]citalopram binding sites in the nonhuman primate brain. Ann N Y Acad Sci 1999;877:700–2.

[21] Anguelova M, Benkelfat C, Turecki G. A systematic review of association studies investigating genes coding for serotonin receptors and the serotonin transporter: II. Suicidal behavior. Mol Psychiatry 2003;8:646–53.

[22] Lin PY, Tsai G. Association between serotonin transporter gene promoter polymorphism and suicide: results of a meta-analysis. Biol Psychiatry 2004;55:1023–30.

[23] Gerra G, Garofano L, Santoro G, et al. Association between low-activity serotonin transporter genotype and heroin dependence: behavioral and personality correlates. Am J Med Genet B Neuropsychiatr Genet 2004;126:37–42.

[24] Retz W, Retz-Junginger P, Supprian T, et al. Association of serotonin transporter promoter gene polymorphism with violence: relation with personality disorders, impulsivity, and childhood ADHD psychopathology. Behav Sci Law 2004;22:415–25.

[25] Hallikainen T, Saito T, Lachman HM, et al. Association between low activity serotonin transporter promoter genotype and early onset alcoholism with habitual impulsive violent behavior. Mol Psychiatry 1999;4:385–8.

[26] Olivier B, van OR. 5-HT1B receptors and aggression: a review. Eur J Pharmacol 2005;526:207–17.

[27] Davidson RJ, Putnam KM, Larson CL. Dysfunction in the neural circuitry of emotion regulation—a possible prelude to violence. Science 2000;289:591–4.

[28] Stanley M, Mann JJ. Increased serotonin-2 binding sites in frontal cortex of suicide victims. Lancet 1983;1:214–6.

[29] Arora RC, Meltzer HY. Serotonergic measures in the brains of suicide victims: 5-HT2 binding sites in the frontal cortex of suicide victims and control subjects. Am J Psychiatry 1989;146:730–6.

[30] Mann JJ, Stanley M, McBride PA, et al. Increased serotonin$_2$ and β-adrenergic receptor binding in the frontal cortices of suicide victims. Arch Gen Psychiatry 1986;43:954–9.

[31] Arango V, Ernsberger P, Marzuk PM, et al. Autoradiographic demonstration of increased serotonin 5-HT2 and beta-adrenergic receptor binding sites in the brain of suicide victims. Arch Gen Psychiatry 1990;47:1038–47.

[32] Pandey GN, Dwivedi Y, Rizavi HS, et al. Higher expression of serotonin 5-HT(2A) receptors in the postmortem brains of teenage suicide victims. Am J Psychiatry 2002;159: 419–29.

[33] Hrdina PD, Demeter E, Vu TB, et al. 5-HT uptake sites and 5-HT$_2$ receptors in brain of antidepressant- free suicide victims/depressives: Increase in 5- HT$_2$ sites in cortex and amygdala. Brain Res 1993;614:37–44.

[34] Stockmeier CA. Involvement of serotonin in depression: evidence from postmortem and imaging studies of serotonin receptors and the serotonin transporter. J Psychiatr Res 2003;37:357–73.

[35] Owen F, Cross AJ, Crow TJ, et al. Brain 5-HT$_2$ receptors and suicide. Lancet 1983;2:1256.

[36] Crow TJ, Cross AJ, Cooper SJ, et al. Neurotransmitter receptors and monoamine metabolites in the brains of patients with Alzheimer-type dementia and depression, and suicides. Neuropharmacology 1984;23:1561–9.

[37] Owen F, Chambers DR, Cooper SJ, et al. Serotonergic mechanisms in brains of suicide victims. Brain Res 1986;362:185–8.

[38] Cheetham SC, Crompton MR, Katona CLE, et al. Brain 5-HT$_2$ receptor binding sites in depressed suicide victims. Brain Res 1988;443:272–80.

[39] Lowther S, De Paermentier F, Crompton MR, et al. Brain 5-HT$_2$ receptors in suicide victims: violence of death, depression and effects of antidepressant treatment. Brain Res 1994;642:281–9.

[40] Arranz B, Eriksson A, Mellerup E, et al. Brain 5-HT1A, 5-HT1D, and 5-HT2 receptors in suicide victims. Biol Psychiatry 1994;35:457–63.

[41] Stockmeier CA, Dilley GE, Shapiro LA, et al. Serotonin receptors in suicide victims with major depression. Neuropsychopharmacology 1997;16:162–73.

[42] Rosel P, Arranz B, San L, et al. Altered 5-HT$_{2A}$ binding sites and second messenger inositol triphosphate (IP$_3$) levels in hippocampus but not in frontal cortex from depressed suicide victims. Psychiatry Res 2000;99:173–81.

[43] Pandey GN. Altered serotonin function in suicide. Evidence from platelet and neuroendocrine studies. Ann N Y Acad Sci 1997;836:182–200.

[44] Pandey GN, Dwivedi Y, Pandey SC, et al. Low phosphoinositide-specific phospholipase C activity and expression of phospholipase C beta1 protein in the prefrontal cortex of teenage suicide subjects. Am J Psychiatry 1999;156:1895–901.

[45] Malone KM, Ellis SP, Currier D, et al. Platelet 5-HT2A receptor subresponsivity and lethality of attempted suicide in depressed in-patients. Int J Neuropsychopharmacol 2007;10(3): 335–43.

[46] Beskow J, Gottfries CG, Roos BE, et al. Determination of monoamine and monoamine metabolites in the human brain: post mortem studies in a group of suicides and in a control group. Acta Psychiatr Scand 1976;53:7–20.

[47] Lloyd KG, Farley IJ, Deck JHN, et al. Serotonin and 5-hydroxyindoleacetic acid in discrete areas of the brainstem of suicide victims and control patients. Adv Biochem Psychopharmacol 1974;11:387–97.

[48] Pare CMB, Yeung DPH, Price K, et al. 5-Hydroxytryptamine, noradrenaline, and dopamine in brainstem, hypothalamus, and caudate nucleus of controls and of patients committing suicide by coal-gas poisoning. Lancet 1969;2:133–5.

[49] Bourne HR, Bunney WE Jr, Colburn RW, et al. Noradrenaline, 5-hydroxytryptamine, and 5-hydroxyindoleacetic acid in hindbrains of suicidal patients. Lancet 1968;2:805–8.

[50] Shaw DM, Camps FE, Eccleston EG. 5-Hydroxytryptamine in the hind-brain of depressive suicides. Br J Psychiatry 1967;113:1407–11.

[51] Du L, Faludi G, Palkovits M, et al. Frequency of long allele in serotonin transporter gene is increased in depressed suicide victims. Biol Psychiatry 1999;46:196–201.

[52] Ono H, Shirakawa O, Nishiguchi N, et al. Serotonin 2A receptor gene polymorphism is not associated with completed suicide. J Psychiatr Res 2001;35:173–6.

[53] Crawford J, Sutherland GR, Goldney RD. No evidence for association of 5-HT2A receptor polymorphism with suicide. Am J Med Genet 2000;96:879–80.

[54] Bondy B, Kuznik J, Baghai T, et al. Lack of association of serotonin-2A receptor gene polymorphism (T102C) with suicidal ideation and suicide. Am J Med Genet 2000;96:831–5.

[55] Arias B, Gasto C, Catalan R, et al. The 5-HT(2A) receptor gene 102T/C polymorphism is associated with suicidal behavior in depressed patients. Am J Med Genet 2001;105:801–4.

[56] Du L, Bakish D, Lapierre YD, et al. Association of polymorphism of serotonin 2A receptor gene with suicidal ideation in major depressive disorder. Am J Med Genet 2000;96:56–60.

[57] Tan EC, Chong SA, Chan AO, et al. No evidence for association of the T102C polymorphism in the serotonin type 2A receptor with suicidal behavior in schizophrenia. Am J Med Genet 2002;114:321–2.

[58] Ertugrul A, Kennedy JL, Masellis M, et al. No association of the T102C polymorphism of the serotonin 2A receptor gene (HTR2A) with suicidality in schizophrenia. Schizophr Res 2004;69:301–5.

[59] Khait VD, Huang YY, Zalsman G, et al. Association of serotonin 5-HT2A receptor binding and the T102C polymorphism in depressed and healthy Caucasian subjects. Neuropsychopharmacology 2005;30:166–72.

[60] Correa H, De Marco L, Boson W, et al. Analysis of T102C 5HT2A polymorphism in Brazilian psychiatric inpatients: relationship with suicidal behavior. Cell Mol Neurobiol 2002;22:813–7.

[61] Zalsman G, Frisch A, Bromberg M, et al. Family-based association study of serotonin transporter promoter in suicidal adolescents: no association with suicidality but possible role in violence traits. Am J Med Genet 2001;105:239–45.

[62] Li D, Duan Y, He L. Association study of serotonin 2A receptor (5-HT2A) gene with schizophrenia and suicidal behavior using systematic meta-analysis. Biochem Biophys Res Commun 2006;340:1006–15.

[63] Huang Y, Grailhe R, Arango V, et al. Relationship of psychopathology to the human serotonin$_{1B}$ genotype and receptor binding kinetics in postmortem brain tissue. Neuropsychopharmacology 1999;21:238–46.

[64] Stefulj J, Buttner A, Skavic J, et al. Serotonin 1B (5HT-1B) receptor polymorphism (G861C) in suicide victims: association studies in German and Slavic population. Am J Med Genet B Neuropsychiatr Genet 2004;127:48–50.

[65] Nishiguchi N, Shirakawa O, Ono H, et al. No evidence of an association between 5HT1B receptor gene polymorphism and suicide victims in a Japanese population. Am J Med Genet 2001;105:343–5.

[66] Rujescu D, Giegling I, Sato T, et al. Lack of association between serotonin 5-HT1B receptor gene polymorphism and suicidal behavior. Am J Med Genet B Neuropsychiatr Genet 2003;116:69–71.

[67] Hong CJ, Pan GM, Tsai SJ. Association study of onset age, attempted suicide, aggressive behavior, and schizophrenia with a serotonin 1B receptor (A-161T) genetic polymorphism. Neuropsychobiology 2004;49:1–4.

[68] Tsai SJ, Hong CJ, Yu YW, et al. Association study of serotonin 1B receptor (A-161T) genetic polymorphism and suicidal behaviors and response to fluoxetine in major depressive disorder. Neuropsychobiology 2004;50:235–8.

[69] Bouwknecht JA, Hijzen TH, van der GJ, et al. Absence of 5-HT(1B) receptors is associated with impaired impulse control in male 5-HT(1B) knockout mice. Biol Psychiatry 2001;49:557–68.

[70] Lappalainen J, Long JC, Eggert M, et al. Linkage of antisocial alcoholism to the serotonin 5-HT1B receptor gene in 2 population. Arch Gen Psychiatry 1998;55:989–94.

[71] Soyka M, Preuss UW, Koller G, et al. Association of 5-HT1B receptor gene and antisocial behavior in alcoholism. J Neural Transm 2004;111:101–9.

[72] Lemonde S, Turecki G, Bakish D, et al. Impaired repression at a 5-hydroxytryptamine 1A receptor gene polymorphism associated with major depression and suicide. J Neurosci 2003;23:8788–99.

[73] Huang YY, Battistuzzi C, Oquendo MA, et al. Human 5-HT1A receptor C(-1019)G polymorphism and psychopathology. Int J Neuropsychopharmacol 2004;7:441–51.

[74] Ohtani M, Shindo S, Yoshioka N. Polymorphisms of the tryptophan hydroxylase gene and serotonin 1A receptor gene in suicide victims among Japanese. Tohoku J Exp Med 2004;202:123–33.

[75] Nishiguchi N, Shirakawa O, Ono H, et al. Lack of an association between 5-HT1A receptor gene structural polymorphisms and suicide victims. Am J Med Genet 2002;114:423–5.

[76] Stefulj J, Buttner A, Kubat M, et al. 5HT-2C receptor polymorphism in suicide victims. Association studies in German and Slavic populations. Eur Arch Psychiatry Clin Neurosci 2004;254:224–7.

[77] Okamura K, Shirakawa O, Nishiguchi N, et al. Lack of an association between 5-HT receptor gene polymorphisms and suicide victims. Psychiatry Clin Neurosci 2005;59:345–9.

[78] Turecki G, Sequeira A, Gingras Y, et al. Suicide and serotonin: study of variation at seven serotonin receptor genes in suicide completers. Am J Med Genet B Neuropsychiatr Genet 2003;118:36–40.

[79] Giegling I, Hartmann AM, Moller HJ, et al. Anger- and aggression-related traits are associated with polymorphisms in the 5-HT-2A gene. J Affect Disord 2006;96:75–81.

[80] Serretti A, Mandelli L, Giegling I, et al. HTR2C and HTR1A gene variants in German and Italian suicide attempters and completers. Am J Med Genet B Neuropsychiatr Genet 2007;144:291–9.

[81] Underwood MD, Khaibulina AA, Ellis SP, et al. Morphometry of the dorsal raphe nucleus serotonergic neurons in suicide victims. Biol Psychiatry 1999;46:473–83.

[82] Boldrini M, Underwood MD, Mann JJ, et al. More tryptophan hydroxylase in the brainstem dorsal raphe nucleus in depressed suicides. Brain Res 2005;1041:19–28.

[83] Bonkale WL, Murdock S, Janosky JE, et al. Normal levels of tryptophan hydroxylase immunoreactivity in the dorsal raphe of depressed suicide victims. J Neurochem 2004;88:958–64.

[84] Bonkale WL, Turecki G, Austin MC. Increased tryptophan hydroxylase immunoreactivity in the dorsal raphe nucleus of alcohol-dependent, depressed suicide subjects is restricted to the dorsal subnucleus. Synapse 2006;60:81–5.

[85] Bach-Mizrachi H, Underwood MD, Kassir SA, et al. Neuronal tryptophan hydroxylase mRNA expression in the human dorsal and median raphe nuclei: major depression and suicide. Neuropsychopharmacology 2006;31:814–24.

[86] Ono H, Shirakawa O, Kitamura N, et al. Tryptophan hydroxylase immunoreactivity is altered by the genetic variation in postmortem brain samples of both suicide victims and controls. Mol Psychiatry 2002;7:1127–32.

[87] Manuck SB, Flory JD, Ferrell RE, et al. Aggression and anger-related traits associated with a polymorphism of the tryptophan hydroxylase gene. Biol Psychiatry 1999;45:603–14.

[88] New AS, Gelernter J, Yovell Y, et al. Tryptophan hydroxylase genotype is associated with impulsive-aggression measures: a preliminary study. Am J Med Genet 1998;81: 13–7.

[89] Jönsson EG, Goldman D, Spurlock G, et al. Tryptophan hydroxylase and catechol-O-methyltransferase gene polymorphisms: relationships to monoamine metabolite concentrations in CSF of healthy volunteers. Eur Arch Psychiatry Clin Neurosci 1997;247:297–302.

[90] Galfalvy H, Huang YY, Oquendo MA, et al. Increased risk of suicide attempt in mood disorders and TPH1 genotype. Submitted.

[91] Lalovic A, Turecki G. Meta-analysis of the association between tryptophan hydroxylase and suicidal behavior. Am J Med Genet 2002;114:533–40.

[92] Rujescu D, Giegling I, Sato T, et al. Genetic variations in tryptophan hydroxylase in suicidal behavior: analysis and meta-analysis. Biol Psychiatry 2003;54:465–73.

[93] Bellivier F, Chaste P, Malafosse A. Association between the TPH gene A218C polymorphism and suicidal behavior: a meta-analysis. Am J Med Genet B Neuropsychiatr Genet 2004;124:87–91.

[94] Li D, He L. Further clarification of the contribution of the tryptophan hydroxylase (TPH) gene to suicidal behavior using systematic allelic and genotypic meta-analyses. Hum Genet 2006;119:233–40.

[95] Nielsen DA, Virkkunen M, Lappalainen J, et al. A tryptophan hydroxylase gene marker for suicidality and alcoholism. Arch Gen Psychiatry 1998;55:593–602.

[96] Roy A, Rylander G, Forslund K, et al. Excess tryptophan hydroxylase 17 779C allele in surviving cotwins of monozygotic twin suicide victims. Neuropsychobiology 2001;43: 233–6.

[97] Mann JJ, Malone KM, Nielsen DA, et al. Possible association of a polymorphism of the tryptophan hydroxylase gene with suicidal behavior in depressed patients. Am J Psychiatry 1997;154:1451–3.

[98] Rujescu D, Giegling I, Bondy B, et al. Association of anger-related traits with SNPs in the TPH gene. Mol Psychiatry 2002;7:1023–9.

[99] Hennig J, Reuter M, Netter P, et al. Two types of aggression are differentially related to serotonergic activity and the A779C TPH polymorphism. Behav Neurosci 2005;119: 16–25.

[100] Nolan KA, Volavka J, Lachman HM, et al. An association between a polymorphism of the tryptophan hydroxylase gene and aggression in schizophrenia and schizoaffective disorder. Psychiatr Genet 2000;10:109–15.

[101] Staner L, Uyanik G, Correa H, et al. A dimensional impulsive-aggressive phenotype is associated with the A218C polymorphism of the tryptophan hydroxylase gene: a pilot study in well-characterized impulsive inpatients. Am J Med Genet 2002;114:553–7.

[102] Zill P, Buttner A, Eisenmenger W, et al. Single nucleotide polymorphism and haplotype analysis of a novel tryptophan hydroxylase isoform (TPH2) gene in suicide victims. Biol Psychiatry 2004;56:581–6.

[103] Zhou Z, Roy A, Lipsky R, et al. Haplotype-based linkage of tryptophan hydroxylase 2 to suicide attempt, major depression, and cerebrospinal fluid 5-hydroxyindoleacetic acid in 4 populations. Arch Gen Psychiatry 2005;62:1109–18.

[104] Lopez de Lara C, Brezo J, Rouleau G, et al. Effect of tryptophan hydroxylase-2 gene variants on suicide risk in major depression. Biol Psychiatry 2007;62:72–80.

[105] De Luca V, Hlousek D, Likhodi O, et al. The interaction between TPH2 promoter haplotypes and clinical-demographic risk factors in suicide victims with major psychoses. Genes Brain Behav 2006;5:107–10.

[106] De Luca V, Voineskos D, Wong GW, et al. Promoter polymorphism of second tryptophan hydroxylase isoform (TPH2) in schizophrenia and suicidality. Psychiatry Res 2005;134: 195–8.

[107] Mann JJ, Currier D, Murphy L, et al. No association between a TPH2 promoter polymorphism and mood disorders or monoamine turnover. J Affect Disord 2008;106:117–21.

[108] Lim JE, Pinsonneault J, Sadee W, et al. Tryptophan hydroxylase 2 (TPH2) haplotypes predict levels of TPH2 mRNA expression in human pons. Mol Psychiatry 2007;12:491–501.

[109] Canli T, Congdon E, Gutknecht L, et al. Amygdala responsiveness is modulated by tryptophan hydroxylase-2 gene variation. J Neural Transm 2005;112:1479–85.

[110] Reuter M, Ott U, Vaitl D, et al. Impaired executive control is associated with a variation in the promoter region of the tryptophan hydroxylase 2 gene. J Cogn Neurosci 2007;19: 401–8.

[111] Sabol SZ, Hu S, Hamer D. A functional polymorphism in the monoamine oxidase A gene promoter. Hum Genet 1998;103:273–9.

[112] Manuck SB, Flory JD, Ferrell RE, et al. A regulatory polymorphism of the monoamine oxidase-A gene may be associated with variability in aggression, impulsivity, and central nervous system serotonergic responsivity. Psychiatry Res 2000;95:9–23.

[113] Jonsson EG, Norton N, Gustavsson JP, et al. A promoter polymorphism in the monoamine oxidase A gene and its relationships to monoamine metabolite concentrations in CSF of healthy volunteers. J Psychiatr Res 2000;34:239–44.

[114] Williams RB, Marchuk DA, Gadde KM, et al. Serotonin-related gene polymorphisms and central nervous system serotonin function. Neuropsychopharmacology 2003;28: 533–41.

[115] Meyer-Lindenberg A, Buckholtz JW, Kolachana B, et al. Neural mechanisms of genetic risk for impulsivity and violence in humans. Proc Natl Acad Sci U S A 2006;103:6269–74.

[116] Huang YY, Cate SP, Battistuzzi C, et al. An association between a functional polymorphism in the monoamine oxidase a gene promoter, impulsive traits and early abuse experiences. Neuropsychopharmacology 2004;29:1498–505.

[117] Kunugi H, Ishida S, Kato T, et al. A functional polymorphism in the promoter region of monoamine oxidase-A gene and mood disorders. Mol Psychiatry 1999;4:393–5.

[118] Ono H, Shirakawa O, Nishiguchi N, et al. No evidence of an association between a functional monoamine oxidase a gene polymorphism and completed suicides. Am J Med Genet 2002;114:340–2.

[119] Gerra G, Garofano L, Bosari S, et al. Analysis of monoamine oxidase A (MAO-A) promoter polymorphism in male heroin-dependent subjects: behavioural and personality correlates. J Neural Transm 2004;111:611–21.

[120] Ho LW, Furlong RA, Rubinsztein JS, et al. Genetic associations with clinical characteristics in bipolar affective disorder and recurrent unipolar depressive disorder. Am J Med Genet 2000;96:36–42.

[121] Courtet P, Jollant F, Castelnau D, et al. Suicidal behavior: relationship between phenotype and serotonergic genotype. Am J Med Genet C Semin Med Genet 2005;133:25–33.

[122] Brunner HG, Nelen M, Breakefield XO, et al. Abnormal behavior associated with a point mutation in the structural gene for monoamine oxidase A. Science 1993;262:578–80.

[123] Cases O, Seif I, Grimsby J, et al. Aggressive behavior and altered amounts of brain serotonin and norepinephrine in mice lacking MAOA. Science 1995;268:1763–6.

[124] Jacob CP, Muller J, Schmidt M, et al. Cluster B personality disorders are associated with allelic variation of monoamine oxidase A activity. Neuropsychopharmacology 2005;30:1711–8.

[125] Passamonti L, Fera F, Magariello A, et al. Monoamine oxidase-a genetic variations influence brain activity associated with inhibitory control: new insight into the neural correlates of impulsivity. Biol Psychiatry 2006;59:334–40.

[126] Fan J, Fossella J, Sommer T, et al. Mapping the genetic variation of executive attention onto brain activity. Proc Natl Acad Sci U S A 2003;100:7406–11.

[127] Caspi A, Sugden K, Moffitt TE, et al. Influence of life stress on depression: moderation by a polymorphism in the 5-HTT gene. Science 2003;301:386–9.

[128] Uher R, McGuffin P. The moderation by the serotonin transporter gene of environmental adversity in the aetiology of mental illness: review and methodological analysis. Mol Psychiatry 2008;13:131–46.

[129] Gibb BE, McGeary JE, Beevers CG, et al. Serotonin transporter (5-HTTLPR) genotype, childhood abuse, and suicide attempts in adult psychiatric inpatients. Suicide Life Threat Behav 2006;36:687–93.

[130] Roy A, Hu XZ, Janal MN, et al. Interaction between childhood trauma and serotonin transporter gene variation in suicide. Neuropsychopharmacology 2007;32:2046–52.

[131] Reif A, Rosler M, Freitag CM, et al. Nature and nurture predispose to violent behavior: serotonergic genes and adverse childhood environment. Neuropsychopharmacology 2007;32:2375–83.

[132] Caspi A, McClay J, Moffitt TE, et al. Role of genotype in the cycle of violence in maltreated children. Science 2002;297:851–4.

[133] Foley DL, Eaves LJ, Wormley B, et al. Childhood adversity, monoamine oxidase a genotype, and risk for conduct disorder. Arch Gen Psychiatry 2004;61:738–44.

[134] Nilsson KW, Sjoberg RL, Damberg M, et al. Role of monoamine oxidase A genotype and psychosocial factors in male adolescent criminal activity. Biol Psychiatry 2006;59: 121–7.

[135] Ducci F, Enoch MA, Hodgkinson C, et al. Interaction between a functional MAOA locus and childhood sexual abuse predicts alcoholism and antisocial personality disorder in adult women. Mol Psychiatry 2006;11:858–66.

[136] Haberstick BC, Lessem JM, Hopfer CJ, et al. Monoamine oxidase A (MAOA) and antisocial behaviors in the presence of childhood and adolescent maltreatment. Am J Med Genet B Neuropsychiatr Genet 2005;135:59–64.

[137] Huizinga D, Haberstick BC, Smolen A, et al. Childhood maltreatment, subsequent antisocial behavior, and the role of monoamine oxidase A genotype. Biol Psychiatry 2006;60: 677–83.

[138] Arborelius L, Hawks BW, Owens MJ, et al. Increased responsiveness of presumed 5-HT cells to citalopram in adult rats subjected to prolonged maternal separation relative to brief separation. Psychopharmacology (Berl) 2004;176:248–55.

[139] Kaufman J, Birmaher B, Perel J, et al. Serotonergic functioning in depressed abused children: clinical and familial correlates. Biol Psychiatry 1998;44:973–81.

[140] Pine DS, Coplan JD, Wasserman GA, et al. Neuroendocrine response to fenfluramine challenge in boys: associations with aggressive behavior and adverse rearing. Arch Gen Psychiatry 1997;54:839–46.

[141] Rinne T, Westenberg HG, Den Boer JA, et al. Serotonergic blunting to meta-chlorophenylpiperazine (m-CPP) highly correlates with sustained childhood abuse in impulsive and autoaggressive female borderline patients. Biol Psychiatry 2000;47: 548–56.

[142] Bennett AJ, Lesch KP, Heils A, et al. Early experience and serotonin transporter gene variation interact to influence primate CNS function. Mol Psychiatry 2002;7:118–22.

[143] Firk C, Markus CR. Review: serotonin by stress interaction: a susceptibility factor for the development of depression? J Psychopharmacol 2007;21:538–44.

[144] O'Hara R, Schroder CM, Mahadevan R, et al. Serotonin transporter polymorphism, memory and hippocampal volume in the elderly: association and interaction with cortisol. Mol Psychiatry 2007;12:544–55.

[145] Wand GS, McCaul M, Yang X, et al. The mu-opioid receptor gene polymorphism (A118G) alters HPA axis activation induced by opioid receptor blockade. Neuropsychopharmacology 2002;26:106–14.

[146] Smith GS, Lotrich FE, Malhotra AK, et al. Effects of serotonin transporter promoter polymorphisms on serotonin function. Neuropsychopharmacology 2004;29:2226–34.

[147] Barr CS, Newman TK, Shannon C, et al. Rearing condition and rh5-HTTLPR interact to influence limbic-hypothalamic-pituitary-adrenal axis response to stress in infant macaques. Biol Psychiatry 2004;55:733–8.

[148] Arango V, Underwood MD, Mann JJ. Fewer pigmented locus coeruleus neurons in suicide victims: preliminary results. Biol Psychiatry 1996;39:112–20.

[149] Ordway GA, Smith KS, Haycock JW. Elevated tyrosine hydroxylase in the locus coeruleus of suicide victims. J Neurochem 1994;62:680–5.

[150] Pandey GN, Dwivedi Y. Noradrenergic function in suicide. Arch Suicide Res 2007;11: 235–46.

[151] Fernandez-Pastor B, Mateo Y, Gomez-Urquijo S, et al. Characterization of noradrenaline release in the locus coeruleus of freely moving awake rats by in vivo microdialysis. Psychopharmacology (Berl) 2005;180:570–9.

[152] Sequeira A, Mamdani F, Lalovic A, et al. Alpha 2A adrenergic receptor gene and suicide. Psychiatry Res 2004;125:87–93.

[153] Martin-Guerrero I, Callado LF, Saitua K, et al. The N251K functional polymorphism in the alpha(2A)-adrenoceptor gene is not associated with depression: a study in suicide completers. Psychopharmacology (Berl) 2006;184:82–6.

[154] Persson M-L, Wasserman D, Geijer T, et al. Tyrosine hydroxylase allelic distribution in suicide attempters. Psychiatry Res 1997;72:73–80.

[155] DeLuca V, Strauss J, Kennedy JL. Power based association analysis (PBAT) of serotonergic and noradrenergic polymorphisms in bipolar patients with suicidal behaviour. Prog Neuropsychopharmacol Biol Psychiatry 2008;32:197–203.

[156] Hattori H, Shirakawa O, Nishiguchi N, et al. No evidence of an association between tyrosine hydroxylase gene polymorphisms and suicide victims. Kobe J Med Sci 2006;52: 195–200.

[157] Lachman HM, Papolos DF, Saito T, et al. Human catechol-O-methyltransferase pharmacogenetics: description of a functional polymorphism and its potential application to neuropsychiatric disorders. Pharmacogenetics 1996;6:243–50.

[158] Chen J, Lipska BK, Halim N, et al. Functional analysis of genetic variation in catechol-O-methyltransferase (COMT): effects on mRNA, protein, and enzyme activity in postmortem human brain. Am J Hum Genet 2004;75:807–21.

[159] Kia-Keating BM, Glatt SJ, Tsuang MT. Meta-analyses suggest association between COMT, but not HTR1B, alleles, and suicidal behavior. Am J Med Genet B Neuropsychiatr Genet 2007;144:1048–53.

[160] Lachman HM, Nolan KA, Mohr P, et al. Association between catechol O-methyltransferase genotype and violence in schizophrenia and schizoaffective disorders. Am J Psychiatry 1998;155:835–7.

[161] Kotler M, Barak P, Cohen H, et al. Homicidal behavior in schizophrenia associated with a genetic polymorphism determining low catechol O-methyltransferase (COMT) activity. Am J Med Genet 1999;88:628–33.

[162] Strous RD, Bark N, Parsia SS, et al. Analysis of a functional catechol-O-methyltransferase gene polymorphism in schizophrenia: evidence for association with aggressive and antisocial behavior. Psychiatry Res 1997;69:71–7.

[163] Nolan KA, Volavka J, Czobor P, et al. Suicidal behavior in patients with schizophrenia is related to COMT polymorphism. Psychiatr Genet 2000;10:117–24.

[164] Rujescu D, Giegling I, Gietl A, et al. A functional single nucleotide polymorphism (V158M) in the COMT gene is associated with aggressive personality traits. Biol Psychiatry 2003;54:34–9.

[165] Zammit S, Jones G, Jones SJ, et al. Polymorphisms in the MAOA, MAOB, and COMT genes and aggressive behavior in schizophrenia. Am J Med Genet B Neuropsychiatr Genet 2004;128:19–20.

[166] Wei J, Hemmings GP. Lack of evidence for association between the COMT locus and schizophrenia. Psychiatr Genet 1999;9:183–6.

[167] Liou YJ, Tsai SJ, Hong CJ, et al. Association analysis of a functional catechol-o-methyltrans-ferase gene polymorphism in schizophrenic patients in Taiwan. Neuropsychobiology 2001;43:11–4.

[168] Russ MJ, Lachman HM, Kashdan T, et al. Analysis of catechol-O-methyltransferase and 5-hydroxytryptamine transporter polymorphisms in patients at risk for suicide. Psychiatry Res 2000;93:73–8.

[169] Jones G, Zammit S, Norton N, et al. Aggressive behaviour in patients with schizophrenia is associated with catechol-O-methyltransferase genotype. Br J Psychiatry 2001;179: 351–5.

[170] Hallikainen T, Lachman H, Saito T, et al. Lack of association between the functional variant of the catechol-o-methyltransferase (COMT) gene and early-onset alcoholism associated with severe antisocial behavior. Am J Med Genet 2000;96:348–52.

[171] Baud P, Courtet P, Perroud N, et al. Catechol-O-methyltransferase polymorphism (COMT) in suicide attempters: a possible gender effect on anger traits. Am J Med Genet B Neuro-psychiatr Genet 2007;144:1042–7.

[172] Ono H, Shirakawa O, Nushida H, et al. Association between catechol-O-methyltransfer-ase functional polymorphism and male suicide completers. Neuropsychopharmacology 2004;29:1374–7.

[173] Heim C, Nemeroff CB. The role of childhood trauma in the neurobiology of mood and anx-iety disorders: preclinical and clinical studies. Biol Psychiatry 2001;49:1023–39.

[174] Dailly E, Chenu F, Renard CE, et al. Dopamine, depression and antidepressants. Fundam Clin Pharmacol 2004;18:601–7.

[175] Bowden C, Cheetham SC, Lowther S, et al. Reduced dopamine turnover in the basal gan-glia of depressed suicides. Brain Res 1997;769:135–40.

[176] Bowden C, Theodorou AE, Cheetham SC, et al. Dopamine D_1 and D_2 receptor binding sites in brain samples from depressed suicides and controls. Brain Res 1997;752: 227–33.

[177] Roy A, Ågren H, Pickar D, et al. Reduced CSF concentrations of homovanillic acid and ho-movanillic acid to 5-Hydroxyindoleacetic acid ratios in depressed patients: relationship to suicidal behavior and dexamethasone nonsuppression. Am J Psychiatry 1986;143: 1539–45.

[178] Roy A, Karoum F, Pollack S. Marked reduction in indexes of dopamine metabolism among patients with depression who attempt suicide. Arch Gen Psychiatry 1992;49:447–50.

[179] Engstrom G, Alling C, Blennow K, et al. Reduced cerebrospinal HVA concentrations and HVA/5-HIAA ratios in suicide attempters. Monoamine metabolites in 120 suicide attemp-ters and 47 controls. Eur Neuropsychopharmacol 1999;9:399–405.

[180] Nordström P, Samuelsson M, Åsberg M, et al. CSF 5-HIAA predicts suicide risk after attempted suicide. Suicide Life Threat Behav 1994;24:1–9.

[181] Placidi GP, Oquendo MA, Malone KM, et al. Aggressivity, suicide attempts, and depres-sion: relationship to cerebrospinal fluid monoamine metabolite levels. Biol Psychiatry 2001;50:783–91.

[182] Soderstrom H, Blennov K, Manhem A, et al. CSF studies in violent offenders. 1. 5-HIAA as a negative and HVA as a positive predictor of psychopathy. J Neural Transm 2001;108: 869–78.

[183] Soderstrom H, Blennow K, Sjodin A-K, et al. New evidence for an association between the CSF HVA:5-HIAA ratio and psychopathic traits. J Neurol Neurosurg Psychiatry 2003;74: 918–21.

[184] Johann M, Putzhammer A, Eichhammer P, et al. Association of the -141C Del variant of the dopamine D2 receptor (DRD2) with positive family history and suicidality in German alco-holics. Am J Med Genet B Neuropsychiatr Genet 2005;132:46–9.

[185] Finckh U, Rommelspacher H, Kuhn S, et al. Influence of the dopamine D2 receptor (DRD2) genotype on neuroadaptive effects of alcohol and the clinical outcome of alcoholism. Phar-macogenetics 1997;7:271–81.

[186] Persson ML, Geijer T, Wasserman D, et al. Lack of association between suicide attempt and a polymorphism at the dopamine receptor D4 locus. Psychiatr Genet 1999;9: 97–100.

[187] Zalsman G, Frisch A, Lev-Ran S, et al. DRD4 exon III polymorphism and response to risperidone in Israeli adolescents with schizophrenia: a pilot pharmacogenetic study. Eur Neuropsychopharmacol 2003;13:183–5.

[188] Coryell W, Schlesser M. The dexamethasone suppression test and suicide prediction. Am J Psychiatry 2001;158:748–53.

[189] Mann JJ, Currier D, Stanley B, et al. Can biological tests assist prediction of suicide in mood disorders? Int J Neuropsychopharmacol 2006;9:465–74.

[190] Szigethy E, Conwell Y, Forbes NT, et al. Adrenal weight and morphology in victims of completed suicide. Biol Psychiatry 1994;36:374–80.

[191] Dorovini-Zis K, Zis AP. Increased adrenal weight in victims of violent suicide. Am J Psychiatry 1987;144:1214–5.

[192] Dumser T, Barocka A, Schubert E. Weight of adrenal glands may be increased in persons who commit suicide. Am J Forensic Med Pathol 1998;19:72–6.

[193] Nemeroff CB, Krishnan KR, Reed D, et al. Adrenal gland enlargement in major depression. A computed tomographic study. Arch Gen Psychiatry 1992;49:384–7.

[194] Nemeroff CB, Owens MJ, Bissette G, et al. Reduced corticotropin releasing factor binding sites in the frontal cortex of suicide victims. Arch Gen Psychiatry 1988;45:577–9.

[195] Secunda SK, Cross CK, Koslow S, et al. Biochemistry and suicidal behavior in depressed patients. Biol Psychiatry 1986;21:756–67.

[196] Brown RP, Mason B, Stoll P, et al. Adrenocortical function and suicidal behavior in depressive disorders. Psychiatry Res 1986;17:317–23.

[197] Modestin J, Ruef C. Dexamethasone suppression test (DST) in relation to depressive somatic and suicidal manifestations. Acta Psychiatr Scand 1987;75:491–4.

[198] Roy A, Pickar D, Linnoila M, et al. Cerebrospinal fluid monoamine and monoamine metabolite levels and the dexamethasone suppression test in depression. Relationship to life events. Arch Gen Psychiatry 1986;43:356–60.

[199] Roy A. Hypothalamic-pituitary-adrenal axis function and suicidal behavior in depression. Biol Psychiatry 1992;32:812–6.

[200] Norman WH, Brown WA, Miller IW, et al. The dexamethasone suppression test and completed suicide. Acta Psychiatr Scand 1990;81:120–5.

[201] Black DW, Monahan PO, Winokur G. The relationship between DST results and suicidal behavior. Ann Clin Psychiatry 2002;14:83–8.

[202] Targum SD, Rosen L, Capodanno AE. The dexamethasone suppression test in suicidal patients with unipolar depression. Am J Psychiatry 1983;140:877–9.

[203] Mathew SJ, Coplan JD, Goetz RR, et al. Differentiating depressed adolescent 24 h cortisol secretion in light of their adult clinical outcome. Neuropsychopharmacology 2003;28: 1336–43.

[204] Cleare AJ, Murray RM, O'Keane V. Reduced prolactin and cortisol responses to d-fenfluramine in depressed compared to healthy matched control subjects. Neuropsychopharmacology 1996;14:349–54.

[205] Duval F, Mokrani MC, Correa H, et al. Lack of effect of HPA axis hyperactivity on hormonal responses to d- fenfluramine in major depressed patients: implications for pathogenesis of suicidal behaviour. Psychoneuroendocrinology 2001;26:521–37.

[206] Malone KM, Corbitt EM, Li S, et al. Prolactin response to fenfluramine and suicide attempt lethality in major depression. Br J Psychiatry 1996;168:324–9.

[207] Brunner J, Stalla GK, Stalla J, et al. Decreased corticotropin-releasing hormone (CRH) concentrations in the cerebrospinal fluid of eucortisolemic suicide attempters. J Psychiatr Res 2001;35:1–9.

[208] Träskman-Bendz L, Ekman R, Regnell G, et al. HPA-related CSF neuropeptides in suicide attempters. Eur Neuropsychopharmacol 1992;2:99–106.

[209] Wust S, Van Rossum EF, Federenko IS, et al. Common polymorphisms in the glucocorticoid receptor gene are associated with adrenocortical responses to psychosocial stress. J Clin Endocrinol Metab 2004;89:565–73.

[210] Wasserman D, Sokolowski M, Rozanov V, et al. The CRHR1 gene: a marker for suicidality in depressed males exposed to low stress. Genes Brain Behav 2008;7:14–9.

[211] Hishimoto A, Shirakawa O, Nishiguchi N, et al. Association between a functional polymorphism in the renin-angiotensin system and completed suicide. J Neural Transm 2006;113:1915–20.

[212] Liu D, Diorio J, Tannenbaum B, et al. Maternal care, hippocampal glucocorticoid receptors, and hypothalamic-pituitary-adrenal responses to stress. Science 1997;277: 1659–62.

[213] Meaney MJ, Diorio J, Francis D, et al. Early environmental regulation of forebrain glucocorticoid receptor gene expression: implications for adrenocortical responses to stress. Dev Neurosci 1996;18:49–72.

[214] Plotsky PM, Meaney MJ. Early, postnatal experience alters hypothalamic corticotropin-releasing factor (CRF) mRNA, median eminence CRF content and stress-induced release in adult rats. Brain Res Mol Brain Res 1993;18:195–200.

[215] Avishai-Eliner S, Eghbal-Ahmadi M, Tabachnik E, et al. Down-regulation of hypothalamic corticotropin-releasing hormone messenger ribonucleic acid (mRNA) precedes early-life experience-induced changes in hippocampal glucocorticoid receptor mRNA. Endocrinology 2001;142:89–97.

[216] Breier AAE. Bennett award paper. Experimental approaches to human stress research: assessment of neurobiological mechanisms of stress in volunteers and psychiatric patients. Biol Psychiatry 1989;26:438–62.

[217] Stein MB, Yehuda R, Koverola C, et al. Enhanced dexamethasone suppression of plasma cortisol in adult women traumatized by childhood sexual abuse. Biol Psychiatry 1997;42: 680–6.

[218] Heim C, Newport DJ, Bonsall R, et al. Altered pituitary-adrenal axis responses to provocative challenge tests in adult survivors of childhood abuse. Am J Psychiatry 2001;158: 575–81.

[219] Heim C, Newport DJ, Heit S, et al. Pituitary-adrenal and autonomic responses to stress in women after sexual and physical abuse in childhood. J Am Med Assoc 2000;284:592–7.

[220] Bradley RG, Binder EB, Epstein MP, et al. Influence of child abuse on adult depression: moderation by the corticotropin-releasing hormone receptor gene. Arch Gen Psychiatry 2008;65:190–200.

[221] Blomeyer D, Treutlein J, Esser G, et al. Interaction between CRHR1 gene and stressful life events predicts adolescent heavy alcohol use. Biol Psychiatry 2008;63:146–51.

Psychiatr Clin N Am 31 (2008) 271–291

PSYCHIATRIC CLINICS
OF NORTH AMERICA

Completed Suicide in Childhood

Kanita Dervic, MD[a],*, David A. Brent, MD[b],
Maria A. Oquendo, MD[c]

[a]Department of Child and Adolescent Psychiatry/University Hospital,
Medical University of Vienna, Waehringer Guertel 18–20, 1090 Vienna, Austria
[b]Division of Child and Adolescent Psychiatry, Western Psychiatric Institute and Clinic,
University of Pittsburgh Medical Center, 3811 O'Hara Street, Room 311 BFT,
Pittsburgh, PA 15213, USA
[c]Division of Molecular Imaging and Neuropathology, New York State Psychiatric Institute,
Columbia University, 1051 Riverside Drive, Office #2725, New York, NY 10032, USA

U nderstanding and counteracting the problem of suicide among children and young adolescents aged 14 years and younger are challenging for every society. As King and Apter [1] stated, the tragic irony is that in an era when medical progress has significantly decreased rates of death and illness among young individuals, many lose their lives through suicide. In the United States, suicide is the third cause of death in the population aged 14 years and younger [2]. In 2004 in the United States, the suicide rate per 100,000 for children aged 10 to 14 was 1.3 [2]; this represents a threefold increase during the past 25 years, considering that it was 0.4 in 1979 [3]. Youngsters aged 14 years and younger are often referred to as children; however, the terms *children* and *young adolescents* seem more appropriate [4,5], given that the onset of puberty often occurs during this time [6,7]. Suicide before puberty is rare, and most suicides occur after 12 years of age [8]. In the United States, the suicide rate for children aged 5 to 9 years was 0.01/100,000 [2] in 2004.

Suicide in childhood is not a random phenomenon. It occurs in vulnerable children [8]. Childhood suicide is associated with severe personal and social pathology [9]. In a series of studies, Pfeffer [9,10] reported on psychosocial and biologic factors related to suicidal behavior in childhood and on its clinical assessment and treatment. Bridge and colleagues [11] proposed a model of early onset of suicidal behavior, in which vulnerability begins with parental risk factors (ie, mood disorder, impulsive aggression, suicide attempt) and depicts transmission of risk factors from parents to children.

This article 1) briefly reviews studies of representative samples of completed suicides in children and early adolescents aged 14 years and younger, 2) summarizes important information on suicide in childhood and early adolescence, and 3) discusses implications for future research and suicide prevention.

*Corresponding author. *E-mail address:* kanita.dervic@meduniwien.ac.at (K. Dervic).

0193-953X/08/$ – see front matter
doi:10.1016/j.psc.2008.01.006

LITERATURE REVIEW

Only a few studies investigated suicides in the population aged 14 years and younger, either as a separate population or as a subsample of a larger study (Table 1). Available studies included investigations of available records on suicide (eg, coroner, educational, medical, psychiatric, social service) (n = 4) [4,5,12,13], epidemiologic studies of suicide trends in childhood and early adolescence (n = 4) [14–17], and a few medical autopsy studies that investigated suicides aged 14 years and younger (n = 4) [18–21]. However, the latter investigated small and selected/nonrepresentative samples, because not every suicide is subject to a medical autopsy. Therefore these data should be interpreted cautiously and are not reviewed here. Furthermore, only one study used the psychologic autopsy method to investigate suicides aged 14 years and younger [22], but the methodology of this study differs somewhat from psychologic autopsy studies, because families and friends were interviewed in only approximately one third of suicides, and were not interviewed personally by the researchers [22]. Most youth psychologic autopsy studies group children, young adolescents, and older adolescents together, and therefore information on the youngest subsample cannot be extracted. One exception is a study by Brent and colleagues [23] in which the subsample of suicides aged 15 years and younger was investigated separately and compared with controls matched for age, gender, race, country of origin, and socioeconomic status and with older adolescents (≥16 years). Although the suicides in this study [23] are somewhat older (mean age, 14.6 years) than the population discussed in this article, they are nearest to the population investigated (see Table 1). Furthermore, two psychologic autopsy studies [24,25] compared child and young adolescent suicides subsample with older adolescent suicides in some aspects (see Table 1).

DATA SYNTHESIS AND DISCUSSION OF THE FINDINGS IN THE CONTEXT OF RELATED RESEARCH

Age and Gender

Suicide before puberty is rare, most probably because depression and substance abuse before puberty are also rare [24]. Suicides in the group aged 14 years and younger occur predominantly among 13- to 14-year-olds [26] and are more common among boys [16]. The most recent World Health Organization (WHO) [27] suicide statistics on the population aged 14 years and younger (Table 2) show that the mean suicide rate per 100,000 was 0.59/100,000 (range 3.1–0). The mean male suicide rate was 0.8/100,000 (range 4.9–0) and mean female rate 0.39/100,000 (range 2.7–0). Previous studies have reported male–female ratios between 5:1 [22], 3:1 [5,16], and 2:1 [4] for this population. The male–female ratio (mean) in the latest WHO reported statistics (see Table 2) was 2:1. Furthermore, the gender ratio increases dramatically with age in many countries, and these increases reflect proportionally more men. However, some countries report that suicide among girls aged 14 years and younger are more common than in the same-aged boys (ie, Georgia, Norway, Slovenia, and Tajikistan in Europe; Colombia, Ecuador, El Salvador, Nicaragua, Puerto Rico, and Trinidad and Tobago in the Region of Americas; China/Hong Kong SAR and Republic of Korea in Western-Pacific Region) (see Table 2).

Racial Distribution

Pfeffer [9] reported that in the racially diverse United States population, the rate for suicide among both genders aged 5 to 14 year is highest for whites than non-whites.

Suicide Trends

Studies are scarce investigating suicide trends in the group aged 14 years and younger over a longer period. According to Centers for Disease Control and Prevention (CDC) [2] data, suicide rates for children and young adolescents in the United States are increasing, whereas no changes in suicide trends are reported in the United Kingdom [14] and Australia [15]. In contrast, Austria reported decreasing suicide rates among individuals aged 14 years and younger [16].

Suicide Methods

Reports from different countries for children and young adolescents aged 14 years and younger show that most suicides in this age group occur through hanging [5,12,13,16,22]. Previously in the United States, most suicides in this population were committed using firearms [3], which is the most common suicide method in all age groups [28]. However, beginning in 1997, firearm suicides in the United States among individuals aged 14 years and younger were surpassed by suicides through suffocation (mostly hanging) [29]. The study by Shaffer [4] in 1974 showed that most child and young adolescent suicides occurred through carbon monoxide gas, which was the predominant suicide method in England and Wales at that time [30]. Similarly, in Austria hanging was the most common suicide method in the general population and children and young adolescents aged 14 years and younger [16].

Suicide Notes and Suicide Intent

Between 14% and 46% child and young adolescents suicides aged 14 years and younger left a suicide note [4,5,22]. Shaffer [4] reported that half of the notes available expressed hostile affect. Less suicide intent was reported [12,22,23,31] among child and young adolescent suicides compared with older adolescents.

Sociocultural Differences

According to latest WHO statistics on suicide in the population aged 14 years and younger, the highest total (3.1/100,000) and male (4.9/100,000) suicide rate was reported in Kazakhstan, whereas the highest female suicide rate was reported in Guyana (2.7/100,000) (see Table 1). The lowest suicide rates were reported for African and Eastern Mediterranean Region (0–0.5/100,000). However, only a few countries from this region reported suicide rates, and the effects of underreporting and fear of stigma [32] should be considered when

Table 1
Reviewed studies on suicide in children and early adolescents aged 14 years and younger

Study type	Country	N	Age range (y)	Controls	Predominant suicide method	Most common precipitant	Disorders	OR for controls
Investigation of available records								
Shaffer [4]	England and Wales	30	12–14	No	Monoxide gas poisoning (>40%)	Disciplinary crisis (36%)	Emotional/affective symptoms (13%) Antisocial symptoms (17%) Mixed emotional and antisocial symptoms (57%)	NA
Beautrais [5]	New Zealand	61	9–14	No	Hanging (>3/4)	Family arguments and disciplinary events	Mental health problems in 23%	NA
Hoberman and Garfinkel [12]	USA	21	≤14	No	Hanging (>1/2)	School problems (1/3)	Impulsive Angry Nervous	NA
Thompson [13]	Canada (Manitoba)	16	6–14	No	Hanging (for 12–14-year-olds)	—	—	NA
Psychologic autopsy studies								
Groholt et al, [22] (one third with psychologic autopsy)	Norway	12	12–14	Students matched for age and gender (self-report survey), and adolescent suicides aged 15–19 y	Hanging (93%)	Parent-child conflict	Affective disorders (33%) Disruptive disorders 8% No past suicide attempt No substance abuse No alcohol/drugs intoxication at time of death	11.0[a] 2.0[a] 0.3[a] — —

Study	Country	N	Age	Controls	Firearms (>3/4)	Parent-child conflict		
Brent et al, [23]	USA	35	≤15	Controls matched for age, gender, race, country of origin, and SES	Firearms (>3/4)	Parent-child conflict	Any mood disorder (42.9%)	20.3
							Anxiety disorders (22.9%)	8.0
							Substance abuse (5.9%)	4.4
							Conduct/Antisocial disorder (17.1%)	5.6
							Past suicide attempt (35.5%)	32.0
Marttunen et al, [25]b	Finland	13	13–16	Suicides aged 17–19 y	—	—	Compared with older suicides: Less alcohol abuse (18%) Less adjustment disorder (6%) Less personality disorder (12%)	—
Shaffer et al, [24]b	United States	19	5–14	Older adolescent suicides	—	—	Compared with older suicides: Less substance abuse (12%) in suicides aged 13–15 No substance abuse in suicides ≤12	—

(continued on next page)

Table 1
(continued)

Epidemiologic studies	Country	Age	Trends (suicide rates per 100,000)
McClure [14]	Great Britain (England and Wales) 1970–1998	10–14	Stable
Dudley et al, [15]	Australia (New South Wales) 1964–1988	10–14	Stable
Dervic et al, [16] Pritchard and Hansen [17]	Austria 1970–2001 United States Canada Australia Japan England and Wales Germany Netherlands Italy France Spain Two cutoff points: suicide rates in 1974–1976 and 1997–1999	10–14 5–14	Decreasing (total) (boys: decreasing; girls: stable) Increasing for boys in the U.S. and Canada; Stable for girls in all investigated countries

Abbreviations: NA, non applicable; OR, odds ratio; SES, socioeconomic status.
^aStudents matched for age and gender.
^bThese psychologic autopsy studies compared children with older adolescents in some aspects.

interpreting the findings. Also, several European (eg, Iceland, Portugal) and Latin American (eg, Dominican Republic, Jamaica) countries reported no suicides in this young population (see Table 2). In Europe, 13 top-ranked countries in terms of suicides among children and young adolescents aged 14 years and younger are from Eastern Europe. Social changes may influence suicide rates in the youngest population (ie, a cohort effect that was described for older adolescents) [10,33]. However, which social changes might contribute to youth suicide trends is unclear [34]. Shared risk factors for suicide (eg, poverty, exposure to violence, poor access to health care, family history) should also be considered regarding regional differences in suicide rates. Furthermore, predominant attitudes toward suicide in the society (eg, viewing suicide as legitimate and understandable) [8,35] should not be neglected in this young population. Investigations of specific regional factors within a country [36] also deserve attention. For example, in Austria, the federal state with the highest total suicide rate (Carinthia) also has the highest suicide rate among children and young adolescents aged 14 years and younger [16].

Prior Suicidal Behavior (Ideation, Threats, Attempt)

More than one third of suicides aged 14 years and younger had previous suicidal ideas/threats/behavior [4,5]. Similarly, in the case-control psychologic autopsy study by Brent and colleagues [23], suicides aged 15 years and younger had significantly more prior suicide attempts than controls (35% versus 0, respectively).

Precipitants

In general, suicides among children and young adolescents seem to have fewer precipitants than older adolescents [22,23]. The most common precipitants were disciplinary events [4,5] and family arguments [5]. Some precipitants were described as minor, but they occurred in the context of actual or anticipated transition/disruptions in family or school environment [5]. Compared with older adolescents, no romantic disappointment precipitants were recorded in children and early adolescents aged 14 years and younger [22]. Furthermore, suicides in children and young adolescents aged 14 years and younger are characterized by brief stress–suicide interval [22]; this may also be the case for teenage suicides [8].

Family History of Suicidal Behavior

Approximately 10% of child and young adolescent suicides had a family history of suicide [4,5]. This finding is consistent with the report from Pfeffer and colleagues [37] that, unlike community controls, children who attempted suicide had a higher prevalence of suicide and suicide attempts among parents and siblings. Also, greater family loading may be related to earlier onset of suicidal behavior [38].

Psychopathology

Approximately one half of children and adolescents aged 14 years and younger who committed suicide had a detectable psychiatric disorder (Fig. 1) [4,5,22], with

Table 2
WHO data on suicides in the population aged 14 years and younger worldwide (last update 2007; accessed September 2007)

Country	Year	Suicide rate (per 100,000)		
		Total	Male	Female
African region				
Zimbabwe	1990	0.5	0.5	0.5
Mauritius	2004	0	0	0
Sao Tome and Principe	1987	0	0	0
Seychelles	1985	0	0	0
Eastern Mediterranean region				
Syrian Arab Republic	1981	0	0.1	0
Bahrain	1988	0	0	0
Egypt	1987	0	0	0
Iran	1991	0	0	0
Jordan	1979	0	0	0
Kuwait	2002	0	0	0
European region				
Kazakhstan	2003	3.1	4.9	1.2
Bosnia and Herzegovina	1991	2.6	4.0	1.1
Russian Federation	2004	2.3	3.6	1.0
Slovenia	2004	2.0	1.9	2.1
Lithuania	2004	1.6	2.7	0.5
Turkmenistan	1998	1.5	2.4	0.5
Ukraine	2004	1.4	2.2	0.5
Kyrgyzstan	2004	1.3	1.7	0.9
Belarus	2003	1.2	1.8	0.5
Romania	2004	1.2	2.2	0.3
Bulgaria	2004	1.1	1.3	0.8
Republic of Moldavia	2004	1.0	1.1	0.8
Uzbekistan	2003	0.9	1.4	0.4
Croatia	2004	0.8	1.2	0.4
Finland	2004	0.8	1.2	0.3
Latvia	2004	0.8	1.6	0
Poland	2004	0.8	1.1	0.4
Albania	2003	0.7	1.3	0
Czech Republic	2004	0.7	0.9	0.6
Estonia	2005	0.7	1.4	0
Hungary	2003	0.7	1.4	0
Sweden	2002	0.6	0.7	0.5
Belgium	1997	0.5	1.0	0
Ireland	2005	0.5	0.7	0.4
Netherlands	2004	0.5	0.7	0.2
Norway	2004	0.5	0	1.0
Serbia and Montenegro	2002	0.5	1.1	0
Austria	2005	0.4	0.6	0.2
France	2003	0.4	0.7	0.2
Denmark	2001	0.3	0.6	0
Germany	2004	0.3	0.4	0.2
Slovakia	2002	0.3	0.6	0
Spain	2004	0.3	0.5	0.1

(continued on next page)

Table 2
(continued)

| Country | Year | Suicide rate (per 100,000) | | |
		Total	Male	Female
Tajikistan	2001	0.3	0.2	0.3
Armenia	2003	0.2	0.4	0
Azerbaijan	2002	0.2	0.4	0
Greece	2004	0.2	0.4	0
Israel	2003	0.2	0.5	0
Italy	2002	0.2	0.2	0.2
Georgia	2001	0.1	0	0.3
Switzerland	2004	0.1	0.2	0
United Kingdom of Great Britain and Northern Ireland	2004	0.1	0.1	0
Iceland	2004	0	0	0
Luxembourg	2004	0	0	0
Macedonia FYR	2003	0	0	0
Malta	2004	0	0	0
Portugal	2003	0	0	0
Region of the Americas				
Guyana	2003	2.7	2.7	2.7
Ecuador	2004	2.1	2.1	2.2
Trinidad and Tobago	2000	1.2	0.8	1.6
Suriname	2000	1.1	2.1	0
Argentina	2003	0.9	1.1	0.7
Canada	2002	0.9	0.9	0.9
Colombia	1999	0.9	0.8	1.1
El Salvador	2003	0.9	0.4	1.4
Nicaragua	2003	0.9	0.8	0.9
Paraguay	2003	0.9	1.2	0.6
Venezuela	2002	0.9	1.1	0.8
Chile	2003	0.8	1.4	0.3
Mexico	2003	0.7	0.8	0.5
Uruguay	2001	0.7	1.1	0.4
United States	2002	0.6	0.9	0.3
Costa Rica	2004	0.5	0.5	0.5
Cuba	2004	0.5	0.6	0.3
Panama	2003	0.5	0.9	0
Guatemala	2003	0.4	0.4	0.4
Brazil	2002	0.3	0.3	0.3
Puerto Rico	2002	0.2	0	0.3
Peru	2000	0.1	0.1	0.1
Antigua and Barbuda	1995	0	0	0
Bahamas	2000	0	0	0
Barbados	2001	0	0	0
Belize	2001	0	0	0
Dominican Republic	2001	0	0	0
Haiti	2003	0	0	0
Honduras	1970	0	0	0
Jamaica	1990	0	0	0
Saint Kitts and Nevis	1995	0	0	0
Saint Lucia	2002	0	0	0

(continued on next page)

Table 2
(continued)

Country	Year	Suicide rate (per 100,000)		
		Total	Male	Female
Saint Vincent	2003	0	0	0
Southeast Asia region				
Thailand	2002	0.6	0.6	0.5
India[a]	2002	2880	1306	1574
Sri Lanka[a]	1991	83	48	35
Western-Pacific region				
China (mainland, selected rural areas)	1999	1.2	1.3	1.0
China (mainland, selected rural and urban areas)	1999	0.8	0.9	0.8
Singapore	2003	0.8	0.8	0.8
New Zealand	2000	0.7	1.0	0.3
China, Hong Kong SAR	2004	0.6	0.5	0.8
Republic of Korea	2004	0.6	0.6	0.7
Australia	2003	0.5	0.5	0.5
China (mainland, selected urban areas)	1999	0.4	0.5	0.4
Japan	2004	0.4	0.4	0.4
Philippines	1993	0	0	0

[a]Only numbers of suicides available.

the most prominent being affective disorders, which pose a suicide risk very early [22]. Mood disorders and poor social adjustment seem to be among the strongest predictors of suicidal behavior in childhood [39]. Recently, in a study of suicidal youth aged 9 to 16 years, Foley and colleagues [40] reported that current depression plus anxiety created the greatest risk for suicidal ideation/attempt. In the reviewed studies, up to one third of children and young adolescents who committed suicide [4,22] had emotional/affective disorders and more than one half had mixed emotional and antisocial symptoms [4]. Among somewhat older suicides (mean age, 14.6 years), more than 40% had affective disorder [23]. Furthermore, this age group is rarely exposed to other risk factors such as substance abuse, because the prevalence of substance abuse increases with age [4,22,23].

Onset of puberty considerably increases suicide risk, probably because of increasing prevalence of depression and substance abuse [24]. Pubertal status is reported to be a stronger predictor than chronologic age for several psychiatric conditions, including depression [41,42]. Gonadal hormones have direct modulatory effects on the central nervous system (CNS) [41,43,44], and their activating effect on neurotransmitter systems is believed to be associated with the development of internalizing symptoms [41,44–47]. Furthermore, gonadal hormones also have an organizational effect on CNS [41,43,44,48] and alter the structural and functional potential of the brain [41,43,44,48]. Further research is needed to examine how shifts in the function of neuroendocrine axes at puberty modulate brain processes during adolescence [49]. Specifically, several systems should be targeted to elucidate neurobiologic pathways involved in

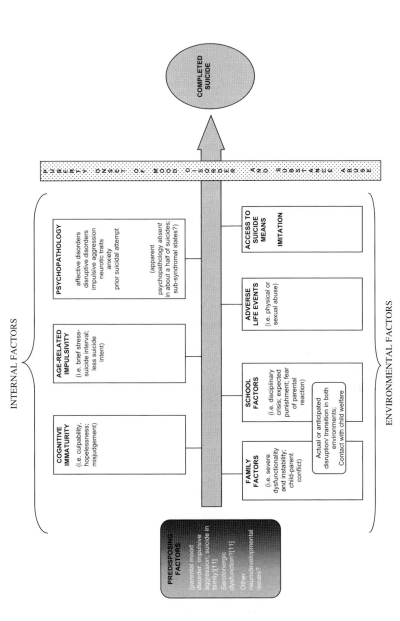

Fig. 1. Risk factors for completed suicide in children and young adolescents aged 14 and under.

onset or development of internalizing of symptoms and reactions to stress during adolescence. For example, investigation of the balance between gonadal hormones and their combined effects on neurotransmitter systems, such as serotonin, and their interaction with hormonal systems, such as the hypothalamic-pituitary-adrenal axis (HPA), would be instructive [41].

A substantial percentage (on average half) of child and adolescent suicides aged 14 years and younger did not have diagnosable psychiatric disorder. No psychiatric symptoms or disorder was found in 13% of suicides in the study by Shaffer [4], 77% in the study by Beautrais [5], and more than 50% in the controlled study Groholt and colleagues [22]. Similarly, in the controlled psychologic autopsy study of suicides aged 15 years and younger, Brent and colleagues [23] found that 40% did not have any detectable psychopathology. In comparison, 90% of youth suicides aged up to 19 years had a psychiatric disorder [24]. These findings deserve attention. In adolescent suicides, those who have no evidence of psychopathology have had disciplinary or legal problems, previous suicidality, family history of psychiatric problems, and particularly greater prevalence of a loaded gun in the home [50].

Furthermore, Brent [50,51] noted that youngsters aged 15 years and younger who had no diagnosable disorders might have had subsyndromal difficulties, excessive stress, and available means. Foley and colleagues [40] noted that suicidal youth aged 16 years and younger who had no diagnosable disorders had subthreshold, most commonly disruptive disorders; disabling relationship difficulties; or psychiatric symptoms with no associated impairment. In this context, distinct developmental differences seem to exist between the psychopathology and suicide risk in children versus other age groups [9]. For example, anxiety or irritability as childhood precursors of depression [11] can be misidentified as temperament traits or age-appropriate behavior. Anxiety states and posttraumatic stress disorder have been neglected and understudied in the context of suicidal behavior in childhood [9]. Furthermore, neuroticism, a personality trait characterized by temperamental tendency to experience a more prolonged and severe range of negative affect in response to stress [11], has been linked with child and adolescent suicidal behavior [11,12,52]. The psychology autopsy method may not be as robust in detecting pediatric psychiatric conditions, especially internalizing conditions, as it is for adult populations.

Developmental Issues

In childhood suicidal behavior, cognitive immaturity and age-related impulsivity have an important role [9]. Suicidal children have poor reality testing, are impulsive, and have problems with emotional and social problem solving [53]. Prepubertal suicidal children were reported to have aberrant cognitive processes [9], particularly hopelessness [54]. Furthermore, Shaffer and colleagues [24] reported that younger adolescents tended to die of suicide under circumstances that suggested they had misjudged the repercussions of a stressful event or crisis. The developmental aspect should not be underestimated, because children were recently shown to have difficulties managing interference from competing distractions, which seem to be related to the immaturity of posterior and anterior cortices [55].

Shaffer [4] reported high intelligence quotient (IQ) in many suicides aged 14 years and younger, and proposed that cognitively precocious youth may be more able than their immature peers to plan and execute lethal suicide attempts. For example, younger children might not have a mastery over suicide means (eg, technical sophistication, careful election of an appropriate and private site) [4], which may protect against suicide. However, this finding was not noted in other studies [9] and also may not apply to impulsive child suicides, which occur without suicide planning and in the context of easy access to suicide means. Suicides in childhood are characterized by a brief stress–suicide interval, less planning, and lower suicide intent [8,11,22]. Rosenthal and Rosenthal [56] reported that among suicidal preschoolers, of whom more than 80% were abused or neglected, greater than one half used methods such as running into fast traffic, jumping from high places, and throwing themselves down stairs.

Neurobehavioral changes triggered by puberty [41,57] may be relevant to suicides in populations aged 14 years and younger. Some neurobehavioral changes, such as drives and emotional changes, occur earlier during puberty [57]. These early changes do not seem to occur synchronously with other maturational processes, such as cognitive development, maturation of self-regulatory capacity, and maturation of judgment. These latter functions are proposed to emerge independently of pubertal processes and continue to evolve long after puberty is complete [57]. Moreover, the ability to integrate the cognitive and affective components of behavior involves neurobiologic systems, which are among the last brain regions to fully mature [57].

Family-Related Factors

Parent–child conflict plays a key role in childhood suicides [12,22,23]. Furthermore, conflicts with parents are more common precipitants and convey higher suicide risk among children and early adolescents compared with older adolescents [22,23]. Children are highly dependent on their caretakers for basic survival [9]. Also, intense family discord is a strong correlate of suicide attempts in prepubertal children [37]. In this context, Sabbath's [58] concept of the *expendable child* highlights children's perceptions of themselves relative to their family context. Children have difficulty differentiating their own actions and feelings from those of their caretakers [9], and negative affects expressed within the family are often internalized by children as feelings of guilt, isolation, and self-destructive fantasies [9], particularly in families with severe instability and tension. Children from these families may be unable to adopt adaptive behavior under family stress and may respond impulsively to family turmoil (eg, suicidal acts) [9]. Moreover, Cohen-Sandler and colleagues [59] suggested that children from abusive homes undertake suicide attempts in an effort to be removed from them. In contrast, because of greater cognitive maturity, adolescents are better able to understand cause and effect relationships of events and their own role in family interactions and problems [9]. Family–child connectedness, parental presence (eg, before school, after school, at bedtime, at dinner), and emotional well-being (eg, feeling loved and wanted) are all protective factors against youth suicidal behavior, even in the presence of increased numbers of risk factors [60,61].

School-Related Factors

Academic failure and fear of parental reaction are common ingredients of an acute suicidal episode in children [9]. Shaffer [4] showed that disciplinary crises had an important role in suicides aged 14 years and younger, whereas in other studies conflicts with parents and family problems outweighed the former [5,22,23]. However, school-related problems (eg, drop-outs, social adjustment, bullying) deserve attention in the context of suicidal behavior in childhood, perhaps particularly regarding suicides who had no apparent psychopathology. Among adolescents, these suicides were associated with disciplinary problems [50], and school drop-outs have an increased risk for suicide attempt [11]. In Shaffer's study [4], many suicides aged 14 years and younger occurred after a period of absence from school. Thompson and colleagues [62] showed that, in a study of potential high school dropouts, the effect of poor school performance on suicidal behavior was mediated by depression, hopelessness, and anxiety. Furthermore, aberrant social adjustment is a hallmark of suicidal children and often an important precipitant [9]. Bullying in school should also not be underestimated for its role in childhood depression and suicidal ideation [63]. Furthermore, disabling relationship difficulties were reported in suicidal children and adolescents who had no diagnosable disorder [40]. Moreover, the case-controlled psychologic autopsy study from Brent and colleagues [50] showed excessive stress to be associated with suicides aged 15 years and younger who had no diagnosable disorder. In this context, perceived connectedness to school (eg, students' perception that teachers care about them, sense of belonging) and academic achievement, measured as grade point average, were reported to be protective against risk for suicidal behavior [61], as was having a nurse or clinic in school, although only for girls [60].

Child Welfare Clients

Between one fifth and one fourth [4,5] of suicides in individuals aged 14 years and younger had contact with welfare institutions, highlighting the complex psychosocial situations in these children. Child welfare/protection clients represent a high-risk group for suicide attempts and severe psychiatric morbidity [64]. Boys in the child welfare system tend to be at higher risk for psychiatric hospitalizations during adolescence (13–17 years of age) compared with girls [64]. Suicidal behavior is linked to several negative influences, and children who become child welfare clients before their teenage years seem to encounter many of them (eg, social disadvantage, family violence, abuse or neglect, parental psychiatric disorder, family disintegration/instability, serious school problems) [64]. Moreover, these risk factors tend to appear in clusters [65]. In this context, older adolescents with "drifting" status (ie, disconnected from major support systems, such as school, family, and work) seem to be at very high risk for suicide [11,26].

Adverse Life-Events

A strong relationship exists between physical and sexual abuse and child suicidal behavior [9,11,66]. The study by Brent and colleagues [23] found that lifetime history of abuse was significantly higher in suicides aged 15 years and younger compared with controls. Early childhood abuse and neglect seem to contribute to the familial transmission of suicidal behavior through compounding genetic vulnerability [67]. Furthermore, a dysregulation of the serotonin system is reported for abused and neglected children [68], which also seems to be related to familial and experiential factors [69]. In a study of young boys [70], the density of 5-HT2A receptors on platelets was inversely related to harsh parenting and frequent parental physical punishment. Furthermore, altered response to fenfluramine challenge was reported for young boys who had aggressive behavior and social circumstances that were conductive to the development of aggressive behavior [71]. More recently, Manuck and colleagues [72] showed that growing up in a socially and economically disadvantaged neighborhood is associated with similar types of changes in serotonin function. Animal studies on rearing show similar findings [73,74]. Moreover, empiric research suggests that early and chronic life events (eg, moves, deaths, losses), particularly within the family context, are associated with prepubertal suicidal behavior and increase risk for future suicidal behavior [39].

Biological Factors

Biological data on suicide in children and early adolescents are scarce. Pfeffer and colleagues [75] reported distinct peripheral serotonin profiles in prepubertal suicide attempters; average tryptophan content in blood was significantly lower in prepubertal psychiatric patients who had recent suicide attempts compared with normal or psychiatric inpatient children who had suicidal ideation. Furthermore, an association was reported between suicidal behavior and plasma cortisol levels in prepubertal children independent of diagnosis [76]. A key risk factor for suicide, aggression is associated with low CSF-5-HIAA in pubertal but not prepubertal boys [77]. In adults, findings from postmortem brain studies suggest that serotonergic abnormalities may be stable trait markers for suicidal behavior, whereas noradrenergic and HPA-axis dysregulation may be partly state-dependent [78,79]. Moreover, spring and autumn suicide peaks have been reported among individuals aged 14 years and younger [16]. In this context, seasonal serotonin changes (ie, platelet [3H]imipramine binding density) in adolescent suicide attempters were reported to reach nadir in late winter/early spring [80]. Adoption, twin, and family studies of suicide and suicidal behavior suggest that suicidal behavior is also highly familial and heritable [81]. Further research on the genetics and neurobiology of early onset suicidal behavior and their interaction with adverse life events (ie, abuse), and neuroimaging studies that provide an opportunity to examine correlates of poor problem solving, emotional reactivity, and impulsivity are needed [11].

Hormonal factors also warrant investigation, given that suicidal behavior increases after puberty [31]. Neuroendocrine changes during puberty seem to be associated with changes in brain organization and cognitive function and with cerebral metabolism [82].

Availability of Suicide Means

Availability of suicide means seems to be the most important factor for impulsive youth suicide attempts [83], particularly given that suicide in individuals aged 14 years and younger is characterized by brief stress–suicide intervals [22] and the availability of suicide means has an important facilitating role in youth suicides [34]. Restricting access to suicide means, including providing means-restriction counseling for parents [11], is an important suicide prevention strategy [26].

Imitation

The role of imitation in suicidal behavior must be considered in vulnerable children and adolescents [11,84,85]. In vulnerable teenagers, suicide can be facilitated through exposure to real or fictional accounts of suicide, including media coverage of suicide [84], and accumulating evidence supports the existence of suicide contagion [86]. The phenomenon of suicide clusters—suicides occurring in close temporal and geographic proximity that often involve previously disturbed young people—is believed to be related to imitation [26,87]. No reports of this exist for children, because suicide clusters occur primarily among teenagers and young adults, and only sporadically beyond 24 years of age [86]. Imitation can also be method-specific [88]. Moreover, among other factors such as availability of means, in the investigation of regional risk factors for suicide [35] (ie, higher child and young adolescent suicide rates in geographic areas with high suicide rates in general population [16]), the possible role of imitation should not be neglected.

SUMMARY

Completed suicide in childhood is associated with an extensive personal and social morbidity [9]. An interplay of psychiatric factors (ie, depression), behavioral components (ie, impulsivity), cognitive immaturity, and environmental–contextual factors (ie, family problems) seems to have an important role in suicides among the youngest population [3,7,23]. Public psychoeducation [89], psychoeducation of gate-keepers [26], and additional training for pediatricians and general practitioners [16,33] regarding childhood suicidal behavior (eg, warning signs, risk factors, referral options) are crucial. The most efficient preventive strategy is early recognition of suicidality, with timely referral to specialized institutions [90]. Pfeffer and colleagues [91] proposed considering three main factors in screening for early-onset suicidal behavior: anxious–impulsive depression, suicidal ideation and acts, and family distress (discord/pathology). However, the lower rate of psychopathology in childhood suicides suggests that screening might be of restricted use, underscoring the importance of restricting suicide means as one of the most efficient suicide prevention strategies in childhood [23,92], and the need to investigate and augment protective factors against suicide in children. Therefore, investigation of protective factors, such as positive parent–child relationship, active parental supervision, positive school–child connectedness, reasons for living, and religious and cultural beliefs [11,61,93–95], should also be advanced. Research data on this topic, particularly those considering developmental distinctions [9], are scarce. Controlled psychologic autopsy studies are needed to investigate the specific psychosocial features of completed suicide in children. Furthermore, developmental neurobiologic and neuroimaging studies might clarify substrates of suicide in this age group.

References

[1] King RA, Apter A, editors. Suicide in children and adolescents. Cambridge (UK): Cambridge University Press; 2003. p. xiii–xiv.
[2] Centers for Disease Control and Prevention (CDC) (2004). Available at: http://webappa. cdc.gov/sasweb/ncipc/mortrate10_sy.html. Accessed September 5, 2007.
[3] Pfeffer CR. Childhood suicidal behavior. A developmental perspective. Psychiatr Clin North Am 1997;20(3):551–62.
[4] Shaffer D. Suicide in childhood and early adolescence. J Child Psychol Psychiatry 1974;15(4):275–91.
[5] Beautrais AL. Child and young adolescent suicide in New Zealand. Aust N Z J Psychiatry 2001;35(5):647–53.
[6] Potter LB, Rosenberg ML, Hammond WR. Suicide in youth: a public health framework. J Am Acad Child Adolesc Psychiatry 1998;37(5):484–7.
[7] Pfeffer CR, Conte HR, Plutchnik R, et al. Suicidal behavior in latency- age children: an empirical study. J Am Acad Child Adolesc Psychiatry 1979;18(4):679–92.
[8] Shaffer D. The epidemiology of teen suicide: an examination of risk factors. J Clin Psychiatry 1988;49(Suppl):36–41.
[9] Pfeffer CR. Assessing suicidal behavior in children and adolescents. In: King RA, Apter A, editors. Suicide in children and adolescents. Cambridge (UK): Cambridge University Press; 2003. p. 211–26.
[10] Pfeffer CR. Suicidal behavior in children: an emphasis on developmental influences. In: Hawton K, van Heeringen K, editors. Suicide and attempted suicide. Baffins Lane, Chichester (England): John Wiley & Sons Ltd.; 2000. p. 237–48.
[11] Bridge JA, Goldstein TR, Brent DA. Adolescent suicide and suicidal behavior. J Child Psychol Psychiatry 2006;47(3–4):372–94.
[12] Hoberman HM, Garfinkel BD. Completed suicide in children and adolescents. J Am Acad Child Adolesc Psychiatry 1988;27(6):689–95.
[13] Thompson T. Childhood and adolescent suicide in Manitoba: a demographic study. Can J Psychiatry 1987;32:264–9.
[14] McClure GM. Suicide in children and adolescents in England and Wales 1970–1998. Br J Psychiatry 2001;178:469–74.
[15] Dudley M, Waters B, Kelk N, et al. Youth suicide in New South Wales: urban-rural trends. Med J Aust 1992;156(2):83–8.
[16] Dervic K, Friedrich E, Oquendo MA, et al. Suicide in Austrian children and young adolescents aged 14 and younger. Eur Child Adolesc Psychiatry 2006;15:427–34.
[17] Pritchard C, Hansen L. Child, adolescent and youth suicide and undetermined deaths in England and Wales compared with Australia, Canada, France, Germany, Italy, Japan and the USA for the 1974–1999 period. Int J Adolesc Med Health 2005;17(3):239–53.
[18] Töero K, Nagy A, Sawaguchi T, et al. Characteristics of suicide among children and adolescents in Budapest. Pediatr Int 2001;43(4):368–71.

[19] Goren S, Gurkan F, Tirasci Y, et al. Suicide in children and adolescents at a province in Turkey. Am J Forensic Med Pathol 2003;24(2):214–7.

[20] Agritmis H, Yayci N, Colak B, et al. Suicidal deaths in childhood and adolescence. Forensic Sci Int 2004;142(1):25–31.

[21] Arslan M, Akcan R, Hilal A, et al. Suicide among children and adolescents: data from Cukurova, Turkey. Child Psychiatry Hum Dev 2007;38(4):271–7.

[22] Groholt B, Ekeberg O, Wichstrom L, et al. Suicide among children and younger and older adolescents in Norway: a comparative study. J Am Acad Child Adolesc Psychiatry 1998;37(5):473–81.

[23] Brent DA, Baugher M, Bridge J, et al. Age- and sex-related risk factors for adolescent suicide. J Am Acad Child Adolesc Psychiatry 1999;38(12):1497–505.

[24] Shaffer D, Gould M, Fisher P, et al. Psychiatric diagnosis in child and adolescent suicide. Arch Gen Psychiatry 1996;53:339–48.

[25] Marttunen MJ, Aro HM, Henriksson MM, et al. Mental disorders in adolescent suicide. DSM-III-R axes I and II diagnoses in suicides among 13- to 19-year-olds in Finland. Arch Gen Psychiatry 1991;48(9):834–9.

[26] Gould MS, Kramer RA. Youth suicide prevention. Suicide Life Threat Behav 2001; 31(Suppl):6–31.

[27] World Health Organization (WHO). Available at: http://www.who.int/mental_health/ prevention/suicide/country_reports/en/index.html. Accessed September 5, 2007.

[28] Gould MS, Shaffer D, Greenberg T. The epidemiology of youth suicide. In: King RA, Apter A, editors. Suicide in children and adolescents. Cambridge (UK): Cambridge University Press; 2003. p. 1–40.

[29] Centers for Disease Control and Prevention (CDC). Methods of suicide among persons aged 10–19 years—United States, 1992–2001. MMWR Morb Mortal Wkly Rep 2004;53(22): 471–4.

[30] Kreitman N. The coal gas story. United Kingdom suicide rates, 1960–1971. Br J Prev Soc Med 1976;30(2):86–93.

[31] Groholt B, Ekeberg O. Suicide in young people under 15 years: problems of classification. Nord J Psychiatry 2003;57(6):411–7.

[32] Dervic K, Oquendo MA, Grunebaum MF, et al. Religious affiliation and suicide attempt. Am J Psychiatry 2004;161:2303–8.

[33] Dervic K, Friedrich E, Prosquill D, et al. Suicide among Viennese minors, 1946–2002. Wien Klin Wochenschr 2006;118:152–9.

[34] Kelleher MJ, Chambers D. Cross cultural variation in child and adolescent suicide. In: King RA, Apter A, editors. Suicide in children and adolescents. Cambridge (UK): Cambridge University Press; 2003. p. 170–97.

[35] Dervic K, Gould MS, Lenz G, et al. Youth suicide risk factors and attitudes in New York and Vienna: a cross-cultural comparison. Suicide Life Threat Behav 2006;36:539–52.

[36] Sonneck G. Krisenintervention und Suizidverhuetung. Wien (Austria): Facultas Universitaetsverlag; 2000.

[37] Pfeffer CR, Normandin L, Kakuma T. Suicidal children grow up: suicidal behavior and psychiatric disorders among relatives. J Am Acad Child Adolesc Psychiatry 1994;33(8): 1087–97.

[38] Brent DA, Oquendo M, Birmaher B, et al. Peripubertal suicide attempts in offspring of suicide attempters with siblings concordant for suicidal behavior. Am J Psychiatry 2003;160(8):1486–93.

[39] Pfeffer CR, Klerman GL, Hurt SW, et al. Suicidal children grow up: rates and psychosocial risk factors for suicide attempts during follow-up. J Am Acad Child Adolesc Psychiatry 1993;32(1):106–13.

[40] Foley DL, Goldston DB, Costello EJ, et al. Proximal psychiatric risk factors for suicidality in youth: the great smoky mountains study. Arch Gen Psychiatry 2006;63(9):1017–24.

[41] Hayward C, Sanborn K. Puberty and the emergence of gender differences in psychopathology. J Adolesc Health 2002;30(Suppl 4):49–58.

[42] Angold A, Costello EJ, Erkanli A, et al. Pubertal changes in hormone levels and depression in girls. Psychol Med 1999;29:1043–53.

[43] Sisk CL, Foster DL. The neural basis of puberty and adolescence. Nat Neurosci 2004;7: 1040–7.

[44] Romeo RD. Puberty: a period of both organizational and activational effects of steroid hormones on neurobehavioural development. J Neuroendocrinol 2003;15:1185–92.

[45] Rubinow DR, Schmidt PJ. Androgens, brain, and behavior. Am J Psychiatry 1996;153: 974–84.

[46] Attali G, Weizman A, Gil-Ad I, et al. Opposite modulatory effects of ovarian hormones on rat brain dopamine and serotonin transporters. Brain Res 1997;756:153–9.

[47] Halbreich U, Lumley LA. The multiple interactional biological processes that might lead to depression and gender differences in its appearance. J Affect Disord 1993;29:159–73.

[48] Sisk CL, Zehr JL. Pubertal hormones organize the adolescent brain and behavior. Front Neuroendocrinol 2005;26:163–74.

[49] Cameron JL. Interrelationships between hormones, behavior, and affect during adolescence: complex relationships exist between reproductive hormones, stress-related hormones, and the activity of neural systems that regulate behavioral affect. Comments on part III. Ann N Y Acad Sci 2004;1021:134–42.

[50] Brent DA, Perper J, Moritz G, et al. Suicide in adolescents with no apparent psychopathology. J Am Acad Child Adolesc Psychiatry 1993;32(3):494–500.

[51] Brent DA. Risk factors for adolescent suicide and suicidal behavior: mental and substance abuse disorders, family environmental factors, and life stress. Suicide Life Threat Behav 1995;25(Suppl):52–63.

[52] Beautrais AL, Joyce PR, Mulder RT. Personality traits and cognitive styles as risk factors for serious suicide attempts among young people. Suicide Life Threat Behav 1999;29(1): 37–47.

[53] Pfeffer CR, Hurt SW, Peskin JR, et al. Suicidal children grow up: ego functions associated with suicide attempts. J Am Acad Child Adolesc Psychiatry 1995;34(10):1318–25.

[54] Kazdin AE, French NH, Unis AS, et al. Hopelessness, depression, and suicidal intent among psychiatrically disturbed inpatient children. J Consult Clin Psychol 1983;51(4):504–10.

[55] Durston S, Casey BJ. What have we learned about cognitive development from neuroimaging? Neuropsychologia 2006;44(11):2149–57.

[56] Rosenthal PA, Rosenthal S. Suicidal behavior by preschool children. Am J Psychiatry 1984;141(4):520–5.

[57] Dahl RE. Adolescent brain development: a period of vulnerabilities and opportunities. Keynote address. Ann N Y Acad Sci 2004;1021:1–22.

[58] Sabbath JC. The suicidal adolescent—the expendable child. J Am Acad Child Psychiatry 1969;8:272–89.

[59] Cohen-Sandler R, Berman AL, King RA. A follow-up study of hospitalized suicidal children. J Am Acad Child Psychiatry 1982;21(4):398–403.

[60] Borowsky IW, Resnick MD, Ireland M, et al. Suicide attempts among American Indian and Alaska native youth: risk and protective factors. Arch Pediatr Adolesc Med 1999;153(6): 573–80.

[61] Borowsky IW, Ireland M, Resnick MD. Adolescent suicide attempts: risks and protectors. Pediatrics 2001;107(3):485–93.

[62] Thompson EA, Mazza JJ, Herting JR, et al. The mediating roles of anxiety depression, and hopelessness on adolescent suicidal behaviors. Suicide Life Threat Behav 2005;35: 14–34.

[63] van der Wal MF, de Wit CA, Hirasing RA. Psychosocial health among young victims and offenders of direct and indirect bullying. Pediatrics 2003;111:1312–7.

[64] Vinnerljung B, Hjern A, Lindblad F. Suicide attempts and severe psychiatric morbidity among former child welfare clients—a national cohort study. J Child Psychol Psychiatry 2006;47(7):723–33.

[65] Rutter M, Dunn J, Plomin R, et al. Integrating nature and nurture: implications of person-environment correlations and interactions for developmental psychopathology. Dev Psychopathol 1997;9(2):335–64.

[66] Pfeffer CR, Trad PV. Sadness and suicidal tendencies in preschool children. J Dev Behav Pediatr 1988;9(2):86–8.

[67] Brent DA, Mann JJ. Familial pathways to suicidal behavior—understanding and preventing suicide among adolescents. N Engl J Med 2006;355(26):2719–21.

[68] Mann JJ. Neurobiology of suicidal behaviour. Nat Rev Neurosci 2003;4(10):819–28.

[69] Kaufman J, Birmaher B, Perel J, et al. Serotonergic functioning in depressed abused children: clinical and familial correlates. Biol Psychiatry 1998;44(10):973–81.

[70] Pine DS, Wasserman GA, Coplan J, et al. Platelet serotonin 2A (5-HT2A) receptor characteristics and parenting factors for boys at risk for delinquency: a preliminary report. Am J Psychiatry 1996;153(4):538–44.

[71] Pine DS, Coplan JD, Wasserman GA, et al. Neuroendocrine response to fenfluramine challenge in boys. Associations with aggressive behavior and adverse rearing. Arch Gen Psychiatry 1997;54:839–46.

[72] Manuck SB, Bleil ME, Petersen KL, et al. The socio-economic status of communities predicts variation in brain serotonergic responsivity. Psychol Med 2005;35:519–28.

[73] Higley JD, Linnoila M. Low central nervous system serotonergic activity is traitlike and correlates with impulsive behavior. A nonhuman primate model investigating genetic and environmental influences on neurotransmission. Ann N Y Acad Sci 1997;836:39–56.

[74] Barr CS, Newman TK, Shannon C, et al. Rearing condition and rh5-HTTLPR interact to influence limbic-hypothalamic-pituitary-adrenal axis response to stress in infant macaques. Biol Psychiatry 2004;55:733–8.

[75] Pfeffer CR, McBride PA, Anderson GM, et al. Peripheral serotonin measures in prepubertal psychiatric inpatients and normal children: associations with suicidal behavior and its risk factors. Biol Psychiatry 1998;44(7):568–77.

[76] Pfeffer CR, Stokes P, Shindledecker R. Suicidal behavior and hypothalamic-pituitary-adrenocortical axis indices in child psychiatric inpatients. Biol Psychiatry 1991;29(9):909–17.

[77] Kruesi MJ, Rapoport JL, Hamburger S, et al. Cerebrospinal fluid monoamine metabolites, aggression, and impulsivity in disruptive behavior disorders of children and adolescents. Arch Gen Psychiatry 1990;47(5):419–26.

[78] Mann JJ, Arango V. Abnormalities of brain structure and function in mood disorders. In: Charney DS, Nestler EJ, Bunney BS, editors. The Neurobiology of mental illness. New York: Oxford University Press; 1999. p. 385–93.

[79] Pfeffer CR. Diagnosis of childhood and adolescent suicidal behavior: unmet needs for suicide prevention. Biol Psychiatry 2001;49(12):1055–61.

[80] Pine DS, Trautman PD, Shaffer D, et al. Seasonal rhythm of platelet [3H]imipramine binding in adolescents who attempted suicide. Am J Psychiatry 1995;152(6):923–5.

[81] Brent DA, Mann JJ. Family genetic studies, suicide, and suicidal behavior. Am J Med Genet C Semin Med Genet 2005;133(1):13–24.

[82] Yurgelun-Todd D. Emotional and cognitive changes during adolescence. Curr Opin Neurobiol 2007;17(2):251–7.

[83] Brent DA, Perper JA, Goldstein CE, et al. Risk factors for adolescent suicide. A comparison of adolescent suicide victims with suicidal inpatients. Arch Gen Psychiatry 1988;45(6):581–8.

[84] Gould MS. Suicide and the media. Ann N Y Acad Sci 2001;932:200–21.

[85] Gould MS, Shaffer D. The impact of suicide in television movies. Evidence of imitation. N Engl J Med 1986;315(11):690–4.

[86] Gould MS, Greenberg T, Velting DM, et al. Youth suicide risk and preventive interventions: a review of the past 10 years. J Am Acad Child Adolesc Psychiatry 2003;42:386–405.
[87] Velting DM, Gould MS. Suicide contagion. In: Maris R, Canetto S, Silverman MM, editors. Annual review of suicidology. New York: Guilford; 1997. p. 96–136.
[88] Schmidtke A, Schaller S. Role of mass media in suicide prevention. In: Hawton K, van Heeringen K, editors. Suicide and attempted suicide. Baffins Lane, Chichester (England): John Wiley & Sons Ltd.; 2000. p. 675–98.
[89] Mann JJ, Apter A, Bertolote J, et al. Suicide prevention strategies: a systematic review. JAMA 2005;294:2064–74.
[90] Shaffer D, Craft L. Methods of adolescent suicide prevention. J Clin Psychiatry 1999;60(Suppl 2):70–4.
[91] Pfeffer CR, Jiang H, Kakuma T. Child-adolescent suicidal potential index (CASPI): a screen for risk for early onset suicidal behavior. Psychol Assess 2000;12(3):304–18.
[92] Christoffel KK, Marcus D, Sagerman S, et al. Adolescent suicide and suicide attempts: a population study. Pediatr Emerg Care 1988;4(1):32–40.
[93] Resnick MD, Bearman PS, Blum RW, et al. Protecting adolescents from harm. Findings from the national longitudinal study on adolescent health. JAMA 1997;278(10):823–32.
[94] Osman A, Downs WR, Kopper BA, et al. The reasons for living inventory for adolescents (RFL-A): development and psychometric properties. J Clin Psychol 1998;54:1063–78.
[95] Gutierrez P. 2005 Shneidman award address. Integratively assessing risk and protective factors for adolescent suicide. Suicide Life Threat Behav 2006;36:129–35.

Psychiatr Clin N Am 31 (2008) 293–316

PSYCHIATRIC CLINICS
OF NORTH AMERICA

Impact of Modeling on Adolescent Suicidal Behavior

Beverly J. Insel, DrPH[a,b], Madelyn S. Gould, PhD, MPH[a,b,c,*]

[a]Columbia University, Division of Child & Adolescent Psychiatry (College of Physicians and Surgeons), New York, NY, USA
[b]New York State Psychiatric Institute, New York, NY, USA
[c]Columbia University, Department of Epidemiology (School of Public Health), New York, NY, USA

A dolescent suicide persists as a significant health problem in the United States; it is the third leading cause of death among adolescents. While individual risk factors, such as depression, anxiety, and substance abuse, have long been shown to exert a significant role in the etiology of suicide, mounting evidence supports the role of imitation and modeling in suicide. The importance of modeling on suicide behavior has been suggested by three areas of research: (1) clusters or "outbreaks" of suicide defined by temporal-spatial proximity, (2) personal exposure to the suicidal behavior of adolescent peers, and (3) media influence on subsequent suicide related behavior. A critical review of these three sources of evidence as they relate to adolescents is presented. To identify recently published studies to update our earlier reviews [1,2], we searched the English literature using MEDLINE and PsycINFO database from January 1995 (exclusive of studies discussed in the past reviews); key words included suicide, cluster, modeling, contagion, and imitation. In addition, published and in-press chapters brought to our attention are in the review. While our aim is to evaluate the impact of modeling on adolescent suicide, studies containing all age groups were included when there were a limited number of studies exclusively devoted to adolescents (eg, media).

TERMINOLOGY

A succinct review of nomenclature is presented to facilitate an understanding of information presented since the terms "clusters," "contagion," and "imitation" are often used indiscriminately in the literature [3]. A suicide "cluster" refers to an excessive number of suicides occurring in close temporal and/or geographic proximity. Suicide "contagion" is the process by which one suicide facilitates the occurrence of a subsequent suicide. Contagion assumes either direct

*Corresponding author. Division of Child & Adolescent Psychiatry, New York State Psychiatric Institute, 1051 Riverside Drive, Unit 72, New York, NY 10032, USA. *E-mail address:* gouldm@childpsych.columbia.edu (M.S. Gould).

0193-953X/08/$ – see front matter
doi:10.1016/j.psc.2008.01.007

awareness through contact or friendship with the suicide victim, word of mouth knowledge, or indirect transmission through the media. The underlying theory to explain the contagion phenomenon is "imitation," the process by which one suicide becomes an influential model for successive suicides.

SOCIAL LEARNING AND NEUROBIOLOGY

Two diverse paradigms, social learning theory and neurobiological approaches, may facilitate an understanding of suicide modeling phenomena. In social learning theory, behavioral scientists have constructed a basis on which aspects of the suicide contagion process can be understood. According to this theory, most human behavior is learned observationally through modeling [4]. Exposure to a behavior is necessary for imitation to occur, whether it occurs by direct contact with an affected person in one's social group or by indirect contact through the media. Imitative learning is influenced by a number of factors, including the characteristics of the model and the consequences or rewards associated with the observed act. Specifically, models who possess engaging qualities or have high status are more likely to be imitated. Similarly, behaviors that are portrayed as resulting in gains, including notoriety, are more effective in prompting imitation. The likelihood of imitative behavior is augmented if the observer can identify with the model via shared characteristics or similar past experiences [4,5]. Moreover, the occurrence of suicides within a community or exposure to suicides in the media may foster familiarity and acceptance of the idea of suicide as a natural or normative phenomenon instead of a pathologic, rare event [6]. Thus, social learning theory describes the social processes and context that may underlie the development of suicide contagion.

The neurobiological paradigm may clarify the greater susceptibility to suicide imitation among adolescents and young adults than among other age groups. For example, the incidence of cluster suicides is higher among this population than among any other age group [7]. Cognitive or executive inhibitory control of behavior comprises the ability to inhibit inappropriate or impulsive behaviors and to interrupt or modify unacceptable behaviors [8]. These complex cognitive functions continue to develop throughout adolescence [9] as evidenced by their poorer performance on tasks of cognitive inhibitory control compared with adults [10]. This provides compelling grounds for the hypothesis that the lack of fully mature response inhibitory networks can predispose adolescents and young adults to imitative suicidal behavior compared with older age groups. This hypothesis is supported by several areas of research; functional magnetic resonance imaging studies showing that the ventrolateral prefrontal cortex involved in response inhibition continues to mature throughout adolescence and behavioral measures of task performance demonstrating that inhibitory control improves throughout normal maturation [11].

CLUSTER SUICIDES

Suicide cluster phenomena have been recognized among civilized cultures since history has been recorded [12,13]. Early research provided only descriptive accounts of suicide "epidemics" that relied heavily on anecdotal accounts of suicide behavior, usually case history methodology (see Reference [14]). Collectively, these studies reinforced the concept that exposure to another individual's suicide, assuming temporal, geographic, and/or interpersonal proximity, could at least in some individuals, precipitate imitative suicidal behavior. Nevertheless, the interpretability of the findings of the earlier studies has been seriously hampered because of their frequent lack of a comparison group and increased presence of selection bias. During the past 2 decades, research in cluster suicide has shifted methodologically and qualitatively from descriptive to inferential studies, reflective of the development and application of statistical techniques such as the Scan statistic, the Knox procedure, and Poisson distribution modeling [3,15] to detect statistically significant clustering effects. These techniques employ, most typically, discrete time intervals to define a unit of frequency of suicide within a finite assessment period, geographic boundaries to delimit spatial variables, and comparison of observed and expected frequencies.

Before we discuss the updated literature, a synopsis of prior review findings on cluster suicides is presented. First, past studies indicated that cluster suicide is predominantly a phenomenon of adolescents and young adults [7,16,17]. Specifically, Gould and colleagues [7] found that the relative risk of suicide following exposure to a suicide was two to four times higher among 15- to 19-year-olds than among other age groups. Second, there appeared to be no significant difference in gender distributions of cluster suicides and noncluster suicides [18]. Third, cluster suicides occurred in variety of populations, including community samples and selected samples, such as incarcerated individuals and psychiatric inpatients [1]. To summarize, the earlier literature showed that there is sufficient evidence to support the existence of suicide clusters but they are rare events, mainly a phenomenon of the young, and do not account for the preponderance of suicides (constituting 1% to 5% of youth suicides).

To identify recently published studies, we used the previously described database and key words, as well as the following a priori inclusion criteria. We included studies that contained adolescents and young adults among the sample population rather than relying on studies that had exclusively adolescent samples because only a few adolescent studies existed. Moreover, although statistical techniques have been implemented to standardize the identification of suicide cluster, studies continue to provide only a descriptive analysis of suicide clusters. Thus, studies were eligible if they were descriptive in nature or used standard statistical techniques to detect clustering. We identified eight studies of cluster suicides: three descriptive in nature and five employing accepted inferential statistical methods for clustering (Table 1).

The three descriptive studies of suicide clusters occurred in diverse adolescent settings and populations: a United States adolescent inpatient psychiatric ward [19], a Swedish population-based community [20], and a Canadian indigenous population [21]. Two of the three descriptive studies suggested the occurrence of actual suicide clustering [20,21]. Johansson and colleagues [20]

Table 1
Recent studies of epidemic or cluster suicide[a]

Citation	Population/period	Source of study/method	Support of time-space clustering
Descriptive studies			
King et al [19]	USA. Date not published	57 adolescents admitted to an acute psychiatric inpatient unit were assessed for suicidality.	No
Johansson et al [20]	Sweden, 1981–2000	88 adolescent suicides autopsied at the Department of Forensic Medicine.	Yes
Wilkie et al [21]	Canada, 1995–1995	6 suicides and 19 suicide attempts (12–25 years old) among Manitoba community.	Yes
Inferential studies			
Hourani et al [22]	US Navy, 1990–1995	362 (44% aged 15–24) Navy personnel suicides. The Knox technique tested the significance of time-space clustering.	Yes
McKenzie & Keane [23]	England and Wales, 1993–2002	Data included young offender institutions for prisoners younger than 18. Used Knox procedure for time-space clustering.	Yes
Silviken, et al [24]	Norway, 1970–1998	89 (30% aged 15–24, 27% aged 25–34) indigenous Sami suicides in Arctic Norway. Assumed a Poisson distribution for incidence rates.	Yes
Hourani et al [25]	US Marine Corps, 1990–1996	213 (67% ≤ 24 years) Marine Corps suicides. Scan statistic tested for evidence of time clustering and Knox procedure for time-space clustering, assumed a Poisson distribution.	Yes for time No for time-space
Wissow, et al [26]	Southwest US, 1990–1995	23 suicides and 22 serious attempts among reservation residents (aged 13–28). Assumed a Poisson distribution. Scan statistic examined time-clustering.	Marginal
Exeter & Boyle [27]	Scotland, for 3 periods; 1980–1982, 1990–1992, and 1999–2001	Residences of suicides (15–44 years) were aggregated into 10,058 small geographic zones. Spatial scan statistic tested for geographic clustering.	No

[a] Not included in Velting and Gould 1997 [1].

identified two clusters of adolescent suicide completers that occurred within a well-defined geographic area and temporal period. Additionally, the adolescents knew one another and employed similar suicide methods. A study conducted in a selected sample of residents of an isolated northern Manitoba First Nations community [21] also provided suggestion of clustering of suicide attempters and completers that occurred within a period of 3 months. Gender differences were observed: 4 of the 6 suicide completers were males and 11 of the 19 suicide attempters were females. However, King and associates [19] found that suicidal behavior of adolescent inpatients did not cluster in time, although the adolescents experienced a significant increase in suicidal ideation during their inpatient psychiatric stay. The lack of clustering of suicidal behavior among psychiatric inpatients may reflect a true phenomenon or the inability to distinguish a real cluster from the baseline suicidal "noise" in the setting.

Of the six inferential statistical studies (see Table 1), three clearly provided evidence of time-space clustering [22–24]. A fourth study indicated time clustering only [25] and a fifth study offered marginal evidence of time-space clustering [26]. The remaining investigation [27] identified a significant spatial cluster of suicides in Glasgow for three periods, but attributed the clustering to socioeconomic deprivation.

The environmental context of the suicide can encourage clustering. For instance, a small community may be particularly susceptible to suicide clustering since knowledge of a suicide can spread quickly when more people know one another. Two studies observed suicide clusters in military units [22,25] and one study detected clustering in a prison environment [23]. Two other studies identified possible suicide clustering in isolated indigenous populations: indigenous Sami in Arctic Norway [24] and Native Americans in the southwest United States [26]. Another study detected clustering in a prison sample, which included young offender institutions for prisoners younger than 18 as part of the sample [23].

The body of research strongly suggests that suicide clustering is a true phenomenon among young people. The paucity of studies that examine the occurrence of a suicide cluster may reflect the rarity of the event. Unfortunately, the limited number of studies hinders the identification of patterns, such as gender differential effects. Nevertheless, a recent finding suggests that young males may be more at risk for clustering of completed suicides, while young females may be more at risk for clustering of suicide attempts, which is consistent with the general epidemiology of suicide that shows while more females attempt suicide, more males complete the act. Observed differences between specific study findings may be a function of their sample characteristics, such as gender, age, and source of population, among others. Moreover, varying statistical methodologies can contribute to these differences since variation in temporal and spatial parameters used in statistical tests can influence the significance of the statistical results of suicide clustering. To date, the mechanisms underlying cluster suicides have not been unequivocally identified.

MEDIA INFLUENCES

Whereas research on cluster suicides underscores the plausibility of direct modes (eg, person-to-person) of transmission of suicide clustering, studies investigating the media influences on subsequent suicide examine the indirect pathways of transfer. Past research on media-related suicides has generally been classified into two lines of inquiry: (1) studies examining the effects of nonfictional descriptions of suicides (eg, newspapers, television news reports) and (2) studies evaluating the influences of fictional portrayals of suicides (eg, soap operas, televised dramatizations, movies). Most of the past research examining the imitative effects of media suicide accounts has been largely supportive of a contagion hypothesis [1,2,28]. In our current review, we did not impose an age exclusion criteria on the literature since studies that examine the effect of media coverage on suicide did not exclusively focus on adolescents.

Modeling From Nonfictional Suicide Stories

The association between exposure to media coverage of real-life suicides and subsequent self-injurious behavior has been investigated for over 3 decades. Recent research examining the effects of nonfictional suicide stories remains largely supportive of the modeling hypothesis. Of the eight original studies reviewed in this section [29–36] (Table 2 for a summary of these studies), six of the studies indicated substantial imitative effects [29–34]. Etzersdorfer and colleagues [29] showed that the magnitude of the increase following a suicide story was proportional to the amount, duration, and prominence of media coverage. Specifically, they observed a "dose-response" association between the regional distribution of newspapers' coverage of celebrity suicide by firearms in Austria and an increase in firearm suicides. Imitative effects attributable to media coverage of suicide transcend national boundaries and cultural distinction. Recent studies that support the influence of nonfictional suicide accounts come from a range of Western countries [29–33] and locales as diverse as Hong Kong [34] and Israel [35].

While most studies investigating nonfictional suicide stories have tested the hypothesis that suicide rates *increase* following exposure to media reports, another methodological strategy is to examine whether a *decrease* in suicide rates occurred following implementation of media guidelines for news reporting. This strategy tests one of Hill's casual criteria [57], referred to as cessation (experiment or evidence of recovery), in which diminishment of an exposure should reduce an adverse outcome. Niederkrotenthaler and Sonneck [30] employed this strategy to test the impact of the Austrian media guidelines introduced in 1987 on the annual suicide numbers and the numbers of Viennese subway suicides. They found a significant overall reduction of suicides. The substantial suicide decline occurred in areas having the highest coverage rates of newspapers. Moreover, the data revealed a sharp decrease of Viennese subway suicides following implementation of the guidelines.

Mixed support for the imitative effect is provided by one study that examined the effect of television broadcast of documentary about a suicidal adolescent girl [35]. In this study, a significant decrease in the mean age of suicide attempters and completers occurred during the week before the broadcast, the period for which the documentary was heavily promoted with repeatedly broadcasting the charismatic young suicide victim. The decrease in the mean age of suicide victims suggests that younger persons who identified with the victim were more susceptible to its imitative effect than older persons. Nevertheless, the study found no increase in suicide rates after the broadcast.

Romer and colleagues [32] explicitly examined age as of a moderator of the imitative effect. They found that persons younger than 25 were susceptible to the effects of local television news. Moreover, young persons were also sensitive to newspaper suicide reporting even though the sampled newspapers (eg, *Los Angeles Times*, *The New York Times*) focused on older suicide victims. Based on this observation, the authors posited that among young persons, exposure to nonfictional suicide stories might reduce restraints on suicidal behavior (disinhibition) rather than provide an identifiable model.

Three reviews of nonfictional suicidal stories [37–39] provided substantial evidence for a suicidal imitative effect. Applying Hill's causal criteria [57], Pirkis and Blood [37] critically examined the validity of the association between nonfiction reporting of suicide (newspapers, television, and books) and actual suicidal behavior in 42 English-language studies. They concluded that the evidence supports a causal association between the nonfictional media reporting of suicide and subsequent suicidal behavior, stating that the data satisfied Hill's criteria of consistency, strength of association, temporality, specificity, and coherence. In a quantitative review of 419 published findings from 55 empiric studies on nonfictional media stories of completed suicides or attempts, Stack [39] determined several features of nonfictional stories that augmented an imitative effect. First, regarding the suicide model, stories about celebrity suicides and female victims were significantly more likely to report an imitative effect than other suicide stories. Second, the source of information also played a role; studies based on newspaper reporting were more likely to report an imitative effect than studies based on televised stories. Third, studies that provided a negative description of the suicide, defined by Stack [39] as including a victim's physical disfigurement and pain, stating that suicide is wrong, and offering alternative solutions, were substantially more likely to *reduce* an imitative effect. Similar conclusions were derived by Stack [38] in his earlier review.

While the body of research has been supportive of the hypothesis that suicides depicted in the media facilitate imitation, Mercy and colleagues [36] have provided a dissenting voice. They found less exposure to media accounts of suicidal behavior in a sample of young adults who made a nearly lethal suicide attempt compared with nonattempters. However, the interpretability of the observed protective effect was limited [58]: (1) the media exposure was derived from an aggregate of different types of media stories; (2) the timing of the exposure was a 30-day interval before the suicide attempt, in contrast to most other studies that examined shorter intervals after exposure; (3) suicide attempters may have had less exposure to media generally (eg, read fewer books,

Table 2
Studies examining media influences on subsequent imitative suicides

Citation	Country studied	Source of study/method	Support of modeling
Nonfictional			
Etzersdorfer et al [29]	Austria	Comparison of firearm suicides before and after publicized suicide of a wellknown hotel owner by firearm in areas having different coverage rate of newspapers	Yes
Niederkrotenthaler and Sonneck [30]	Austria	Examined the impact of media guidelines on overall annual suicide rates and numbers of Viennese subway suicides to regional differences in newspapers coverage	Yes
Pirkis and Blood [37]	—	Review of English-language 42 studies that examined the nonfiction reporting of suicide (newspapers, television, and books) according to Hill's causal criteria	Yes
Pirkis et al [31]	Australia	Examined the association between various nonfictional media sources (newspapers, news and current affairs shows on television and radio) and suicide rates	Yes
Shoval et al [35]	Israel	Examined the effect of a television documentary on an adolescent female suicide on national suicide rates	Somewhat
Stack [38]	—	Review of 42 empiric studies on the impact of publicized nonfictional suicide stories (published 1974–1996)	Yes
Stack [39]	—	Review of 55 empiric research studies on nonfictional media stories of suicides (published 1967–2001)	Yes
Tousignant et al [33]	Canada	Examined associations between suicide of a television male reporter and subsequent suicide rates	Yes
Yip et al [34]	Hong Kong	Examined associations between suicide of a male pop star and subsequent suicide rates	Yes
Fiction			
Hawton et al [40]	United Kingdom	Examined association between a drug overdose in a television drama and deliberate self-poisoning rates	Yes

Pirkis and Blood [41]	—	Review of 34 studies that examined the association between fictional portrayal of suicide (movies, television, music, and plays) and subsequent actual suicidal behavior	No
Fiction and nonfiction combined			
Mercy et al [36]	US	Assessed exposure to accounts of suicidal behavior in the media (movies, television shows or videos, news articles, and books) in suicide attempters and controls	No
Romer et al [32]	US	Assessed associations between coverage of suicides (newspapers, television news and shows and movies) and suicide rates	Yes
Content analysis			
Fekete et al [42]	Germany, US, Hungary, Japan, Austria, Finland	Content analysis of newspaper suicide reports from countries with different suicide rates	Not Applicable
Frey et al [43]	Switzerland	Compared content of Swiss print media before and after implementation of guidelines; focused on frequency, form, and content (explanatory model of suicide, prevention, therapy mentioned)	Not Applicable
Gould et al [44]	US	Content analysis of 151 articles from a database of 1851 newspaper suicide stories	Not Applicable
Jamieson et al [45]	US	Content analysis of 3 years of reporting practices of suicide in The New York Times newspaper	Not Applicable
Jamieson et al [46]	US	Content Analysis of US movies on suicide over a 55-year period.	Not Applicable
Kuess and Hatzinger [47]	Austria	Examined the content of newspaper suicide articles from 1984–1985	Not Applicable
Michel et al [48]	Switzerland	Comparison of the content of newspaper suicide articles before and after guidelines	Not Applicable
Michel et al [49]	Switzerland	Examined the content of 208 newspaper suicide articles over 8 months in 1991	Not Applicable
Pirkis et al [50]	Australia	Examined the extent, nature and quality of media suicide reporting (newspaper, television and radio stories) over 12 months	Not Applicable

(continued on next page)

Table 2
(continued)

Citation	Country studied	Source of study/method	Support of modeling
Weimann and Fishman [51]	Israel	Content analysis of suicide stories in the Israeli Press from 1955–1990	Not applicable
Internet			
Alao et al [52]	US	9 suicide attempters (5 cases aged 19–25) who received information from Web sites or chat rooms	Yes
Becker et al [53]	US	Suicide behavior among two adolescent females who visited suicide Web forums	Yes
Gallagher et al [54]	US	A case of suicidal asphyxiation by a 19-year-old female who obtained instructional material from an Internet site	Yes
Rajagopal [55]	Japan	Cyberspace suicide pact among 9 persons	Yes
Lee et al [56]	Japan	Four cyberspace suicide pacts and 13 deaths in 2 months	Yes

fewer newspapers); (4) the suicide attempters had significantly more proximal stressors, possibly obscuring their recall of media exposure; and (5) nearly half of the suicide attempters were between 25 and 34 years of age, a group not particularly susceptible to imitation.

Recently, investigators have begun to acknowledge the potential impact of the Internet. While research on the Internet and adolescent suicides is in its inchoate stage, it demonstrates the disturbing power of the Internet. Case reports have underscored that youths have turned to the Internet for detailed instructions on suicide methods and have received encouragement to commit suicide [52–54]. The Internet has given rise to the phenomenon of cybersuicide pacts, the formation of suicide pacts that involves strangers meeting over the Internet [55,56].

Modeling from Fictional Suicide Stories

In contrast to the multitude of studies that examined the imitative effects of nonfictional suicide stories, little research has been devoted to the influence of fictional suicide stories. The studies examining the imitative effects of fictional suicide accounts produced somewhat conflicting findings, alternatively providing evidence to either validate or invalidate an imitative hypothesis. Moreover, the conclusions derived from studies on imitative effects of fictional accounts were often open to differing interpretations [1,59,60].

Two recent studies examined the contributions of fictional suicide stories to the suicide contagion process (see Table 2): one was an original study conducted in the United Kingdom [40] and the other was a review [41] undertaken in Australia. Hawton and colleagues [40] assessed whether a drug overdose in a television drama broadcast in the United Kingdom affected the incidence and nature of presentations for self-poisoning at accident and emergency departments. They found increases of 17% and 9% in self-poisoning presentations to hospitals for the first and second weeks, respectively, after the broadcast and then the rates returned to pre–broadcast levels in the third week. The overdoses were specific to the drug depicted in the dramatization. Moreover, this study demonstrated the importance of the interactions between the characteristics of the stories, the viewers' attributes, and the environment. First, the increase in self-poisoning rates was largest in 25- to 34-year-olds, the age group that included the male actor who overdosed in the index episode. Second, females showed somewhat greater increases in self-poisoning than males, probably reflecting the female dominant viewing audience of the television drama.

Pirkis and Blood [41] evaluated the quality of 34 studies that examined the impact of fictional media portrayal of suicide (film, television, music, and plays) and subsequent actual suicidal behavior. They found the studies to be crosssectional, subject to ecological fallacy, and surveyed subjects after viewing or listening to fictional portrayals. Pirkis and Blood [41] concluded that poor-quality studies limit the ability to draw valid internal conclusions and thereby can produce systematically different results among the studies that evaluate the influence of fictional accounts of suicide.

Content Analytic Studies

Despite the substantial research on media influences and the development of several guidelines for the media to follow in presenting suicide story content [61], research on the specific aspects of media stories that facilitate suicide contagion has been markedly limited [48]. Few studies have systematically investigated the specific story elements believed to either facilitate or limit the contagious effects of media accounts of suicide. Most studies that have examined the newspaper characteristics focused on the quantitative aspects, such as the placement of the story and other formatting elements [47,49,62,63]. One study assessed whether *The New York Times* suicide stories published in 1990, 1995, and 1999 conformed to US media suicide guidelines implemented in 2001 [45]. Their content analysis revealed that while the prominence (frequency and placement) of suicide reporting rose, the national suicide rate did not increase. Those few studies that evaluated the qualitative characteristics of newspaper stories [43,48,50,51] either examined a limited number of newspaper articles or appraised a restricted number of newspaper dimensions. The reliability of the newspaper content analyses has only been minimally addressed [43,48,51].

To identify specific features in media suicide reports that may contribute to the initiation of teenage suicide clusters, Gould and colleagues [44] developed a content analytic strategy of qualitative characteristics abstracted from newspaper stories. Using a random subset of 151 articles from a database of 1851 newspaper suicide stories published from 1988 through 1996 in the United States, the content analysis showed that the majority of variables in the content analysis were very reliable and obtained excellent percent agreement; however, the reliability of complicated constructs, such as sensationalizing, glorifying, or romanticizing the suicide, was comparatively low. The data emphasize that before effective guidelines and responsible suicide reporting can ensue, further explication of suicide story constructs is necessary to ensure the implementation and compliance of responsible reporting on behalf of the media.

A content analysis of suicide reports from six countries with different suicide rates (Hungary had the highest suicide rate followed by Japan, Finland, Austria, and Germany; the United States had the lowest suicide rate) was performed to assess whether any differences existed in the characteristics of publicized suicide stories between the countries [42] (see Table 2). They found that attitudes toward suicide varied by country. Specifically, the Hungarian media were more accepting of suicide as demonstrated by its relatively positive presentation and thereby potentially fostering the increased likelihood of imitation. Japanese media presented a positive and heroizing portrayal of the suicide victim, but depicted the negative consequences of suicide. The media of Germany, Finland, and the United States characterized suicide in the most negative terms, portraying the victim and the act in terms of psychopathology and abnormality, and describing the negative consequences of the suicide, thereby potentially reducing the media's potential imitative effect. Several interpretations of Fekete and colleagues' [42] findings are possible since the causal direction of the association between media reporting and suicide rates was not clear because of the cross-sectional study design. The media presentation of suicide may reflect sociocultural attitudes toward suicide or the media presentation may influence the suicide rates, or most likely reflect a bidirectional association in which each influences the other.

Focusing on the fictional presentation of suicide, Jamieson and associates [46] investigated the content of US movies over a 55-year period, 1950 to 2004 (see Table 2). They found that approximately 11% of top-grossing films contained some suicidal enactment, most were depicted by male actors, and 10% of the enacted suicides occurred to persons below age 21. While the rate of suicide depiction remained stable over the years, the explicitness of the portrayal increased. Most importantly, the suicide explicitness in the films over the 55-year period increased in concert with US youth suicide rates.

Summary of Media Effects

Studies clearly show that coverage of nonfictional suicides results in subsequent suicides, but the imitative effect of exposure to fictional depiction of suicides is equivocal. With the advent of comprehensive and reliable content analyses, advances are likely to be made in identifying important stimulus characteristics in media reports. Relevant stimuli include the characteristics of the suicide model, the media portrayal of suicidal behavior, the explanatory paradigm for suicide, consequences of the act, and preventive and educational information. Content analyses can yield empirically based media recommendations to augment existing guidelines. Last, the Internet has been recognized as a burgeoning media source in need of research because of its appeal to youth.

EXPOSURE TO THE SUICIDAL BEHAVIOR OF ADOLESCENT PEERS

Social learning theory contends that an observer is more inclined to imitate a behavior of a model if the observer can identify with the model through shared common characteristics. For adolescents, peer group members often serve as models, replacing family members and other adults; peers function as the most influential group during this developmental period [64]. In contrast to this modeling hypothesis, others posit that adolescents and young adults do not necessarily imitate the behavior of their peers. Rather, through "assortative relating," persons who possess similar personality traits and share similar interests are more likely to form relationships and, thus, belong to the same peer group [65]. Accordingly, persons who are vulnerable to suicide ideation and suicide attempts may belong to the same peer group or "cluster" before the occurrence of a suicidal stimulus by a peer member.

The literature reviewed on the personal exposure to the suicidal behavior of adolescent peers was not restricted by year of publication since this focus of inquiry was not comprehensively reviewed in the past (see References [1,2]). Studies that did not distinguish the influence of suicidal peers from suicidal siblings or other family members were excluded to avoid the confounding effect of family history of suicidality (eg, Reference [66]). Of the 21 studies reviewed in this section (Table 3 for a summary of the reports), 16 revealed substantial imitative effects for exposure to peer suicidal behavior [67–71, 74–83,85] and one study offered mixed support for the impact of suicidal friends and peers [86].

The 16 studies that provided support for an imitative effect of peer suicidal behavior can be categorized into studies that examined the impact of any suicidal behavior (n = 6 [69–71,77,81,82]), those that examined and distinguished between peer attempters or completers (n = 7 [68,74–76,78,79,85]), those that considered the impact of peer attempters only (n = 2 [67,80]), and those that examined completers only (n = 1 [83]).

Of the seven studies that separately examined the influence of exposure to completers and attempters, one study, conducted in a population of Icelandic adolescents, reported a comparable, increased risk of suicide attempt among youths exposed to either friends who attempted or completed suicide [68]. Using a large, nationally representative sample of adolescents, Cerel and colleagues [74] observed that exposure to a completed suicide of a peer was associated with increased odds of both ideation and suicide attempt compared with exposure to a suicide attempt of a peer. The other five studies found that adolescents exposed to attempters were at higher risk of suicidal behavior than those exposed to suicide completers. Specifically, employing the 1988 Navajo Adolescent Health data, Grossman and associates [76] determined that while either having a friend who attempted suicide or one who completed suicide was a predictor of a suicide attempt, only having a friend who attempted suicide was statistically significant. Studying 798 adolescents from two high schools in which a completed suicide occurred 8 months earlier, Hazell and Lewin [78] found that students who had both suicide attempters and completers as friends scored higher on suicidality than friends of attempters only, or completers only, or those who were "unexposed." Moreover, the students exposed to attempters scored higher on suicidality than those exposed to completers only. Nevertheless, the findings of Hazell and Lewin [78] are difficult to interpret and, thereby, to generalize because all students in the study were exposed to a completed suicide. Using data from 23 high schools throughout Hong Kong, Ho and colleagues [79] observed that while both peers of suicide completers and attempters scored significantly higher on suicidality than the unexposed controls, peers of suicide attempters carried a higher risk than peers of suicide completers. Another study conducted in Hong Kong observed that exposure to a suicide attempt was associated with an increased risk of suicidal behaviors, while exposure to a completed suicide was not associated with an elevated risk [85]. Using wave 1 data from the National Longitudinal Study of Adolescent Health (ADD Health), a nationally representative sample of US high school students, Culter and associates [75] found that adolescents who knew friends who had attempted suicide or committed suicide were significantly more likely to attempt suicide than adolescents who did not know suicidal friends. Importantly, stronger causal evidence is provided by the wave 2 data that found that adolescents who did not previously attempt suicide in wave 1 were more likely to attempt suicide if they had a friend who attempted suicide.

Significant gender differences in patterns of the effect of exposure to the suicidal behavior of friends were reported by two studies [68,75]. In a population of Icelandic adolescents, Bjarnason and Thorlindsson [68] found that attempted and completed suicide of a friend had a similar effect for both genders, but suicidal ideation by a friend produced gender differential effects. For male adolescents, the effect of being informed about suicidal ideation was almost identical to the effect of suicide attempt and completion, while for females suicidal ideation by a friend had only a small effect on suicide attempt. Culter and colleagues [75] found that among a sample of US adolescents, girls were more likely to attempt suicide if they knew someone who made an attempt, while boys were substantially more likely to make an attempt if they knew someone who completed suicide than if they knew someone who attempted suicide.

In contrast to the ample body of research suggesting an association between exposure to suicidal behavior of peers and friends and adolescent attempted suicide, a few studies have found no association or an inverse association. Examining students who were exposed to a suicide cluster in their school, Brent and associates [72] observed that 75% of the 12 suicidal students described themselves as a friend or close friend of one of the suicide victims compared with 65% of the 88 nonsuicidal students. The suicidal students were significantly more likely to have been both suicidal in the past and to suffer from an episode of major depression in their lifetime compared with the nonsuicidal students. Brent and colleagues [72] concluded that prior and current psychopathology predicted suicidal behavior following exposure to a suicidal outbreak more than closeness of the relationship to the suicide victim.

Brent and associates [73,86,87] examined the impact of exposure to suicide on the friends of adolescent suicide victims over several years. In the 3-year follow-up of 166 adolescents exposed to suicide and 175 demographically and psychologically matched controls sampled from communities where no adolescent suicide occurred within the past 2 years, they [73] observed that the incidence of suicide attempts during the course of the follow-up was comparable in the exposed and control adolescents. Citing Gould and colleagues [88], the authors stated that only close friends of suicide victims were included as exposed subjects and close friends or acquaintances of the suicide victim might be less likely to engage in imitative suicidal behavior than less close friends. While Brent and colleagues [73] did not observe an increased risk for suicidal behavior among the exposed adolescents, they did find that the exposed youths were at increased risk for depression, anxiety, and posttraumatic stress disorder. These psychiatric disorders are major precursors of suicidal behavior, suggesting that if the duration of the follow-up was extended, the exposed subjects might have experienced signs and symptoms of suicidality. A study conducted by Mercy and associates [36] found that exposure to the suicidal behavior of friends or acquaintances was *protective* against nearly lethal suicide attempts.

Table 3
Studies examining the influences of peers on subsequent imitative suicidal behavior

Citation	Period and population	Methodology/comparison group	Support of modeling
Bearman and Moody [67]	13,465 adolescents in grades 7–12 from National Longitudinal Survey of Adolescent Health, Denver, US, 1994–1995.	Cross-sectional data examined the contribution of having a friend who attempted suicide in the past year to suicidal ideation and attempt.	Yes
Bjarnason and Thorlindsson [68]	7018 adolescents from all schools in Iceland, 1992.	Cross-sectional data examined whether a completed and attempted suicide by a friend and being told about suicidal ideation were correlated with past suicide attempt.	Yes
Blum et al [69]	13,454 American Indian and Alaska Native students, grades 7–12, US, 1989.	Cross-sectional data examined the prevalence of exposure to suicidal peers among high-risk youths (defined as suicide attempted in past year plus current suicide thoughts or multiple attempts regardless of timing) and low-risk youths.	Yes
Borowsky et al [70]	13,110 students in grades 7–12, US, 1995 and 1996.	Longitudinal data examined whether having a friend attempt or complete suicide (assessed at Time 1) predicted suicide attempt in past 12 months (assessed at Time 2).	Yes
Borowsky et al [71]	11,666 American Indian and Alaska native 7–12 grade students, US, 1989.	Cross-sectional data examined whether having a friend who attempted suicide was associated with reporting ever attempting suicide.	Yes
Brent et al [72]	110 students who were exposed to a suicide cluster in their high school, US, Date not published.	Cross-sectional data compared students with and without suicidality on their relationships with suicide victims.	Mixed

Source	Sample	Description	
Brent et al [73]	166 friends and acquaintances of adolescent suicides and 175 matched controls, Pittsburgh, US, 1991–1994.	Cross-sectional data examined long-term sequelae of suicide exposure by comparing suicide behavior among friends and acquaintances of suicide victims with matched controls.	No
Cerel et al [74]	5852 students from Add Health, Denver, US, 1995–1996.	Cross-sectional data compared suicidal risk factors during previous 12 months among adolescents who were exposed to peer suicidal behavior and those who were not exposed to suicidal behaviors.	Yes
Cutler et al [75]	17,004 high school students from Add Health, US, 1996.	Longitudinal data examined whether adolescents who knew friends who attempted suicide or committed suicide were more likely to attempt suicide than adolescents who did not have suicidal friends.	Yes
Grossman et al [76]	7241 students, grades 6–12, from 47 schools on Navajo reservation, US, 1988.	Cross-sectional data compared students reporting suicide attempts with those who did not report such behavior on various potential risk factors.	Yes
Harkavy-Friedman et al [77]	380 students attending high school, New York, US, 1985.	Cross-sectional data compared experience with suicidal behavior among 3 groups of students who were identified as (1) never thought of killing themselves, (2) suicidal ideators, and (3) suicidal attempters.	Yes
Hazell and Lewin [78]	798 students from 2 high schools in which a suicide occurred 8 months earlier, Australia, 1990–1991.	Cross-sectional data compared friends of adolescent suicide attempters and or suicide completers with students who had low exposure to suicide.	Yes
Ho et al [79]	1920 students from high school without history of student suicide in past 3 years, Hong Kong, 1994–1995.	Cross-sectional data compared suicidal behavior among peers of suicide completers and suicide attempters with unexposed youths.	Yes

(continued on next page)

Table 3
(continued)

Citation	Period and population	Methodology/comparison group	Support of modeling
Joiner [65]	138 college undergraduates and their roommates, US, date not listed.	Cross-sectional data compared suicidality among 90 undergraduate roommate pairs who chose to room together with 48 pairs who were assigned to each other.	No
Lewinsohn et al [80]	1508 high school students, Oregon, US, 1987–1989.	Longitudinal data examined individual risk factors and psychosocial factors among attempters and nonattempters to determine factors that uniquely contributed to the prediction of future suicide attempts.	Yes
Manson et al [81]	188 American Indians attending a tribally governed boarding school, US, 1987–1988.	Cross-sectional data examined exposure to suicidal friends among students who reported ever attempting suicide and those who reported having thoughts about killing themselves within the past month.	Yes
Mercy et al [36]	153 victims of attempted suicide from emergency departments and 513 controls (aged 13–34, 53% aged 13–24 years), Houston, US, 1992–1995.	Cross-sectional data compared victims of suicide attempts with controls on exposures to suicidal behavior of others.	No
Prinstein et al [82]	527 adolescents from a New England high school, US, dates not published.	Cross-sectional data examined associations between peer behavior and adolescent suicidal ideation and behavior.	Yes

Wagner et al [83]	1050 adolescents in grades 7–12 from three rural counties of a mid-Atlantic state, US, 1990.	Cross-sectional data examined suicidal risk factors among three groups: (1) those who made a prior suicide attempt, (2) those who never made an attempt but exhibited depressed mood or suicidal ideation, and (3) those who were neither depressed nor suicidal and never made a suicide attempt.	Yes
Watkins and Gutierrez [84]	27 students exposed to a peer suicide and 27 matched unexposed high students, Illinois, US, date not published.	Cross-sectional data compared adolescents exposed to suicide of a peer with those who were not exposed on (1) measures of reasons for living inventory (RFL-A), (2) suicidal ideation (SIQ), and (3) suicidal behavior (SBQ).	No
Wong et al [85]	1361 secondary school students, Hong Kong, 2002–2003.	Cross-sectional data compared characteristics of students who reported that they had engaged in suicidal behaviors in previous 12 months with those who did not report such behaviors (subjects classified as belonging to the "suicidal behaviors" group if reported at least one self-injurious behavior and an affirmative response to an intent question).	Yes/No

In contrast to the postulation by Brent and associates [73], the protective association was only evident when the relationship was described as "not particularly close or distant" as compared with "very close or close." Furthermore, the study findings may have limited generalizability; the cases represented a select population of suicide attempters since they were adolescents and younger adults (aged 13 to 34 years) who were treated for a nearly lethal suicide attempt in emergency departments. Watkins and Gutierrez [84] also found no evidence of increased risk of suicide-related behavior in the students exposed to suicide of a peer compared with unexposed high school students. Nevertheless, although not statistically significant ($P = .08$), Watkins and Gutierrez [84] found that the students who reported being friends with the suicide victim (n = 14) had appreciably higher scores on suicidal ideation and suicidal behavior than those who were classified as acquaintances (n = 13).

Using a quasi-experimental design in a sample of college students and their roommates, Joiner [65] tested whether students' suicidal symptoms were more comparable to their roommate's symptoms if they chose to live with their roommate compared with students who were assigned their roommate. He found that correlation between roommates' suicidality was greater in roommate pairs (n = 90) who chose to room together than in roommate pairs who were assigned to room together (n = 48), providing support for the hypothesis of "assortative relating."

The majority of studies examining exposure to suicidal behavior of adolescent peers have found a significant association with adolescent suicide attempt. While modeling and imitation is a possible mechanism underlying the association between exposure to suicidal peers and subsequent suicidal behavior, we cannot negate the possible contribution of assortative relating regarding the choice of friends that may result in groupings of vulnerable suicidal youths. Assortative relating and the modeling are not mutually exclusive, but may be complementary processes underlying the effect of exposure to suicidal behavior of adolescent peers and friends. Nevertheless, in support of a modeling mechanism are the findings that, in general, exposure to a suicide attempt by a peer appears to be a stronger predictor of suicidal behavior than exposure to a peer's completed suicide. Moreover, the closeness of the relationship appears to modify the association, although direction of its effect is equivocal. The differential effect of these stimulus characteristics (eg, nature of suicidal exposure and closeness of the relationship) is more consistent with a modeling hypothesis. Unfortunately, the vast majority of the studies have employed cross-sectional designs, so that only associations and not causality can be derived.

SUMMARY

The evidence to date suggests that suicide modeling is a real phenomenon, although of a smaller effect size than other psychiatric and psychosocial risk factors for adolescent suicide. Multiple lines of inquiry provide converging evidence, including studies on suicide clusters, media influence on suicide (particularly coverage of nonfictional suicides), and peer influence on suicidality.

Despite variations in study setting and methodology, the body of literature is consistent with a modeling hypothesis. Although advances in documentation of suicide modeling have been made over the past decade, we are still confronted by unresolved issues regarding the underlying mechanisms. Prevention and postvention strategies can be optimized to avert modeling of suicidal behavior only once research addresses the complexities and uncertainties of this phenomenon.

References

[1] Velting DM, Gould MS. Suicide contagion. In: Maris R, Canetto S, Silverman MM, editors. Review of suicidology. New York: Guilford Press; 1997. p. 96–137.
[2] Gould MS. Suicide and the media. In: Hendin H, Mann JJ, editors. The clinical science of suicide prevention. New York: Academy of Sciences; 2001. p. 200–24.
[3] Gould MS, Wallenstein S, Davidson L. Suicide clusters: a critical review. Suicide Life Threat Behav 1989;19(1):17–29.
[4] Bandura A. Self-efficacy: toward a unifying theory of behavioral change. Psychol Rev 1977;84(2):191–215.
[5] Sacks M, Eth S. Pathological identification as a cause of suicide on an inpatient unit. Hosp Community Psychiatry 1981;32(1):36–40.
[6] Rubinstein DH. A stress-diathesis theory of suicide. Suicide Life Threat Behav 1986;16(2): 182–97.
[7] Gould MS, Wallenstein S, Kleinman MH, et al. Suicide clusters, an examination of age-specific effects. Am J Public Health 1990;80(2):211–2.
[8] Kindlon DJ. The measurement of attention. J Child Psychol Psychiatry 1998;3(2):72–8.
[9] Levin HS, Culhane KA, Hartmann J, et al. Developmental changes in performance on tests of purported frontal lobe functioning. Dev Neuropsychol 1991;7(3):377–95.
[10] Rubia K, Smith AB, Woolley J, et al. Progressive increase of frontostriatal brain activation from childhood to adulthood during event-related tasks of cognitive control. Hum Brain Mapp 2006;27(12):973–93.
[11] Stevens MC, Kiehl KA, Pearlson GD, et al. Functional neural networks underlying response inhibition in adolescents and adults. Behav Brain Res 2007;181(1):12–22.
[12] Bakwin H. Suicide in children and adolescents. J Pediatr 1957;50(6):749–69.
[13] Popow NM. The present epidemic of school suicides in Russia. Nevrol Vestnik (Kazan) 1911;18:592–646.
[14] Gould MS, Davidson L. Suicide contagion among adolescents. In: Stiffman AR, Feldman RA, editors. Advances in adolescent mental health. Greenwich (CT): JAI Press; 1988. p. 29–59.
[15] Gibbons RD, Clark DC, Fawcett J. A statistical method for evaluating suicide clusters and implementing cluster surveillance. Am J Epidemiol 1990;132(1 Suppl):S183–91.
[16] Gould MS, Petrie K, Kleinman MH, et al. Clustering of attempted suicide, New Zealand national data. Int J Epidemiol 1994;23(6):1185–9.
[17] Gould MS, Wallenstein S, Kleinman M. Time-space clustering of teenage suicide. Am J Epidemiol 1990;131(1):71–8.
[18] Taiminen TJ, Helenius H. Suicide clustering in a psychiatric hospital with a history of a suicide epidemic: a quantitative study. Am J Psychiatry 1994;151(7):1087–8.
[19] King CA, Franzese R, Gargan S, et al. Suicide contagion among adolescents during acute psychiatric hospitalization. Psychiatr Serv 1995;46(9):915–8.
[20] Johansson L, Lindqvist P, Eriksson A. Teenage suicide cluster formation and contagion: implications for primary care. BMC Fam Pract 2006;7:32.
[21] Wilkie C, Macdonald S, Hildahl K. Community case study: suicide cluster in a small Manitoba community. Can J Psychiatry 1998;43(8):823–8.

[22] Hourani LL, Warrack G, Coben PA. A demographic analysis of suicide among U.S. Navy personnel. Suicide Life Threat Behav 1999;29(4):365–75.

[23] McKenzie N, Keane M. Contribution of imitative suicide to the suicide rate in prisons. Suicide Life Threat Behav 2007;37(5):538–42.

[24] Silviken A, Haldorsen T, Kvernmo S. Suicide among indigenous Sami in Arctic Norway, 1970–1998. Eur J Epidemiol 2006;21(9):707–13.

[25] Hourani LL, Warrack AG, Coben PA. Suicide in the U.S. Marine Corps, 1990 to 1996. Mil Med 1999;164(8):551–5.

[26] Wissow LS, Walkup J, Barlow A, et al. Cluster and regional influences on suicide in a South-western American Indian tribe. Soc Sci Med 2001;53(9):1115–24.

[27] Exeter DJ, Boyle PJ. Does young adult suicide cluster geographically in Scotland? J Epidemiol Community Health 2007;61(8):731–6.

[28] Schmidtke A, Schaller S. The role of mass media in suicide prevention. In: Hawton K, van Heeringen K, editors. The international handbook of suicide and attempted suicide. New York: John Wiley & Sons Ltd.; 2000. p. 675–97.

[29] Etzersdorfer E, Voracek M, Sonneck G. A dose-response relationship between imitational suicides and newspaper distribution. Arch Suicide Res 2004;8(2):137–45.

[30] Niederkrotenthaler T, Sonneck G. Assessing the impact of media guidelines for reporting on suicides in Austria: interrupted time series analysis. Aust N Z J Psychiatry 2007;41(5): 419–28.

[31] Pirkis JE, Burgess PM, Francis C, et al. The relationship between media reporting of suicide and actual suicide in Australia. Soc Sci Med 2006;62(11):2874–86.

[32] Romer D, Jamieson PE, Jamieson KH. Are news reports of suicide contagious? A stringent test in six U.S. cities. J Commun 2006;56(2):253–70.

[33] Tousignant M, Mishara BL, Caillaud A, et al. The impact of media coverage of the suicide of a well-known Quebec reporter: the case of Gaetan Girouard. Soc Sci Med 2005;60(9): 1919–26.

[34] Yip P, Fu K, Yang K, et al. The effects of a celebrity suicide on suicide rates in Hong Kong. J Affect Disord 2006;93(1–3):245–52.

[35] Shoval G, Zalsman G, Polakevitch J, et al. Effect of the broadcast of a television documentary about a teenager's suicide in Israel on suicidal behavior and methods. Crisis 2005; 26(1):20–4.

[36] Mercy JA, Kresnow MJ, O'Carroll PW, et al. Is suicide contagious? A study of the relation between exposure to the suicidal behavior of others and nearly lethal suicide attempts. Am J Epidemiol 2001;154(2):120–7.

[37] Pirkis J, Blood RW. Suicide and the media: Part I. Reportage in nonfictional media. Crisis 2001;22(4):146–54.

[38] Stack S. Media coverage as a risk factor in suicide. J Epidemiol Community Health 2003;57(4):238–40.

[39] Stack S. Suicide in the media, a quantitative review of studies based on non-fictional stories. Suicide Life Threat Behav 2005;35(2):121–33.

[40] Hawton K, Simkin S, Deeks JJ, et al. Effects of a drug overdose in a television drama on presentations to hospital for self poisoning: time series and questionnaire study. BMJ 1999; 318(7189):972–7.

[41] Pirkis J, Blood RW. Suicide and the media: part II. Portrayal in fictional media. Crisis 2001;2(4):155–62.

[42] Fekete S, Schmidtke A, Takahashi Y, et al. Mass media, cultural attitudes, and suicide. Results of an international comparative study. Crisis 2001;22(4):170–2.

[43] Frey C, Michel K, Valach L. Suicide reporting in the Swiss print media: responsible or irresponsible? Eur J Public Health 1997;7(1):15–9.

[44] Gould MS, Midle JB, Insel B, et al. Suicide reporting content analysis: abstract development and reliability. Crisis 2007;28(4):165–74.

[45] Jamieson P, Jamieson KH, Romer D. The responsible reporting of suicide in print journalism. Am Behav Sci 2003;46(12):1643–60.

[46] Jamieson PE, More E, Lee SS, et al. It matters what young people watch: health risk behaviors portrayed in top grossing movies since 1950. In: Jamieson PE, Romer D, editors. The changing portrayal of adolescents in the media and why it matters. New York: Oxford University Press; 2008 [in press].

[47] Kuess S, Hatzinger R. Attitudes toward suicide in the print media. Crisis 1986;7(2): 118–25.

[48] Michel K, Frey C, Wyss K, et al. An exercise in improving suicide reporting in print media. Crisis 2000;21(2):71–9.

[49] Michel K, Frey C, Schlaepfer TE, et al. Suicide reporting in the Swiss print media: frequency, form and content of articles. Eur J Public Health 1995;5(3):199–203.

[50] Pirkis J, Francis C, Blood RW, et al. Reporting of suicide in the Australian media. Aust N Z J Psychiatry 2002;36(2):190–7.

[51] Weimann G, Fishman G. Reconstructing suicide: reporting suicide in the Israeli press. Journalism Mass Comm Q 1995;72(3):551–8.

[52] Alao AO, Soderberg M, Pohl EL, et al. Cybersuicide: review of the role of the Internet on suicide. Cyberpsychol Behav 2006;9(4):489–93.

[53] Becker K, Mayer M, Nagenborg M, et al. Parasuicide online: can suicide websites trigger suicidal behaviour in predisposed adolescents? Nord J Psychiatry 2004;58(2):111–4.

[54] Gallagher KE, Smith DM, Mellen PF. Suicidal asphyxiation by using pure helium gas: case report, review, and discussion of the influence of the Internet. Am J Forensic Med Pathol 2003;24(4):361–3.

[55] Rajagopal S. Suicide pacts and the Internet. BMJ 2004;329(7478):1298–9.

[56] Lee DT, Chan KP, Yip PS. Charcoal burning is also popular for suicide pacts made on the Internet. BMJ 2005;330(7491):602.

[57] Hill AB. The environment and disease: association or causation? Proc R Soc Med 1965;58: 295–300.

[58] Gould M, Jamieson P, Romer D. Media contagion and suicide among the young. Am Behav Sci 2003;46(9):1269–84.

[59] Berman AL. Fictional depiction of suicide in television films and imitation effects. Am J Psychiatry 1988;145(8):982–6.

[60] Phillips DP, Paight DJ. The impact of televised movies about suicide. A replicative study. N Engl J Med 1987;317(13):809–11.

[61] Pirkis J, Blood RW, Beautrais A, et al. Media guidelines on the reporting of suicide. Crisis 2006;27(2):82–7.

[62] Phillips D. The influence of suggestions on suicide; substantive and theoretical implications of the Werther effect. Am Sociol Rev 1974;39(3):340–54.

[63] Phillips D. Suicide, motor vehicle fatalities, and the mass media: evidence toward a theory of suggestion. Am Sociol Rev 1979;84(5):1150–74.

[64] Steinberg L. Autonomy, conflict, and harmony in the family. In: Feldman SS, Elliot GR, editors. At the threshold: the developing adolescent. Cambridge (MA): Harvard University Press; 1990. p. 255–76.

[65] Joiner TE. Contagion of suicidal symptoms as a function of assortative relating and shared relationship stress in college roommates. J Adolesc 2003;26(4):495–504.

[66] Fleming TM, Merry SN, Robinson EM, et al. Self-reported suicide attempts and associated risk and protective factors among secondary school students in New Zealand. Aust N Z J Psychiatry 2007;41(3):213–21.

[67] Bearman PS, Moody J. Suicide and friendships among American adolescents. Am J Public Health 2004;94(1):89–95.

[68] Bjarnason T, Thorlindsson T. Manifest predictors of past suicide attempts in a population of Icelandic adolescents. Suicide Life Threat Behav 1994;24(4):350–8.

[69] Blum RW, Harmon B, Harris L, et al. American Indian–Alaska Native youth health. JAMA 1992;267(12):1637–44.

[70] Borowsky IW, Ireland M, Resnick MD. Adolescent suicide attempts: risks and protectors. Pediatrics 2001;107(3):485–93.

[71] Borowsky IW, Resnick MD, Ireland M, et al. Suicide attempts among American Indian and Alaska Native youth: Risk and protective factors. Arch Pediatr Adolesc Med 1999;153(6): 573–80.

[72] Brent DA, Kerr MM, Goldstein C, et al. An outbreak of suicide and suicidal behavior in a high school. Child Adolesc Psychiatry 1989;28(6):918–24.

[73] Brent DA, Moritz G, Bridge J, et al. Long-term impact of exposure to suicide: a three-year controlled follow-up. J Am Acad Child Adolesc Psychiatry 1996;35(5):646–53.

[74] Cerel J, Roberts TA, Nilsen WJ. Peer suicidal behavior and adolescent risk behavior. J Nerv Ment Dis 2005;193(4):237–43.

[75] Cutler DM, Glaesen EL, Norberg KE. Explaining the rise in youth suicide. In: Gruber J, editor. Risky behavior among youths: an economic analysis. Chicago: University Of Chicago Press; 2001. p. 219–69.

[76] Grossman DC, Milligan BC, Deyo RA. Risk factors for suicide attempts among Navajo adolescents. Am J Public Health 1991;81(7):870–4.

[77] Harkavy Friedman JM, Asnis GM, Boeck M, et al. Prevalence of specific suicidal behaviors in a high school sample. Am J Psychiatry 1987;144(9):1203–6.

[78] Hazell P, Lewin T. Friends of adolescent suicide attempters and completers. J Am Acad Child Adolesc Psychiatry 1993;32(1):76–81.

[79] Ho TP, Leung PW, Hung SF, et al. The mental health of the peers of suicide completers and attempters. J Child Psychol Psychiatry 2000;41(3):301–8.

[80] Lewinsohn PM, Rohde P, Seeley JR. Psychosocial risk factors for future adolescent suicide attempts. J Consult Clin Psychol 1994;62(2):297–305.

[81] Manson SM, Beals J, Dick RW, et al. Risk factors for suicide among Indian adolescents at a boarding school. Public Health Rep 1989;104(6):609–14.

[82] Prinstein MJ, Boergers J, Spirito A. Adolescents' and their friends' health-risk behavior: factors that alter or add to peer influence. J Pediatr Psychol 2001;26(5):287–98.

[83] Wagner BM, Cole RE, Schwartzman P. Psychosocial correlates of suicide attempts among junior and senior high school youth. Suicide Life Threat Behav 1995;25(3):358–72.

[84] Watkins RL, Gutierrez PM. The relationship between exposure to adolescent suicide and subsequent suicide risk. Suicide Life Threat Behav 2003;33(1):21–32.

[85] Wong JPS, Stewart SM, Ho SY, et al. Exposure to suicide and suicidal behaviors among Hong Kong adolescents. Soc Sci Med 2005;61(3):591–9.

[86] Brent DA, Perper J, Moritz G, et al. Psychiatric effects of exposure to suicide among the friends and acquaintances of adolescent suicide victims. J Am Acad Child Adolesc Psychiatry 1992;31(4):629–39.

[87] Brent DA, Perper JA, Moritz G, et al. Stressful life events, psychopathology, and adolescent suicide: a case control study. Suicide Life Threat Behav 1993;23(3):179–87.

[88] Gould MS, Forman J, Kleinman MH. The psychological autopsy of cluster suicide in adolescents. Presented at the Sixth Scientific Meeting of the Society of Research in Child and Adolescent Psychopathology. London, UK. June 1994.

Psychiatr Clin N Am 31 (2008) 317–331

PSYCHIATRIC CLINICS
OF NORTH AMERICA

Suicidal Behavior in Young Women

Enrique Baca-Garcia, MD[a,b,c],
M. Mercedes Perez-Rodriguez, MD[d],
J. John Mann, MD, PhD[a,e], Maria A. Oquendo, MD[f,g,h],*

[a]Columbia University, 1051 Riverside Drive, Box 42, New York, NY 10032, USA
[b]Department of Psychiatry, Universidad Autonoma de Madrid, Calle Arzobispo Morcillo s/n, 28029, Madrid, Spain
[c]Department of Psychiatry, Fundacion Jimenez Diaz University Hospital. Avda. Reyes Católicos, 2. Madrid 28040, Spain
[d]Department of Psychiatry, Ramon y Cajal University Hospital, Carretera de Colmenar Viejo Km 9,100 Madrid 28034, Spain
[e]Molecular Imaging and Neuropathology Division, New York State Psychiatric Institute and Columbia University, 1051 Riverside Drive, Box 42, New York, NY 10032, USA
[f]Molecular Imaging and Neuropathology Division, New York State Psychiatric Institute and Columbia University, 1051 Riverside Drive, Office # 2725, New York, NY 10032, USA
[g]Department of Psychiatry, Columbia University, 1051 Riverside Drive, Office # 2725, New York, NY 10032, USA
[h]Silvio O. Conte Center for the Neurobiology of Mental Disorders, Molecular Imaging and Neuropathology Division, New York State Psychiatric Institute, 1051 Riverside Drive, New York, NY 10032, USA

S uicide prevention is one of the top public health priorities, and an important first step in a public health approach to suicide prevention is to identify groups that may be at increased risk for suicide attempts [1].

In the United States, several sociodemographic groups, such as women [2–5] and young people [2,5–8], have been consistently reported to be at increased risk for attempting suicide. In 2004, suicide was the third leading cause of death for persons aged 10 to 24 years in the United States [9]. Thus, the mental health of young people (aged 12–24 years) has become a global public health challenge [10].

The mental health needs of the young must be contextualized, because youth represents the confluence of several significant experiences. Young people are in the first stages of education or employment and are facing the struggle to find and keep a job and start romantic relationships [10]. Most mental disorders begin in youth but often remain undetected until later life [10], and the reported prevalence of mental disorders among young people ranges from 8% to 57% [11,12]. In addition, whether rates of mental disorders and suicide rates among young people have increased over the past decades is unclear [10].

*Corresponding author. Molecular Imaging and Neuropathology, Division at the New York State Psychiatric Institute and Columbia University, 1051 Riverside Drive, Office #2725, New York, NY 10032. E-mail address: mao4@columbia.edu (M.A. Oquendo).

0193-953X/08/$ – see front matter
doi:10.1016/j.psc.2008.01.002

GENDER AND AGE DIFFERENCES IN EPIDEMIOLOGY OF SUICIDAL BEHAVIORS

Studies in different countries have consistently reported gender differences in the epidemiology of suicidal behaviors. Men seem to have higher rates of completed suicide than women, whereas women have higher rates of suicide attempts than men [2–5,13–15]. This pattern has been reported across different countries, cultures and ethnic groups, with just a few exceptions such as women in China, who have higher rates of completed suicide than men, although the difference may be decreasing [16,17].

Among young people aged 15 to 19 years, rates of suicide are higher in men than women, with some exceptions, such as in China, Cuba, Ecuador, El Salvador, and Sri Lanka, where the female suicide rate is higher [18]. No recent data on deaths and causes of death are available to the World Health Organization (WHO) for more than 25% of the world's population, mainly in Africa, Southeast Asia, and the Middle East. Moreover, the WHO has recently warned that the quality of cause-of-death information is adequate in only 29 of 115 countries that report these statistics to WHO, representing less than 13 % of the world population [19].

Attempted Suicide

Numerous studies report that women have higher rates of suicide attempts than men [2–5,14,15,20]. The rates of attempted suicide are two to three times higher in women than men [21].

Rates of attempted suicide decrease with age in both sexes, with young women showing the highest rates of suicide attempts and the highest ratio of attempted suicides to suicides among all age-by-gender groups [22,23]. Among young adults aged 15 to 24 years, one suicide occurs for every 100 to 200 attempts [24].

In 2005, 16.9% of students in grades 9 through 12 in the United States seriously considered suicide in the previous 12 months (21.8% of women and 12.0% of men), and 8.4% of students reported making at least one suicide attempt in the previous 12 months (10.8% of women and 6.0% of men). All these rates were higher among women than men [25].

In older individuals, the gender differences in rates of suicide attempt tend to disappear and the ratio of attempted suicides to suicides significantly decreases [22].

Various factors may account for the higher rates of suicide attempts among young women. Compared with men, women have higher rates of mood disorders, particularly depression [26–29]. Depression has been reported to be one of the most important risk factors for suicide attempts, and major depressive disorder (MDD) and bipolar disorder are the most common psychiatric disorders associated with attempted and completed suicide [22,30,31]. Moreover, women experience higher rates of borderline personality disorder and domestic violence or physical or sexual abuse, which are linked to increased risk for suicidal ideation and attempts [32–35].

Completed Suicide

The age and gender distribution of completed suicide is almost opposite the distribution of suicide attempts. In most studies, women have consistently lower rates of completed suicide than men [13,14]. In the United States, the rates of completed suicide are approximately four times higher in men than women, with fluctuations across the life cycle, although these gender differences are less prominent in the psychiatric population [22,23].

Suicide rates in the general population of the United States increase with age and are highest in older adults. However, the age distribution of suicide rates is different in men and women, and in populations of different race and ethnicity [22,23].

Several factors have been suggested that may contribute to the gender differences in risk for committing suicide [36]. Women seem to have several protective factors against completed suicide: they are less impulsive than men, have lower rates of alcohol and substance abuse, are more socially embedded, and are more willing to seek and accept help or treatment and more likely to admit the severity of their symptoms [22]. Although women have higher rates of depression and other mood disorders than men [26–29,37], across all ethnic groups, women have suicide rates relative to major depression that are an order of magnitude lower than those of men [37].

Part of the gender discrepancy in suicide completion rates may be explained by the lethality of the method chosen. Men seem to choose highly lethal methods, such as firearms or hanging, whereas overdose and wrist-cutting are the preferred methods for women [22,38,39]. Suicides involving firearms are reported to be more lethal than those involving other methods [40]. In the United States, poisoning was the most common method of suicide for women and firearms the most common for men in 2004 (the last year for which mortality data are available in the United States) [23]. However, from 2003 to 2004, suicide rates and suicides by hanging or suffocation and poisoning increased significantly for women aged 10 to 19 years [9].

Several reasons have been suggested to explain why women tend to choose less lethal methods than men. One theory argues that individuals who use more lethal methods have more desire to kill themselves [40], and therefore women choose less lethal methods because they have lower suicide intent than men. However, some studies have found that women and men report similar levels of intent to die, although women choose less violent methods [41]. Moreover, some authors have suggested that the gender differences in suicide methods are far more complex than previously believed [42]. For example, it has been proposed that women choose suicide methods that will not destroy their external appearance [41,42], which would partially explain their lower rates of suicide using firearms. Consistent with this notion, when women use a firearm to attempt suicide, they are less likely to shoot themselves in the head, thus increasing their chances of survival [42]. However, experts have argued that the fact that women are less experienced in using firearms and less likely to own one explains these lower rates of suicide using firearms

[43]. This finding may be attributed to socialization factors, leading to boys having higher familiarity with guns and violence compared with girls [41]. Another psychologic factor may be that women wish to have a painless and "neat" death, not wanting to traumatize the people who will find their bodies [41]. Finally, some suicidal acts in women are ambivalent and instrumental, with the goal of communicating something or asking for help [44].

The Role of Race and Ethnicity

Although the rates of attempted and completed suicide have been consistently reported to vary across countries, cultures, and ethnic groups [13,15,45], little is known about the relationship between race and ethnicity and suicide attempts. Non-Hispanic whites have been reported to have significantly higher risk for suicide attempts than other ethnic groups [4], such as Blacks [2] and Hispanics [46]. By contrast, two nationwide studies did not find any significant relationship between race/ethnicity and suicide ideation and attempts [2,6]. Another study using nationwide data of the black population [47] reported that suicide attempt rates might be increasing significantly among Blacks, particularly younger individuals.

In 2004, suicide rates among American Indian/Alaska Native adolescents and young adults aged 15 to 24 years (21.0 per 100,000) were more than two times higher than the national average for that age group (10.4 per 100,000). Among women aged 15 to 24 years, the rate of suicide among American Indians/Alaskan Natives (10.6 per 100,000) was almost three times higher than among Whites (3.8 per 100,000) and than the national average for that age group among women (3.6 per 100,000) [23].

Other ethnic groups may be at increased risk for suicide attempts. Hispanic female high school students in grades 9 through 12 reported a higher percentage of suicide attempts (14.9%) than any other ethnic group (White, non-Hispanic [9.3%] or Black, non-Hispanic [9.8%]) [25].

A possible explanation is that young women may have increased risk for suicide attempts, but that predisposition may be buffered by cultural norms and religious beliefs [48] and overall lower rates of psychiatric disorders [49,50] in some ethnic groups, such as Asians, Blacks, and some Hispanic groups. Another explanation may be that the biologic (eg, genetic), psychologic (eg, impulsivity), and environmental (eg, stressors) variables that increase suicide attempt risk are more prevalent among women from some ethno-racial groups than among women of other ethno-racial groups.

Several limitations should be taken into account when considering the findings of studies examining attempted and completed suicide rates in specific ethnic groups. First, some ethnic groups are heterogeneous in terms of ethnicity, geography, acculturation, education, migration patterns, socioeconomic status, and access to health care [51,52]. Second, access to care, which may vary across ethnic groups, may have excluded suicidal behavior not requiring medical attention in some studies [51]. Reports have shown that immigrants may underuse psychiatric services [53]. Additionally, some of the ethnic groups analyzed may be too small ($<$ 5% of the general population) and attempted and completed suicide are sufficiently rare for the differences between races to achieve statistical significance in epidemiologic surveys in the general population [6].

In conclusion, future studies should better delineate the ethno-racial groups at highest risk to further refine the reports of higher prevalence of suicide attempts among young women [2,5]. It is important to learn about the specific contributors or buffers of suicidal risk in different racial and ethnic groups, and cultural differences in beliefs about death and views of suicide [22].

RISK FACTORS FOR SUICIDAL BEHAVIOR IN WOMEN

Suicidal behavior is complex and is probably caused by a combination of factors [32]. According to the stress–diathesis model, the risk for suicidal behaviors is determined by both a state-dependent trigger domain related to stressors (life events, states of depression or psychosis) and a threshold domain (diathesis), or trait-like predisposition to suicidal acts [32,54]. Neither domain alone determines suicide risk, but the combination of risk factors across domains increases the likelihood of suicidal acts, either through increasing the suicidal impulse caused by excess stress or decreasing internal barriers against suicide [32,54].

Many risk factors for suicidal behaviors have been identified. Most of them are additive, with the level of risk increasing with the number of risk factors, but some may act synergistically (the combined risk associated with two co-occurring risk factors being higher than the sum of the risk associated with each of the risk factors taken individually) [22]. Reports have shown that the importance of risk factors for suicidal behaviors are different in depressed men and women [55].

Stressful Life Events

Among the risk factors for suicidal behavior, life events have been extensively studied, but the results have been inconsistent. Although several studies have reported significant associations between recent life events and suicide attempts [56–60], others have found no significant differences in life events between attempters and nonattempters [32,54]. Several methodological differences among the studies may account for the mixed findings (different suicide outcomes: suicide attempts, completed suicide; different control groups: general population sample, nonsuicidal psychiatric patients; different periods over which life events were assessed; and different scales used to measure life events) [61]. Some researchers have reported that specific types or combinations of life events may be associated with attempted or completed suicide [57], whereas others have observed that the additive effect of negative life events is related to suicide risk [60]. The type of suicide triggers, the number of life events related to suicide attempts, and the influence of life events on the suicide attempt have been reported to be different in patients who have different psychiatric diagnoses [62,63]. However, other authors have pointed out that the role of stressful life events on the risk for suicidal behaviors has not been adequately assessed in prospective studies [30].

Women experience higher rates of domestic violence or physical or sexual abuse, which are linked to increased risk for suicidal ideation and attempts [32–35]. Moreover, among individuals who have a history of childhood abuse, those who attempt suicide tend to be younger than nonattempters, suggesting an increased suicidal risk among the young [64].

Mental Disorders

According to the American Psychiatric Association, the presence of a psychiatric disorder and the existence of previous suicide attempts are probably the main risk factors for suicide [22]. Psychologic autopsy studies have consistently reported that approximately 90% of the victims of completed suicide fulfilled the diagnostic criteria for a mental disorder [65–67]. However, most individuals with psychiatric disorders do not commit suicide. For example, although patients who have schizophrenia have high rates of suicide attempt, only 10% are estimated to die because of suicide [68]. Moreover, although a significant proportion of the general population experience relevant stressors and major depressive episodes, only a minor percentage of subjects will perform suicidal acts. This fact has prompted clinicians to search for other risk and protective factors for suicidal behavior [32,54,60].

In addition to the higher rates of mood disorders in women, which likely contribute to risk for suicide attempt, other diagnoses also are associated with increased likelihood of suicidal behavior. Eating disorders are prevalent among female suicide attempters, and suicide attempts are frequent among women who have eating disorders, particularly in those who have bingeing and purging behaviors and those who have comorbid mood disorders, aggression, or impulsivity [69,70]. The high rates of suicide attempts in women who have eating disorders may relate to the presence of borderline personality disorder. Studies have reported that eating disorders are common among individuals who have borderline personality disorder, and that borderline personality disorder is frequently diagnosed among those who have eating disorders [71–73].

Many studies have found an association between alcoholism and suicidality. Individuals who have alcohol use disorders are at increased risk for attempted [74,75] and completed suicide [66,76]. Among young people, those who misuse alcohol may be more likely to report suicidal ideation while experiencing depressive or anxiety disorders [77].

The lower rates of alcohol abuse among women may protect them against completed suicide [22]. In contrast, among alcoholics, suicide attempts are associated with female gender and younger age [74,78,79]. Among young adults aged 18 to 26 years, individuals who had comorbid alcohol use disorders had higher aggression and impulsivity scale scores and were more likely to be tobacco smokers than persons who had no comorbid alcohol use disorders. A trend was seen toward higher lethality of suicide attempts in subjects who had alcohol use disorders [80].

Abuse of other substances is also associated with increased rates of suicide [66], and is particularly common among adolescents and young adults who die by suicide [81,82]. Young women have lower rates of substance abuse than men, which may contribute to their lower rates of completed suicide [22].

Individuals who have personality disorders have approximately a seven times higher risk for suicide than the general population [66]. Compared with men, women experience higher rates of borderline personality disorder, which is linked to increased risk for suicidal ideation and attempts [32,83]. Rates of borderline personality disorder have been reported to be higher among women who attempt suicide compared with men [84].

Hormonal Factors

Although gender differences in mood disorder rates may be mediated by other factors, such as willingness to declare symptoms, culture, and methodological factors, hormonal factors seem to play a relevant role [85]. The cyclic fluctuation of gonadal hormones at menarche marks the onset of gender differences in rates of depression, which continue until menopause. This fact has inspired increasing studies on the association between sexual hormone levels and depression, the findings of which suggest that vulnerability to mood disorders in women is affected by hormonal fluctuations [85].

Increasing studies have described an association between the menstrual cycle and suicide attempts [86–90]. Saunders and Hawton [90] reviewed studies of suicidal behavior and the menstrual cycle and found that 15 of 23 studies reported an association between attempted suicide and menstrual cycle phase, whereas the remaining 8 studies found no association. Many studies have reported an association between the menstrual phase and suicide attempts, with a higher rate of suicide attempts occurring during the menses [86,87,89,90].

The authors' group found evidence of an association between the menses and suicide attempts in three different studies [86,87,89]. Baca-Garcia and colleagues [89] estimated that the probability of attempting suicide during the menses was 1.68 times higher than the overall probability of attempting suicide for any fertile women.

Other studies have suggested that, although the suicide rate in the general population is low postpartum, suicide risk may be increased in teenagers, women who have a history of depression or suicide attempts, and women hospitalized with postpartum psychiatric disorders [22,91].

Several theories have been suggested that may explain the role of the hypothalamic-pituitary-gonadal (HPG) axis in suicidal behaviors. First, the HPG axis may be involved in suicidal behavior through its interaction with the serotonergic system. Low estradiol may contribute to decreased serotonergic neurotransmission and mediate the association between menses and suicidal behaviors [90]. Available evidence suggests that when estrogen levels are low, the brain uses less tryptophan, which would result in serotonergic hypofunction observed in suicidal behavior [92,93]. It has also been reported that estradiol may increase serotonin levels [94–97], and may increase the expression of serotonin transporter (5-HTT) mRNA and the density of the 5-HTT binding sites in several brain areas that seem to be altered in suicide victims [98,99]. Second, the interaction between hormonal and genetic factors may play a significant role in female suicide attempts [100]. Third, low progesterone levels are associated with higher levels of suicidal ideation in female adolescents [101]. Some metabolites of progesterone are anxiogenic, whereas others are anxiolytic [102]. Finally, according to the stress–diathesis model for suicidal behavior [32], low sex hormonal levels could be considered a stressor acting on GABAergic and serotonergic systems, therefore increasing risk for suicide attempts during the menstrual phase. All these hypotheses require further study.

However, cultural, social, biologic, and clinical factors probably modulate the effect of sex hormones on suicidal risk [88,103]. For example, unwanted pregnancy has been suggested as a risk factor for suicide attempts [90].

PROTECTIVE FACTORS FOR SUICIDAL BEHAVIOR IN WOMEN

Protective factors act in the opposite way than risk factors: they decrease the probability of suicidal behaviors. In studies that compare suicide attempters with nonattempters, protective factors against suicidal behaviors are usually the opposite of risk factors.

Although most studies investigating variables associated with suicidal behaviors have focused on risk factors, only a few studies have examined protective factors [48]. The Practice Guideline for the Assessment and Treatment of Suicidal Behaviors published by the American Psychiatric Association [22] lists 10 factors believed to be protective against suicide: (1) children in the home (except among those who have postpartum psychosis or mood disorder), (2) sense of responsibility to family, (3) pregnancy, (4) religiosity, (5) life satisfaction, (6) reality testing ability, (7) positive coping skills, (8) positive problem-solving skills, (9) positive social support, and (10) positive therapeutic relationship.

The Reasons for Living Inventory (RFLI) [104] was developed to assess protective factors for suicidal behaviors. It is based on a cognitive–behavioral theory of suicidality suggesting that individuals who do not act on their suicidal impulses or feelings have different beliefs, expectations, and adaptive ways of thinking that help them resist the suicidal impulses than individuals who yield to suicidal urges and perform suicidal acts. The RFLI [104] measures six factors: (1) survival and coping beliefs, (2) responsibility to family, (3) child-related concerns, (4) fear of suicide, (5) fear of social disapproval, and (6) moral objections to suicide. Several studies reported that individuals who attempted suicide had significantly lower total RFLI scores than nonattempters [32,54,105].

Significant differences exist between levels of adaptive characteristics in women and men. Ellis and Lamis [106] observed that women consistently scored higher than men on the Survival and Coping Beliefs, Responsibility to Family, Child-Related Concerns, and Fear of Suicide subscales of the RFLI.

The protective role of social and cultural factors on suicidal behaviors has been consistently observed in many studies. The effect of sociocultural factors on suicidal risk may mediate part of the large differences in suicide rates that have been observed among different countries. Although the highest annual rates are in Eastern Europe and the former Soviet Union, with several countries reflecting more than 30 suicides per 100,000 individuals, the lowest rates are found in most Latin American and Muslim countries, with fewer than 6.5 per 100,000 individuals. However, some countries outside Europe, such as Guyana, the Republic of Korea, and Sri Lanka, have high suicide rates [16]. Among African American women, the protective effects of religion and extended kin networks might explain the very low rate of suicide [107].

Particularly in women, having children has been reported to have a protective effect against suicidal behaviors [108,109]. Qin and Mortensen [110] found that having young children was protective. In another study, Qin and colleagues [111] found that having a child younger than 2 years significantly decreased the suicide risk in women but not in men. In contrast, Malone and colleagues [54] found that child-related concerns assessed with the RFLI did not differ significantly between suicide attempters and nonattempters.

Although married adults have lower rates of suicide overall, young married couples may have increased suicide risk [22,112]. However, young widows have the highest suicide rates across all marital status groups in women [112].

For women in the general population, pregnancy and the puerperium also seem to be protective for suicidal behaviors [113], although suicide risk may be increased postpartum in teenagers, women who have a history of depression or suicide attempts, and women hospitalized with postpartum psychiatric disorders [22,91].

CONSIDERATIONS FOR TREATING YOUNG WOMEN

Depression, suicide ideation, and attempts among the young are frequently undetected and untreated by health professionals [114,115]. Although women are more willing than men to seek and accept help or treatment [22], young women have been reported to be more likely to receive care from nonspecialty mental health care providers [114].

Regarding pharmacologic treatments, although gender differences exist in the pharmacokinetics of several antidepressants, how they may affect clinical treatment response is unclear [116–118]. For example, women, particularly those who are premenopausal, have been reported to respond better to selective serotonin reuptake inhibitors than to tricyclic antidepressants (TCA) and norepinephrinergic tetracyclic antidepressants (maprotiline), whereas men tend to do the opposite [119–121]. Moreover, women who were taking imipramine (a TCA) tended to experience a significantly slower response than men and had higher rates of withdrawal from the study [120].

A possible explanation for these gender differences in treatment response is that female sex hormones may affect treatment response [120]. Increasing evidence supports the effect of female sex hormones on treatment response. Studies have reported that hormonal therapy could have positive effects in the treatment and prevention of depressive disorders [85,122]. Moreover, oral contraceptive pills may improve depressive symptoms and reduce mood fluctuation across the menstrual cycle [85]. In a study of premenopausal women who had major depressive disorder, those who used combined (estrogen plus progestin) oral contraception pills were significantly less depressed than those who underwent no hormone treatment [123]. Although the report of health risks associated with estrogen plus progestin treatment in postmenopausal women has slowed hormonal therapy research, this promising field requires further investigation [85].

SUMMARY

Suicide is one of the leading causes of death among young people, and suicide ideation and attempts are frequent in both general and clinical populations [8]. Clinicians assessing young patients must examine the presence of suicidal ideation, previous suicide attempts, factors that may interfere with treatment, and risk factors for suicidal behaviors, such as the presence of depression, drug or alcohol abuse, and access to firearms, to determine the level of risk [8,22]. Public health researchers must find out more about the risk factors for suicide among young women and evaluate effective measures for suicide prevention. Prevention strategies should be specifically tailored for this population, taking into account specific risk and protective factors and underlying reasons for suicidal acts [9].

References

[1] The Substance Abuse and Mental Health Services Administration's (SAMHSA) National Mental Health Information Center. Summary of National Strategy for Suicide Prevention: Goals and Objectives for Action. Available at: http://mentalhealth.samhsa.gov/publications/allpubs/SMA01-3518/default.asp#goal11. Accessed September 27, 2007.

[2] Kessler RC, Borges G, Walters EE. Prevalence of and risk factors for lifetime suicide attempts in the National Comorbidity Survey. Arch Gen Psychiatry 1999;56(7):617–26.

[3] Klerman GL. Clinical epidemiology of suicide. J Clin Psychiatry 1987;48(Suppl):33–8.

[4] Moscicki EK, O'Carroll P, Regier DA, et al. Suicide attempts in the Epidemiologic Catchment Area Study. Yale J Biol Med 1988;61(3):259–68.

[5] Spicer RS, Miller TR. Suicide acts in 8 states: incidence and case fatality rates by demographics and method. Am J Public Health 2000;90(12):1885–91.

[6] Kessler RC, Berglund P, Borges G, et al. Trends in suicide ideation, plans, gestures, and attempts in the United States, 1990–1992 to 2001–2003. JAMA 2005;293(20):2487–95.

[7] Kuo WH, Gallo JJ, Tien AY. Incidence of suicide ideation and attempts in adults: the 13-year follow-up of a community sample in Baltimore, Maryland. Psychol Med 2001;31(7): 1181–91.

[8] Posner K, Melvin GA, Stanley B, et al. Factors in the assessment of suicidality in youth. CNS Spectr 2007;12(2):156–62.

[9] Centers for Disease Control and Prevention (CDC). Suicide trends among youths and young adults aged 10–24 years—United States, 1990–2004. MMWR Morb Mortal Wkly Rep 2007;56(35):905–8.

[10] Patel V, Flisher AJ, Hetrick S, et al. Mental health of young people: a global public-health challenge. Lancet 2007;369(9569):1302–13.

[11] Verhulst FC, van der Ende J, Ferdinand RF, et al. The prevalence of DSM-III-R diagnoses in a national sample of Dutch adolescents. Arch Gen Psychiatry 1997;54(4):329–36.

[12] Garland AF, Hough RL, McCabe KM, et al. Prevalence of psychiatric disorders in youths across five sectors of care. J Am Acad Child Adolesc Psychiatry 2001;40(4):409–18.

[13] La Vecchia C, Lucchini F, Levi F. Worldwide trends in suicide mortality, 1955–1989. Acta Psychiatr Scand 1994;90(1):53–64.

[14] Mościcki EK. Gender differences in completed and attempted suicides. Ann Epidemiol 1994;4(2):152–8.

[15] Weissman MM, Bland RC, Canino GJ, et al. Prevalence of suicide ideation and suicide attempts in nine countries. Psychol Med 1999;29(1):9–17.

[16] World Health Organization. Suicide rates per 100,000 by country, year and sex. Geneva: World Health Organization; 2007. Available at: http://www.who.int/mental_health/prevention/suicide_rates/en/index.html. Accessed September 27, 2007.

[17] Yip PS, Liu KY. The ecological fallacy and the gender ratio of suicide in China. Br J Psychiatry 2006;189:465–6.

[18] Wasserman D, Cheng Q, Jiang GX. Global suicide rates among young people aged 15–19. World Psychiatry 2005;4(2):114–20.

[19] World Health Organization. Data and statistics web page. Quality of cause-of-death information: a challenge in large part of the world. Geneva: World Health Organization; 2007. Available at: http://www.who.int/research/cod_info_quality_20071005.pdf. Accessed September 27, 2007.

[20] Baca-Garcia E, Diaz-Sastre C, Basurte E, et al. A prospective study of the paradoxical relationship between impulsivity and lethality of suicide attempts. J Clin Psychiatry 2001;62(7):560–4.

[21] Krug EG, Dahlberg LL, Mercy JA, et al, editors. World report on violence and health. Geneva: World Health Organization; 2002. Available at: http://www.who.int/violence_injury_prevention/violence/world_report/en/full_en.pdf. Accessed September 27, 2007.

[22] American Psychiatric Association. Practice guideline for the assessment and treatment of patients with suicidal behaviors. Arlington (VA): American Psychiatric Association; 2003. Available at: http://www.psych.org/psych_pract/treatg/pg/SuicidalBehavior_05-15-06.pdf. Accessed September 27, 2007.

[23] Centers for Disease Control and Prevention. Web-based Injury Statistics Query and Reporting System. Available at: http://www.cdc.gov/ncipc/wisqars/. Accessed September 27, 2007.

[24] Centers for Disease Control and Prevention. Suicide: facts at a glance. 2007. Available at: http://www.cdc.gov/ncipc/dvp/Suicide/SuicideDataSheet.pdf. Accessed September 27, 2007.

[25] Eaton DK, Kann L, Kinchen SA, et al. Youth risk behavior surveillance—United States, 2005. MMWR Surveill Summ 2006;55(No. SS-5):1–108.

[26] Alonso J, Angermeyer MC, Bernert S, et al. Prevalence of mental disorders in Europe: results from the European Study of the Epidemiology of Mental Disorders (ESEMeD) project. Acta Psychiatr Scand Suppl 2004;109(420):21–7.

[27] Kessler RC, McGonagle KA, Swartz M, et al. Sex and depression in the National Comorbidity Survey. I: Lifetime prevalence, chronicity and recurrence. J Affect Disord 1993;29(2–3):85–96.

[28] Robins LN, Helzer JE, Weissman MM, et al. Lifetime prevalence of specific psychiatric disorders in three sites. Arch Gen Psychiatry 1984;41(10):949–58.

[29] Weissman MM, Leaf PJ, Holzer CE 3rd, et al. The epidemiology of depression. An update on sex differences in rates. J Affect Disord 1984;7(3–4):179–88.

[30] Oquendo MA, Currier D, Mann JJ. Prospective studies of suicidal behavior in major depressive and bipolar disorders: what is the evidence for predictive risk factors? Acta Psychiatr Scand 2006;114(3):151–8.

[31] Chen YW, Dilsaver SC. Lifetime rates of suicide attempts among subjects with bipolar and unipolar disorders relative to subjects with other Axis I disorders. Biol Psychiatry 1996;39(10):896–9.

[32] Mann JJ, Waternaux C, Haas GL, et al. Toward a clinical model of suicidal behavior in psychiatric patients. Am J Psychiatry 1999;156(2):181–9.

[33] Molnar BE, Berkman LF, Buka SL. Psychopathology, childhood sexual abuse and other childhood adversities: relative links to subsequent suicidal behaviour in the US. Psychol Med 2001;31(6):965–77.

[34] Molnar BE, Buka SL, Kessler RC. Child sexual abuse and subsequent psychopathology: results from the National Comorbidity Survey. Am J Public Health 2001;91(5):753–60.

[35] Wunderlich U, Bronisch T, Wittchen HU, et al. Gender differences in adolescents and young adults with suicidal behaviour. Acta Psychiatr Scand 2001;104(5):332–9.

[36] Murphy GE. Why women are less likely than men to commit suicide. Compr Psychiatry 1998;39(4):165–75.

[37] Oquendo MA, Ellis SP, Greenwald S, et al. Ethnic and sex differences in suicide rates relative to major depression in the United States. Am J Psychiatry 2001;158(10):1652–8.

[38] Beautrais AL. Suicide and serious suicide attempts in youth: a multiple-group comparison study. Am J Psychiatry 2003;160(6):1093–9.

[39] Edwards MJ, Holden RR. Coping, meaning in life, and suicidal manifestations: examining gender differences. J Clin Psychol 2001;57(12):1517–34.

[40] Shenassa ED, Catlin SN, Buka SL. Lethality of firearms relative to other suicide methods: a population based study. J Epidemiol Community Health 2003;57(2):120–4.

[41] Denning DG, Convell Y, King D, et al. Method choice, intent, and gender in completed suicide. Suicide Life Threat Behav 2000;30(3):282–8.

[42] Kposowa AJ, McElvain JP. Gender, place, and method of suicide. Soc Psychiatry Psychiatr Epidemiol 2006;41(6):435–43.

[43] Conner KR, Zhong Y. State firearm laws and rates of suicide in men and women. Am J Prev Med 2003;25(4):320–4.

[44] Hawton K. Sex and suicide. Gender differences in suicidal behaviour. Br J Psychiatry 2000;177:484–5.

[45] Shiang J. Does culture make a difference? Racial/ethnic patterns of completed suicide in San Francisco, CA 1987–1996 and clinical applications. Suicide Life Threat Behav 1998;28(4):338–54.

[46] Sorenson SB, Golding JM. Suicide ideation and attempts in Hispanics and non-Hispanic whites: demographic and psychiatric disorder issues. Suicide Life Threat Behav 1988; 18(3):205–19.

[47] Joe S, Baser RE, Breeden G, et al. Prevalence of and risk factors for lifetime suicide attempts among blacks in the United States. JAMA 2006;296(17):2112–23.

[48] Oquendo MA, Dragatsi D, Harkavy-Friedman J, et al. Protective factors against suicidal behavior in Latinos. J Nerv Ment Dis 2005;193(7):438–43.

[49] Grant BF, Stinson FS, Hasin DS, et al. Immigration and lifetime prevalence of DSM-IV psychiatric disorders among Mexican Americans and non-Hispanic whites in the United States: results from the National Epidemiologic Survey on Alcohol and Related Conditions. Arch Gen Psychiatry 2004;61(10):1226–33.

[50] Alegria M, Canino G, Stinson FS, et al. Nativity and DSM-IV psychiatric disorders among Puerto Ricans, Cuban Americans, and non-Latino Whites in the United States: results from the National Epidemiologic Survey on Alcohol and Related Conditions. J Clin Psychiatry 2006;67(1):56–65.

[51] Oquendo MA, Lizardi D, Greenwald S, et al. Rates of lifetime suicide attempt and rates of lifetime major depression in different ethnic groups in the United States. Acta Psychiatr Scand 2004;110(6):446–51.

[52] Fortuna LR, Perez DJ, Canino G, et al. Prevalence and correlates of lifetime suicidal ideation and suicide attempts among Latino subgroups in the United States. J Clin Psychiatry 2007;68(4):572–81.

[53] Perez-Rodriguez MM, Baca-Garcia E, Quintero-Gutierrez FJ, et al. Demand for psychiatric emergency services and immigration. Findings in a Spanish hospital during the year 2003. Eur J Public Health 2006;16(4):383–7.

[54] Malone KM, Oquendo MA, Haas GL, et al. Protective factors against suicidal acts in major depression: reasons for living. Am J Psychiatry 2000;157(7):1084–8.

[55] Oquendo MA, Bongiovi-Garcia ME, Galfalvy H, et al. Sex differences in clinical predictors of suicidal acts after major depression: a prospective study. Am J Psychiatry 2007;164(1):134–41.

[56] Baca-Garcia E, Parra CP, Perez-Rodriguez MM, et al. Psychosocial stressors may be strongly associated with suicide attempts. Stress and Health 2007;23(3):191–8.

[57] Cavanagh JT, Owens DG, Johnstone EC. Life events in suicide and undetermined death in south-east Scotland: a case-control study using the method of psychological autopsy. Soc Psychiatry Psychiatr Epidemiol 1999;34(12):645–50.

[58] Heikkinen M, Aro H, Lönnqvist J. Life events and social support in suicide. Suicide Life Threat Behav 1993;23(4):343–58.

[59] Paykel ES, Prusoff BA, Myers JK. Suicide attempts and recent life events. A controlled comparison. Arch Gen Psychiatry 1975;32(3):327–33.

[60] Phillips MR, Yang G, Zhang Y, et al. Risk factors for suicide in China: a national case-control psychological autopsy study. Lancet 2002;360(9347):1728–36.

[61] Yen S, Pagano ME, Shea MT, et al. Recent life events preceding suicide attempts in a personality disorder sample: findings from the collaborative longitudinal personality disorders study. J Consult Clin Psychol 2005;73(1):99–105.

[62] Baca-Garcia E, Perez-Rodriguez MM, Diaz Sastre C, et al. Suicidal behavior in schizophrenia and depression: a comparison. Schizophr Res 2005;75(1):77–81.

[63] Brodsky BS, Groves SA, Oquendo MA, et al. Interpersonal precipitants and suicide attempts in borderline personality disorder. Suicide Life Threat Behav 2006;36(3):313–22.

[64] Dervic K, Grunebaum MF, Burke AK, et al. Protective factors against suicidal behavior in depressed adults reporting childhood abuse. J Nerv Ment Dis 2006;194(12):971–4.

[65] Arsenault-Lapierre G, Kim C, Turecki G. Psychiatric diagnoses in 3275 suicides: a meta-analysis. BMC Psychiatry 2004;4:37.

[66] Harris EC, Barraclough B. Suicide as an outcome for mental disorders. A meta-analysis. Br J Psychiatry 1997;170:205–28.

[67] Lonnqvist JK, Henriksson MM, Isometsa ET, et al. Mental disorders and suicide prevention. Psychiatry Clin Neurosci 1995;49(Suppl 1):S111–6.

[68] Radomsky ED, Haas GL, Mann JJ, et al. Suicidal behavior in patients with schizophrenia and other psychotic disorders. Am J Psychiatry 1999;156(10):1590–5.

[69] Kent A, Goddard KL, van den Berk PA, et al. Eating disorder in women admitted to hospital following deliberate self-poisoning. Acta Psychiatr Scand 1997;95(2):140–4.

[70] Thompson KM, Wonderlich SA, Crosby RD, et al. The neglected link between eating disturbances and aggressive behavior in girls. J Am Acad Child Adolesc Psychiatry 1999;38(10):1277–84.

[71] Marino MF, Zanarini MC. Relationship between EDNOS and its subtypes and borderline personality disorder. Int J Eat Disord 2001;29(3):349–53.

[72] Zanarini MC, Frankenburg FR, Hennen J, et al. The McLean Study of Adult Development (MSAD): overview and implications of the first six years of prospective follow-up. J Personal Disord 2005;19(5):505–23.

[73] Larsson JO, Hellzén M. Patterns of personality disorders in women with chronic eating disorders. Eat Weight Disord 2004;9(3):200–5.

[74] Gomberg ES. Suicide risk among women with alcohol problems. Am J Public Health 1989;79(10):1363–5.

[75] Petronis KR, Samuels JF, Moscicki EK, et al. An epidemiologic investigation of potential risk factors for suicide attempts. Soc Psychiatry Psychiatr Epidemiol 1990;25(4):193–9.

[76] Inskip HM, Harris EC, Barraclough B. Lifetime risk of suicide for affective disorder, alcoholism and schizophrenia. Br J Psychiatry 1998;172:35–7.

[77] Carballo JJ, Bird H, Giner L, et al. Pathological personality traits and suicidal ideation among older adolescents and young adults with alcohol misuse: a pilot case-control study in a primary care setting. Int J Adolesc Med Health 2007;19(1):79–89.

[78] Preuss UW, Schuckit MA, Smith TL, et al. Comparison of 3190 alcohol-dependent individuals with and without suicide attempts. Alcohol Clin Exp Res 2002;26(4):471–7.

[79] Roy A, Lamparski D, DeJong J, et al. Characteristics of alcoholics who attempt suicide. Am J Psychiatry 1990;147(6):761–5.

[80] Sher L, Sperling D, Stanley BH, et al. Triggers for suicidal behavior in depressed older adolescents and young adults: do alcohol use disorders make a difference? Int J Adolesc Med Health 2007;19(1):91–8.

[81] Brent DA, Perper JA, Moritz G, et al. Psychiatric risk factors for adolescent suicide: a case-control study. J Am Acad Child Adolesc Psychiatry 1993;32(3):521–9.

[82] Fowler RC, Rich CL, Young D. San Diego Suicide Study. II. Substance abuse in young cases. Arch Gen Psychiatry 1986;43(10):962–5.

[83] Skodol AE, Bender DS. Why are women diagnosed borderline more than men? Psychiatr Q 2003;74(4):349–60.

[84] Persson ML, Runeson BS, Wasserman D. Diagnoses, psychosocial stressors and adaptive functioning in attempted suicide. Ann Clin Psychiatry 1999;11(3):119–28.

[85] Ancelin ML, Scali J, Ritchie K. Hormonal therapy and depression: are we overlooking an important therapeutic alternative? J Psychosom Res 2007;62(4):473–85.

[86] Baca-García E, Sánchez-González A, González Diaz-Corralero P, et al. Menstrual cycle and profiles of suicidal behaviour. Acta Psychiatr Scand 1998;97(1):32–5.

[87] Baca-Garcia E, Diaz-Sastre C, de Leon J, et al. The relationship between menstrual cycle phases and suicide attempts. Psychosom Med 2000;62(1):50–60.

[88] Baca-Garcia E, Diaz-Sastre C, Saiz-Ruiz J, et al. Influence of psychiatric diagnoses on the relationship between suicide attempts and the menstrual cycle. Psychosom Med 2001;63(3):509–10.

[89] Baca-Garcia E, Diaz-Sastre C, Ceverino A, et al. Association between the menses and suicide attempts: A replication study. Psychosom Med 2003;65(2):237–44.

[90] Saunders KE, Hawton K. Suicidal behaviour and the menstrual cycle. Psychol Med 2006;36(7):901–12.

[91] Appleby L, Mortensen PB, Faragher EB. Suicide and other causes of mortality after postpartum psychiatric admission. Br J Psychiatry 1998;173:209–11.

[92] Carretti N, Florio P, Bertolin A, et al. Serum fluctuations of total and free tryptophan levels during the menstrual cycle are related to gonadotrophins and reflect brain serotonin utilization. Hum Reprod 2005;20(6):1548–53.

[93] Kamali M, Oquendo MA, Mann JJ. Understanding the neurobiology of suicidal behavior. Depress Anxiety 2001;14(3):164–76.

[94] Berman NEJ, Puri V, Chandrala S, et al. Serotonin in trigeminal ganglia of female rodents: relevance to menstrual migraine. Headache 2006;46(8):1230–45.

[95] Fink G, Sumner BE, McQueen JK, et al. Sex steroid control of mood, mental state and memory. Clin Exp Pharmacol Physiol 1998;25(10):764–75.

[96] Gundlah C, Lu N, Bethea C. Ovarian steroid regulation of monoamine oxidase-A and B mRNAs in the macaque dorsal raphe and hypothalamic nuclei. Psychopharmacology (Berl) 2002;160(3):271–82.

[97] Hiroi R, McDevitt RA, Neumaier JF. Estrogen selectively increases tryptophan hydroxylase-2 mRNA expression in distinct subregions of rat midbrain raphe Nucleus: association between gene expression and anxiety behavior in the open field. Biol Psychiatry 2006;60(3):288–95.

[98] Arango V, Underwood MD, Boldrini M, et al. Serotonin 1A receptors, serotonin transporter binding and serotonin transporter mRNA expression in the brainstem of depressed suicide victims. Neuropsychopharmacology 2001;25(6):892–903.

[99] McQueen JK, Wilson H, Fink G. Estradiol-17 beta increases serotonin transporter (SERT) mRNA levels and the density of SERT-binding sites in female rat brain. Brain Res Mol Brain Res 1997;45(1):13–23.

[100] Baca-Garcia E, Vaquero C, Diaz-Sastre C, et al. A pilot study on a gene-hormone interaction in female suicide attempts. Eur Arch Psychiatry Clin Neurosci 2003;253(6):281–5.

[101] Martin CA, Mainous AG, Mainous RO, et al. Progesterone and adolescent suicidality. Biol Psychiatry 1997;42(10):956–8.
[102] Dubrovsky BO. Steroids, neuroactive steroids and neurosteroids in psychopathology. Prog Neuropsychopharmacol Biol Psychiatry 2005;29(2):169–92.
[103] Dahlen ER, Canetto SS. The role of gender and suicide precipitant in attitudes toward nonfatal suicide behavior. Death Stud 2002;26(2):99–116.
[104] Linehan MM, Goodstein JL, Nielsen SL, et al. Reasons for staying alive when you are thinking of killing yourself: the reasons for living inventory. J Consult Clin Psychol 1983;51(2):276–86.
[105] Lizardi D, Currier D, Galfalvy H, et al. Perceived reasons for living at index hospitalization and future suicide attempt. J Nerv Ment Dis 2007;195(5):451–5.
[106] Ellis JB, Lamis DA. Adaptive characteristics and suicidal behavior: a gender comparison of young adults. Death Stud 2007;31(9):845–54.
[107] Gibbs JT. African-American suicide: a cultural paradox. Suicide Life Threat Behav 1997;27(1):68–79.
[108] Hoyer G, Lund E. Suicide among women related to number of children in marriage. Arch Gen Psychiatry 1993;50(2):134–7.
[109] Warshaw MG, Dolan RT, Keller MB. Suicidal behavior in patients with current or past panic disorder: five years of prospective data from the Harvard/Brown Anxiety Research Program. Am J Psychiatry 2000;157(11):1876–8.
[110] Qin P, Mortensen PB. The impact of parental status on the risk of completed suicide. Arch Gen Psychiatry 2003;60(8):797–802.
[111] Qin P, Agerbo E, Westergård-Nielsen N, et al. Gender differences in risk factors for suicide in Denmark. Br J Psychiatry 2000;177(6):546–50.
[112] Luoma JB, Pearson JL. Suicide and marital status in the United States, 1991–1996: is widowhood a risk factor? Am J Public Health 2002;92(9):1518–22.
[113] Harris EC, Barraclough BM. Suicide as an outcome for medical disorders. Medicine (Baltimore) 1994;73(6):281–96.
[114] Cheung AH, Dewa CS. Mental health service use among adolescents and young adults with major depressive disorder and suicidality. Can J Psychiatry 2007;52(4):228–32.
[115] Wang PS, Berglund P, Kessler RC. Recent care of common mental disorders in the United States: prevalence and conformance with evidence-based recommendations. J Gen Intern Med 2000;15(5):284–92.
[116] Frackiewicz EJ, Sramek JJ, Cutler NR. Gender differences in depression and antidepressant pharmacokinetics and adverse events. Ann Pharmacother 2000;34(1):80–8.
[117] Thase ME, Entsuah R, Cantillon M, et al. Relative antidepressant efficacy of venlafaxine and SSRIs: sex-age interactions. J Womens Health (Larchmt) 2005;14(7):609–16.
[118] Yonkers KA, Brawman-Mintzer O. The pharmacologic treatment of depression: is gender a critical factor? J Clin Psychiatry 2002;63(7):610–5.
[119] Baca E, Garcia-Garcia M, Porras-Chavarino A. Gender differences in treatment response to sertraline versus imipramine in patients with nonmelancholic depressive disorders. Prog Neuropsychopharmacol Biol Psychiatry 2004;28(1):57–65.
[120] Kornstein SG, Schatzberg AF, Thase ME, et al. Gender differences in treatment response to sertraline versus imipramine in chronic depression. Am J Psychiatry 2000;157(9):1445–52.
[121] Martenyi F, Dossenbach M, Mraz K, et al. Gender differences in the efficacy of fluoxetine and maprotiline in depressed patients: a double-blind trial of antidepressants with serotonergic or norepinephrinergic reuptake inhibition profile. Eur Neuropsychopharmacol 2001;11(3):227–32.
[122] Zanardi R, Rossini D, Magri L, et al. Response to SSRIs and role of the hormonal therapy in post-menopausal depression. Eur Neuropsychopharmacol 2007;17(6–7):400–5.
[123] Young EA, Kornstein SG, Harvey AT, et al. Influences of hormone-based contraception on depressive symptoms in premenopausal women with major depression. Psychoneuroendocrinology 2007;32(7):843–53.

Psychiatr Clin N Am 31 (2008) 333–356

PSYCHIATRIC CLINICS
OF NORTH AMERICA

ELSEVIER
SAUNDERS

Suicidal Behavior in Elders

Yeates Conwell, MD[a,b,*], Caitlin Thompson, PhD[a,b]

[a]University of Rochester School of Medicine, 300 Crittenden Boulevard, Rochester, NY 14642, USA
[b]University of Rochester Center for the Study and Prevention of Suicide (CSPS), 300 Crittenden Boulevard, Rochester, NY 14642, USA

I n the United States, as in many countries of the world, older adults are at greater risk for suicide than other age groups. This article provides an overview of suicide in later life and a foundation on which to base decisions about the design and implementation of preventive interventions. Ultimately, implementation of effective suicide prevention strategies and reduction of self-inflicted deaths by older people will depend on information obtained at each of four stages of the preventive intervention research cycle, depicted in Fig. 1. First is the definition of the scope of the problem: rates of suicide in the older population and their patterns over time and space. Second is the characterization of suicide in older adults, with particular reference to risk and protective factors. These in turn suggest potential pathogenic mechanisms and indicate where one can obtain the most efficient access to older adults at risk, or who may be targets of preventive interventions. With this information, those interventions can be designed and preliminary testing conducted for their refinement before they are implemented on a larger scale. With effective surveillance tools established to evaluate the impact of the intervention, the cycle then starts afresh.

This article first considers special challenges to suicide prevention in older adults, and then reviews the information available to inform each of these steps in the late-life suicide preventive intervention research cycle.

CHALLENGES TO LATE-LIFE SUICIDE PREVENTION

Developing suicide prevention strategies in older adults is particularly challenging because of a range of factors at the individual, provider, systems, and even social/cultural levels. To the extent that suicide prevention relies on timely and effective detection and treatment of mental disorders, older adults face multiple barriers to the acquisition of care [1]. At the service system level, discriminatory barriers still exist in access to mental health care. Medicare recipients are

This work was supported by Grant #T32MH20061 and #P20 MH071897 from the National Institute of Mental Health.

*Corresponding author. E-mail address: yeates_conwell@urmc.rochester.edu (Y. Conwell).

0193-953X/08/$ – see front matter
doi:10.1016/j.psc.2008.01.004

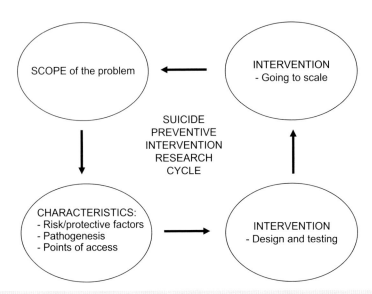

Fig. 1. The suicide preventive intervention research cycle.

required to pay 50% of charges for mental health services, rather than a 20% copay for physical health conditions. Older adults tend not to use mental health services, but rather seek care from primary care providers. Affective syndromes may be milder in older adults, expressed as physical symptoms [2]. Their presentations are further complicated by comorbid medical illness and the multiple medications prescribed to treat them. Older adults are reluctant to talk about emotional problems and are less likely to report depression and suicidal ideation to others [3,4]. Although doctors see many older people in a typical primary care practice, they often lack specialized training in geriatric care, the information and decision support needed to optimize quality of care, and the time necessary to diagnose affective disorders and assess suicide risk among so many competing demands [5,6].

Consequently, fewer than half of older people with clinically significant mood disorders are diagnosed with depression in primary care, and of those, a minority undergo treatment for their illness. Among those who are treated, few receive the intervention at sufficient doses and duration to be effective [7]. Many primary care providers fear that giving the older patient a psychiatric diagnosis or referral for mental health care will be stigmatizing for the patient, and therefore avoid the issue altogether. Underlying many of these barriers is bias against aging and mental illness and promulgation of the attitude that such feelings are "normal" among older people who experience multiple losses, physical illness, and functional decline.

Characteristics of suicidal behavior in older adults also present special challenges to its prevention. Available data indicate that 8 to 40 suicides are attempted for each completed suicide in the general population [8]. In younger adult groups, that ratio may be as high as 200:1 [9]. Among older adults, however, a far higher proportion of suicidal acts are fatal; for every completed suicide, an estimated two to four attempts occur [10]. Several factors may account for this important observation. Older adults in general (and those at risk for suicide in particular) tend to be frailer, and are therefore more likely to die as a result of any self-inflicted injury. Second, older adults are more likely than younger people to live alone, and are therefore less likely to be found in sufficient time to be rescued after an attempt. Finally, older people tend to use more immediately lethal means to kill themselves than younger age groups, and also implement their suicidal acts in a manner more likely to result in death [11]. In 2004, 52% of suicides in the United States were by firearm: 57% of men and 32% of women [12]. Among those older than 65 years, however, more than 72% of suicides were by firearm. These observations indicate the importance of performing screening and assessment to identify seniors who have suicidal thoughts and implementing aggressive clinical interventions to protect and treat them. However, because of the various barriers, fewer opportunities are available to detect and treat older adults at high risk for suicide. Greater emphasis may need to be placed, therefore, on interventions to prevent the development of suicidal states.

SCOPE OF THE PROBLEM: THE EPIDEMIOLOGY OF SUICIDE IN LATER LIFE

Each year in the United States approximately 32,000 deaths result from suicide, of which more than 5000 (14%) are among people older than 65 years [12]. Fig. 2 illustrates the complex relationships among suicide risk, age, gender, and race. At each point in the life course, suicide rates are higher for men than women and for whites than non-whites. One notable exception is American Indian youth, who have higher rates of suicide than their white counterparts. The rise in suicide risk for older adults in the United States is solely accounted for by the dramatic increase in rates among older white men to 48.7/100,000, which is more than four times the nation's overall age-adjusted rate of 11.1/100,000.

Countries that report statistics to the World Health Organization have considerable variability in associations among age, gender, and suicide risk. Fig. 3, for example, illustrates rates reported to the World Health Organization for Canada (2002) and rural China (1999) [13]. In Canada, the highest rates are seen among young adult and middle-aged men and women, respectively. In rural China, suicide risk for men and women is comparable, with rates rising to more than 100/100,000 in the oldest age groups of both genders. These variations may reflect reporting differences among countries, but cultural factors clearly play an important role.

Suicide rates among people older than 65 years declined substantially over the 20th century, a change ascribed to improved economic well-being of seniors who have social security, Medicare legislation, improved access to health care and effective treatments for depressive illness [14], and other undetermined

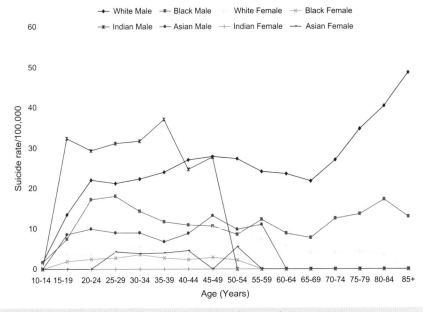

Fig. 2. Suicide rates by age, race, and gender in the United States in 2004.

factors [15]. Between 2000 and 2004, that trend continued, with the overall late-life suicide rate decreasing from 15.1 to 14.3 per 100,000 [12].

Required reporting of cause of death to the Centers for Disease Control and Prevention constitutes an effective surveillance mechanism for completed suicide in the United States, but no mechanism exists for suicide attempts or ideation. Instead, epidemiologic data must be derived from population-based

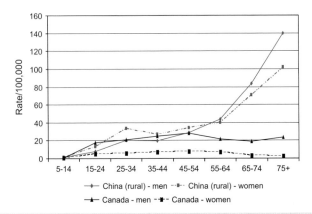

Fig. 3. Suicide rates by age and gender for Canada (2002) and rural China (1999).

surveys. These studies consistently show that rates of suicidal ideation and a history of suicide attempts are lower in elders than younger adult populations [4,16]. Variation in methodology among studies, lack of standardized definitions, and few well-validated measures of suicidal ideation and behavior limit the ability to draw firmer conclusions.

The presence of a history of either suicide attempts or suicidal ideation increases risk for subsequent suicidal behavior and completed suicide in older adults, just as at earlier points in the life course [17–19]. Therefore, interventions designed to prevent suicidal ideation and behavior may be effective in reducing completed suicides. It would be a mistake, however, to assume that ideation or attempts were close proxies for suicide. Rates of ideation and attempts are far higher in younger adults and women, whereas completed suicide rates are highest in older men; approximately 75% of older adults who commit suicide have never made a prior attempt [20]. The remainder of this article, therefore, focuses on the available evidence to inform the design of preventive interventions that target completed suicide.

RISK AND PROTECTIVE FACTORS
Much of what we know about risk factors for suicide in later life is derived from "psychological autopsies" (PAs), a research method in which mental and physical health status and social circumstances are reconstructed from records and interviews with next of kin and other knowledgeable informants [21]. Findings from several PAs of older adult suicides were recently published [22–26], including a handful that used matched comparison groups [19,27–33], allowing factors associated with suicide case status to be identified and quantified. These findings map well onto the multiaxial system of psychiatry's Diagnostic and Statistical Manual of Mental Disorders [34], forming a framework for the subsequent discussion.

AXIS I: MAJOR PSYCHIATRIC ILLNESS
Table 1 lists the distribution of psychiatric diagnoses among older adults who committed suicide and underwent PA. Affective illness was the most common disorder, present in 54% to 87% of cases. Major affective disorder accounted for most of these affective syndromes. The prevalence of substance use disorders varied widely, from 3% to 46%, reflecting the different age groups, locations, and dates of studies; those conducted more recently and in Western countries tend to have higher rates. Primary psychotic illnesses, including schizophrenia, schizoaffective illness, and delusional disorder, play a smaller role in suicide in later life, as do anxiety disorders and other diagnoses. Overall, between 71% and 95% of elderly suicide decedents had a diagnosable Axis I condition.

Table 2 lists results from case-control psychological autopsy (PA) studies for which the inclusion of a demographically matched comparison group enables calculation of odds ratios, which indicate the strength of association between major psychiatric illnesses and suicide in older adults. The odds of a subject

Table 1
Axis I diagnoses made by psychologic autopsy in studies of late life suicide

| Study | Location | Age (y) | Sample size | Diagnosis (%) | | | | | | |
				Major depression	Other mood disorder	Alcohol use disorder	Other drug use disorder	Nonaffective psychosis	No diagnosis[a]
Barraclough [22]	West Sussex, UK	≥65	N = 30	87		3		0	13
Beautrais [31]	New Zealand	≥55	N = 31 20 men (64.5%) 11 women (35.5%)	86		14		—	9
Carney et al. [23]	San Diego, US	≥60	N = 49 29 men (59.2%) 20 women (40.8%)	54		22		—	14
Chiu et al. [27]	Hong Kong	≥60	N = 70 32 men (45.7%) 38 women (54.3%)	53 46.9% 57.9%	26 34.4% 18.4%	3 6.3% 0%	—	9 9.4% 7.9%	14 12.5% 15.8%
Clark [24]	Chicago, US	≥65	N = 54	54	11	19		0	24

Study	Location	Age	N							
Conwell et al. [25]	Monroe County, US	55–74	N = 36 28 men (77.8%) 8 women (22.2%)	47	17	43		3	6	8
		75–92	N = 14 9 men (64.3%) 5 women (35.7%)	57	21	27		7	0	29
Harwood et al. [32]	Central England, UK	≥60	100	63		5		5	4	23
Henriksson et al. [26]	Finland	≥60	43 34 men (54.1%) 39 women (45.9%)	44	21		25		5	12
Waern et al. [28]	Goteborg, Sweden	≥65	N = 85 46 men (54.1%) 39 women (45.9%)	46	36		27	8	8	5

aIncludes cases with insufficient data to allow diagnosis.

Table 2
Odds ratios for suicide by Axis I diagnosis in controlled psychologic autopsy studies of older adults

Odds ratio	Harwood et al. [32]	Beautrais [31]	Waern et al. [28]	Chiu et al. [27]
Any Axis I diagnosis	—	43.9	113.1	50.0
Any mood disorder	4.0	184.6	63.1	59.2
Major depressive episode	—	—	28.6	36.3
Substance use disorder	ns	4.4	43.1	ns
Anxiety disorder	—	—	3.6	ns
Schizophrenic spectrum	ns	—	10.7	>1.0
Dementia/delirium	0.2	—	ns	ns

Abbreviation: ns, not significant.

in these studies having any Axis I diagnosis was between 44 and 113 times higher among older suicides than matched controls [27,28,31]. The association with mood disorders, and major depression in particular, was especially high. The lower (but still significant) odds ratio for any mood disorder reported by Harwood and colleagues [32] is easily explained by the greater likelihood of affective illness in the population of older adults who died of natural causes in the hospital that they selected for comparison.

Two of the four studies that examined diagnoses of substance use disorder found a significant association with suicide case status, and one of two studies reported a significant relationship between anxiety disorders and suicide in older adults. Similarly, schizophrenic spectrum disorders were significantly associated with suicide in two of three studies, although at low odds ratios.

The devastating effects of dementia on patient and family and its close association with mood disorders, suicidal ideation, and suicide attempts all suggest that risk for suicide is high in people with the disease. However, of four case-control studies that attempted to diagnose dementia or delirium using the PA method, only one reported a significant association. Harwood and colleagues [32] found that dementia/delirium had a protective effect (odds ratio <1.0). This counterintuitive finding likely reflects the special characteristics of their comparison group, because hospitalized patients who die of natural causes are more likely to be cognitively impaired before death than those commit suicide and were not hospitalized. Until further research can address this critical question, optimal clinical practice should assume that any older adult with dementia or delirium is at increased risk for suicide.

AXIS II: PERSONALITY TRAITS AND DISORDERS

Investigators have long noted associations between late-life suicides and traits such as timidity and shy seclusiveness [35], hostility, and a rigid, independent style [35,36]. Only one case-control PA study examined whether personality disorders elevate risk in this age group. Harwood and colleagues [32] found that levels of anankastic (obsessional) and anxious traits significantly distinguished suicides from natural deaths, but personality disorder per se did not.

Using an informant-report version of the NEO Personality Inventory, Duberstein and colleagues [37] also examined personality traits in individuals older than 50 years who committed suicide and a matched, living comparison group [38]. Of the five domains of personality measured (neuroticism, extroversion, openness to experience [OTE], agreeableness, and conscientiousness), high neuroticism and low OTE distinguish the groups. Low OTE is associated with muted affective and hedonic responses, a constricted range of interests, and a strong preference for the familiar over the novel. These investigators posit that patients who have low OTE are at risk for suicide because they are less well-equipped socially and psychologically to manage the challenges of aging and more likely to not be recognized as being in distress and in need of intervention [39].

Hopelessness, shown by Beck and colleagues [40,41] to be a significant predictor of suicidal ideation, intent, and eventual suicide in mixed-age samples, may have special relevance in elderly individuals [42,43], including as a trait characteristic or marker of suicide risk. Szanto and colleagues [44] have shown that hopelessness remains significantly elevated after resolution of major depression in older adults who have a lifetime history of suicide attempts. Hopelessness, therefore, may have specific implications in designing preventive interventions using cognitive behavioral strategies, although their relevance and applicability to suicide and older adults remains largely unexplored.

AXIS III: PHYSICAL ILLNESS
Because physical illnesses are so common in older adults, the relative risk for suicide associated with them, and their usefulness in identifying any individual in need of acute intervention, is low. Furthermore, the association between physical illnesses and suicide in later life could be partly explained by the mediating effect of depression (physical illness causes depression and depression increases risk for suicide).

Studies linking death records with disease registries have found significant associations between suicide and HIV/AIDS, Huntington's disease, multiple sclerosis, renal disease, peptic ulcer disease, spinal cord injury, and systemic lupus erythematosus [45]. Studies have also found consistent associations between suicide and malignant neoplasms (other than skin cancer), and more variable associations with heart and lung disease; epilepsy and other central nervous system (CNS) disorders; and genitourinary and gastrointestinal illnesses [46,47]. In general, the relative risk for suicide is 1.5 to 4 times higher if an individual has one of these illnesses. Compared with the strength of association between suicide and psychiatric illness, the added risk for medical illness is small. However, older adults may have multiple comorbid medical conditions, and as the number of illnesses increases so does their cumulative risk. Juurlink and colleagues [46] linked prescription records for all residents of Ontario, Canada, aged 65 years and older with provincial coroners' reports of suicide to conduct a case-control analysis of risk associated with specific medical conditions. They found that patients who had three physical illnesses had approximately a threefold increase in the estimated relative risk for suicide compared with subjects who had no diagnosis, whereas older adults who had seven or more illnesses had an approximately nine times greater risk for suicide.

AXIS IV: LIFE EVENT STRESSORS AND SOCIAL CIRCUMSTANCES

The life events associated with suicide in older adults are those typically associated with aging: bereavement, financial stressors associated with retirement and living on reduced means, family discord and loss of social support, and the social and psychological impacts of physical illness. Controlled PA studies again help define whether these stressors are present before suicide more often in older adults than in the general older adult population.

In her PA study of older adults in New Zealand, Beautrais [31] found that elders who committed suicide were more likely to have experienced serious relationship and financial problems in the past year than controls. In Sweden, Rubenowitz and colleagues [33] found, using multivariate analyses, that suicides were more likely than controls to have experienced family discord and financial trouble in the 2 years preceding death, and that after accounting for mental illness, family discord continued to distinguish the groups. In their PA study of individuals older than 50 years who committed suicide in Western New York State, Duberstein and colleagues [29] reported that family discord and employment change distinguished suicides from controls even after adjusting for sociodemographic characteristics and mental disorders that developed in the prior year. Conceptualizing social support as a protective factor, Turvey and colleagues [48] analyzed prospectively collected data in the Established Populations' for Epidemiologic Studies of the Elderly database. They found that having a greater number of friends and relatives with whom to confide was associated with significantly reduced suicide risk in these older adults. Miller [49] reported that matched community controls were significantly more likely than elderly men who committed suicide to have had a confidant, and Barraclough [22] used census data for comparison with elder suicides to conclude that cases were more likely to live alone than their peers in the community. The weight of the evidence indicates that, like psychological and medical factors, social stressors place older adults at risk, whereas robust social supports seem to be a buffer against suicide.

Beautrais [31] used her New Zealand PA study data to estimate the population attributable risk (PAR) for suicide in later life associated with major affective illness and low social support. The PAR statistic estimates the portion of an adverse outcome that may be avoided if a risk factor could be eliminated. She found that if all late-life major depressive episodes could be prevented, suicide rates among older adults would drop by almost 75%. If all seniors could be assured adequate social support, suicides would drop by 27%. These findings have clear implications for the design of preventive interventions in late life.

AXIS V: FUNCTIONING

Measurement of functional status is a core component of comprehensive clinical assessment in geriatric medicine and psychiatry because it is often a sensitive indicator of underlying physical and psychological problems. Defining associations between functional decrements and suicidal behavior in older adults, therefore, may also help identify those in need of further assessment and intervention. Typical measurements include activities of daily living (ADLs), such as dressing and feeding oneself, and higher-order skills, such as using the telephone or managing one's finances (called *instrumental activities of daily living*, or IADLs).

Only a few controlled studies of late-life suicide, however, have examined the construct of functional capacity. Conwell and colleagues [19] compared functional status among adults aged 60 and older enrolled in primary care practices who had taken their own lives, with a matched sample of living primary care patients. Along with measures of physical health, ADL and IADL scales significantly distinguished the groups. However, after controlling for the presence of mood disorders, neither physical health nor functional variables remained significant predictors of suicide status. Tsoh and colleagues [50] examined IADLs among 66 elderly suicide attempters, 67 suicide completers, and 91 community-dwelling comparison subjects aged 65 years or older, and found that both attempters and completers had significantly greater functional impairment than the nonsuicidal group. Further studies that include more refined measurement of functional capacity in discreet domains are needed.

OTHER FACTORS AND POTENTIAL MECHANISMS

Another potential risk factor with implications for prevention is access to lethal means. Older adults tend to act on suicidal thoughts with greater lethality of intent and implementation, and use more immediately lethal means, particularly firearms. In his PA study of older men who took their own lives, Miller [49] observed that, although no difference was seen between men who completed suicides and controls in the proportion who owned a firearm, a significantly greater proportion of men who completed suicide had acquired the weapon within the past week. In the authors' controlled PA study in Western New York State, they found that the presence of a handgun (but not a rifle) in the home significantly increased risk for suicide in elderly men but not women [51]. Among those who kept a gun, storing the weapon loaded and unlocked were also independent predictors of suicide case status.

Among the exciting advances in suicide research in recent decades are the observed associations between suicidal behavior and a range of neurobiological parameters. The most consistent findings suggest that abnormalities in central serotonergic function predispose individuals to act impulsively and aggressively in the face of dysphoria, hopelessness, and emergent suicidal ideation in the depressed state [52]. Noradrenergic, dopaminergic, and other neurobiological systems have also been implicated [53]. The dramatic rise in suicide rates concomitant with age among men in the United States and among men and women in many other countries raises the question of whether aging-related changes in neurobiological systems may contribute. However, few studies have examined these questions in older adults because high rates of medication use and medical comorbidity in elderly individuals who commit suicide complicate the interpretation of findings.

Several investigators have explored whether measures of brain structure or neuropsychological function distinguish those at greater risk for suicide. For example, underlying vascular disease may predispose to depression [54,55], but also result in abnormalities in frontal executive function that could impair a person's capacity to manage stress effectively [55]. Keilp and colleagues [56] found that adult suicide attempters performed poorly on frontal executive tasks relative to controls, whereas King and colleagues [57] made a similar observation in older adults who attempted suicide. Ahearn and colleagues [58] reported that elderly depressives with lifetime histories of suicide attempts had significantly more subcortical gray matter hyperintensities on MRI than carefully matched depressives with no previous suicide attempt history, further supporting the hypothesis that underlying vascular disease may predispose to late-life suicidal acts.

Elucidation of neurobiological mechanisms for the expression of suicidal behavior has exciting implications for the design of preventive interventions. Currently, however, their value for older adults is heuristic.

POINTS OF ACCESS: WHERE TO FIND SENIORS AT RISK

This article next consider where preventive interventions can be most effectively implemented: what settings provide the greatest access to older adults, both those at high risk and those amenable to interventions designed to prevent development of risk states? Fig. 4 illustrates the primary targets. Given the strong link between suicide and psychiatric illness, mental health providers and clinics would be a logical starting point. However, older adults rarely use these services. Instead, they are far more likely to visit a primary care provider, including during periods of high risk. Studies have repeatedly found that two thirds or more of older adults who killed themselves had been in a primary care provider's office in the past 30 days of life and up to a half within 1 week of their suicide, many with symptomatic affective disorders [19,59]. Given that a large proportion of the population at risk is seen in these settings, primary care is the most obvious venue for which to develop and implement preventive interventions.

Any health care delivery setting in which older adults who have chronic physical illness and functional decline receive services may offer important opportunities for preventive interventions, including community-based long-term care. Bruce and colleagues [60], for example, found high rates of major affective disorder among older adults who used visiting nurse services. Reported rates of suicide in nursing homes are not as high as one might expect given the prevalence of psychiatric illness among their residents [61,62], a finding that might be explained by underreporting and the level of supervision and restricted access

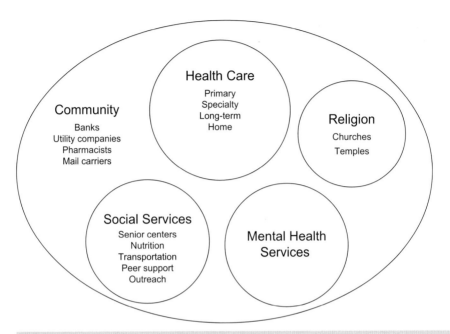

Fig. 4. Points of access to older adults at risk for suicide.

to lethal means characteristic of residential long-term care. At the same time, rates of indirect self-destructive behaviors (acts that cause self harm leading indirectly over time to one's death) are high [61].

The observation that life stressors and social isolation contribute independently to risk for suicide in later life, whereas social support may help protect against the emergence of suicidal states, indicates other potential venues for preventive interventions. The aging services network consists of a well-organized infrastructure of 655 Area Agencies on Aging connected and partially funded through an amendment to the Older Americans Act of 1973. Together they constitute an extensive, federally mandated and funded social service system designed to address the needs of older people experiencing social stressors that are associated with increased suicide risk. Faith communities may offer important opportunities to access older people at risk, as may other community "gatekeepers," or service providers who are likely to interact with senior citizens and, therefore, with training may identify those in distress and refer them for evaluation and care [63].

APPROACHES TO PREVENTION

With knowledge of the epidemiology of suicide in older adults and the settings best suited for case finding, the next step in the prevention research cycle involves the design and testing of preventive interventions. These may be characterized as addressing suicide at one or more of three levels: indicated, selective, and universal [64]. Table 3 provides a definition and general example for each, and Table 4 lists published studies in which the impact of an intervention on suicidal ideation or completed suicide in older adults was the specific outcome of interest. The authors are not aware of any studies with attempted suicide as the targeted outcome.

Two studies represent indicated preventive interventions. Both targeted older adults in primary care practices who had symptomatic affective illness, and were based on the collaborative, stepped-care model in which expertise in the diagnosis and treatment of affective illness is incorporated into the practice. The Prevention of Suicide In Primary Care Elderly: Collaborative Trial (PROSPECT study) compared usual care by the primary care providers with algorithm-driven antidepressant treatment; interpersonal psychotherapy when indicated; physician, patient, and family education about the illness; and care management by a depression specialist (social worker, nurse, or psychologist) [65]. In a sample of 598 subjects older than 60 years who had depression, Bruce and colleagues [65] found that rates of suicidal ideation declined significantly faster in the intervention than comparison condition.

Unützer and colleagues [66] took a similar approach with the Improving Mood: Promoting Access to Collaborative Treatment (IMPACT) study. They compared a collaborative depression care management intervention with usual care of 1801 patients aged 60 years or older who had major depression, dysthymic disorder, or both. As in PROSPECT, the IMPACT intervention included a depression care manager collaborating with a psychiatrist and primary care provider to offer patient and family education, facilitation of antidepressant treatment, and the option of brief problem-solving psychotherapy. In addition to significantly greater improvements in depressive symptoms, intervention subjects had significantly lower rates of suicidal ideation than controls for up to 24 months [67].

Unfortunately, neither trial could assess the effectiveness of the intervention on suicidal behavior. Furthermore, given that approximately 70% of subjects in each trial were women and therefore at far lower risk for completed suicide than men, the impact that collaborative care models may have on late-life suicide at the population level remains to be established. Nonetheless, the most appropriate clinical position is certainly that screening for depressive illness in older adults should be routine and its diagnosis and treatment assertively pursued. When suicidal ideation is detected, aggressive indicated interventions should be initiated.

Examples of selective and universal preventive interventions applied to late-life suicide are also rare. The Telehelp/Telecheck service evaluated by DeLeo and colleagues [68] represents a selective late-life suicide preventive intervention because the targeted population is older adults who are socially isolated and functionally impaired. Telehelp/Telecheck, based in Padua, Italy, provided telephone-based outreach, evaluation, and support services to more than 18,600 seniors with a mean age of 80 years; 84% were women. Over 11 years of service delivery, significantly fewer suicides occurred among clients than

Table 3
Levels of preventive intervention

Intervention	Target population	Prevention objectives	Examples
Indicated	Individuals who have detectable symptoms or other proximal risk factors for suicide	Treat individuals who have precursor signs and symptoms to prevent development of disorder or the expression of suicidal behavior	Increase screening/treatment in primary care settings for elders who have depression, anxiety, and substance misuse Improve providers' assessment and restriction of access to lethal means
Selective	Asymptomatic or presymptomatic individuals or subgroups who have distal risk factors for suicide, or who have a higher-than-average risk for developing mental disorders or other more proximal risk factors	Prevent suicide-related morbidity and mortality through addressing specific characteristics that place elders at risk	Promote church-based and community programs to contact and support isolated elders for those experiencing social isolation Focus medical and social services on reducing disability and enhancing independent functioning; increase access to home care and rehabilitation service; and improve access to pain management and palliative care services; treat elders with chronic pain syndromes more effectively for those who are medically ill, functionally impaired Provide gatekeeper training Link outreach and gatekeeper services to comprehensive evaluation and health management services in a continuum of care
Universal	Entire population, not identified based on individual risk	Implement broadly directed initiatives to prevent suicide-related morbidity and mortality through reducing risk and enhancing protective factors	Implement strategies to provide more accessible, acceptable, and affordable mental health care to elders Education of the general public, clergy, the media, and health care providers concerning normal aging, ageism and stigma regarding mental illness, and depression and suicidal behaviors Restrict access to lethal means

Table developed in collaboration with Kerry Knox, PhD, and Eric D. Caine, MD.

Table 4
Studies of elderly suicide prevention programs

Study	Intervention type	Target population	Intervention	Age (y)	Sample size	Outcomes
Bruce et al.[a] [65]	Indicated	Depressed elderly patients from primary care practices	Interpersonal psychotherapy and/or citalopram monitored by depression care manager who collaborated with primary care provider	60–94	N = 598 Intervention: n = 320 Usual care: n = 278	Rates of suicidal ideation declined faster in intervention patients than in usual care patients
Unützer et al.[a] [67]	Indicated	Depressed elderly patients from primary care practices	1-year treatment group: depression care manager provided who assessed depression, collaborated with primary care provider on antidepressant medication management, offered 12-month course of Problem Solving Treatment	≥60	N = 1801 Intervention: n = 906 Usual care: n = 895	Significantly lower rates of suicidal and death ideation compared with usual care group at 6, 12, 18, and 24 months
Deleo et al.[b] [68]	Selective	Elderly users of telephone helpline and emergency response service	Telehelp: 24-hour emergency alarm service. Telecheck: twice-weekly support and needs assessment telephone calls	≥65	N = 18,641	Observed completed suicide rate significantly lower for clients than expected. Significantly fewer observed suicides in women than expected. No difference between observed and expected suicide rates in men

Oyama et al.[b] [72]	Multi-level	All elderly in rural area	Community-based suicide prevention program: 7-year depression screening with follow-up by primary care providers 10-year implementation of public education on depression and suicide in elderly	≥65	N = 998 to 1260/year	64% suicide risk reduction of completed suicides among women in intervention compared with baseline No significant change in risk reduction for men
Oyama et al.[b] [74]	Multi-level	All elderly in rural area	10-year community-based suicide prevention program: mental health workshops for elderly Depression screening with follow-up by primary care providers Public education on depression and suicide in elderly	≥65	N = 12,782	70% risk reduction in completed suicides among women in intervention compared with baseline No significant change in risk for men
Oyama et al.[b] [75]	Multi-level	All elderly in rural area	Community-based suicide prevention program: depression screening with follow-up by primary care providers Group activities with public health nurses: social, voluntary, leisure, exercise	≥65	N = 403–463	74% risk reduction in completed suicides among women in intervention compared with baseline No significant change in risk for men

(continued on next page)

Table 4
(continued)

Study	Intervention type	Target population	Age (y)	Intervention	Sample size	Outcomes
Oyama et al.[b] [73]	Universal + selective	All elderly in rural area	≥65	8-year community-based suicide prevention program: mental health workshops for elderly Group activities to increase relationships Psychoeducation and self-assessment of depression	N = 1407–1739	76% risk reduction in completed suicides among women in intervention compared with baseline No significant change in risk for men
Oyama et al.[b] [71]	Multi-level	All elderly in rural area	≥65	10-year community-based suicide prevention program: depression screening with follow-up in mental health care or psychiatric treatment Psychoeducation on depression	N = 1121–1505	76% risk reduction in completed suicides among women in intervention compared with baseline Psychoeducation on depression

[a] Randomized controlled trials.
[b] Well-designed controlled and uncontrolled studies.

would have been expected in the elder population of that region. In subsequent analyses, however, no specific effect of the intervention on suicide in men could be shown; the intervention seemed to be effective in reducing suicide only in elderly women.

Experience in the United Kingdom indicates that means restriction may be an effective universal approach to preventing suicide. Hawton and colleagues [69] reported that after legislation limited the pack size of paracetamol and salicylates sold over the counter, morbidity and mortality from overdose with these medications decreased significantly.

One study was found that suggests a specific effect of means restriction on suicide among older adults. Ludwig and Cooke [70] examined whether implementation of the Brady Handgun Violence Prevention Act in the United States in 1994 was associated with changes in total and firearm-specific homicide and suicide rates in the general adult (≥ 21 years) and later late (≥ 55 years) populations. The Brady Act required that licensed firearm dealers observe a waiting period and initiate a background check before selling a handgun. States that already had this legislation established constituted the control group, whereas states newly instituting the legislation served as the experimental condition. Changes in rates of homicide and suicide in experimental and control states were not significantly different, except for firearm suicides among persons aged 55 years or older, which showed a significant reduction in the intervention states. Consistent with Miller's [49] observation that older male suicides were more likely than controls to have purchased the gun used to kill themselves in the week preceding death, the observed effect of the Brady legislation was much stronger in states that had instituted waiting periods and background checks than in states that only changed background check requirements. In the United States, where older men are at far higher risk than other groups and more than 75% die of self-inflicted gunshot wounds, these findings are particularly notable. Because of the complex social and political implications of gun control legislation, however, this promising approach to late-life suicide prevention will be difficult to test.

A basic tenet of prevention science is that interventions that combine approaches are more likely to have an effect at the population level than any single preventive intervention. Oyama and colleagues [71–75] recently reported results of a series of five studies that test, in a quasi-experimental design, combinations of universal, selective, and indicated preventive interventions referred to in Table 4 as a multilayered approach. Subjects included all residents aged 65 years and older who lived in small towns in rural Japan. Implemented over 5- to 10-year periods, these complex interventions typically included public education and socialization programs for seniors held in community centers; either a self-assessment or structured screening for depression; and follow-up referral with primary care or mental health care providers for those who screened positive. The investigators measured changes in the relative risk for suicide in older adults before and after the program's implementation and relative to a neighboring reference town of similar size and character. In all five of these separate studies, a significant reduction (64%–76%) was seen in the risk for suicide in elderly women. However, only one of the five towns showed a significant risk reduction for men [71].

SUMMARY

Suicide is a major public health concern for older adults, who have higher rates of completed suicide than any other age group in most countries of the world. Older men are at greatest risk. Reduction of suicide-related morbidity and mortality in this age group hinges on systematic and methodological study at each point in the suicide preventive intervention research cycle. Improvements in systems for surveillance of late-life suicidal behavior, particularly attempted suicide, are needed to further develop the foundation on which to evaluate differences in the elderly subgroup, over time, and in different locations, and to better assess changes in response to interventions.

PA studies of completed suicide in later life are limited by their retrospective approach, reliance on proxy informants, and typically small sample sizes. Nonetheless, recent efforts that have included standardized measures and matched comparison samples have greatly increased understanding of the factors that contribute to, and to a lesser extent serve as a buffer against, suicide risk in later life. Psychiatric illness, and particularly late-life affective disorder, is the most potent of these factors. A past history of attempts is less common than among younger adults, but vitally important for clinicians to be aware of in their patients. Comorbid general medical conditions, often including pain and role function decline, also seem to contribute as independent risk factors and because of their close association with depression in older adults. Social dependency or isolation and family discord and bereavement should also be included as a component of routine risk assessment. Neuroticism and low OTE, along with a rigid coping style, may predispose to the emergence of suicidal states under certain stressful circumstances.

The U.S. Preventive Services Task Force does not recommend routine screening for suicidal ideation in primary care [76]. However, routine screening for depression using one of the readily available and easily applied screening tools is appropriate for older adults [7,77,78]. When depression is suspected, or when words or actions by the older person may suggest thoughts of suicide (eg, withdrawal, nihilistic, morbid comments), further inquiry about suicidal thoughts and intent pursued in a nonjudgmental and supportive manner is necessary. When suicide risk is appreciable, aggressive intervention should be performed, including any measures necessary to maintain safety until the crisis passes. As in other age groups, reduction of intolerable pain will help resolve thoughts of suicide.

Ultimately, however, the most effective approach to reducing suicide deaths among older people requires development of strategies that prevent onset of the suicidal state. Preliminary data suggest that selective preventive interventions targeting groups of older adults at risk for suicide because of their social isolation, recent losses, pain, or functional impairment may be effective for older women. Universal prevention through education programs to reduce stigma associated with seeking help, improve access to quality health care, and remove access to immediately lethal means may also be useful approaches. Although the most effective strategy is likely one that combines indicated, selective, and universal strategies, older men—the group at highest risk in this country—remain resistant to any intervention tested. A more refined understanding of gender differences in late-life suicide is needed to inform subsequent steps in the development of preventive interventions.

References

[1] Wells KB, Miranda J, Bauer MS, et al. Overcoming barriers to reducing the burden of affective disorders. Biol Psychiatry 2002;52(6):655–75.

[2] Heithoff K. Does the ECA underestimate the prevalence of late-life depression? J Am Geriatr Soc 1995;43(1):2–6.

[3] Duberstein PR, Conwell Y, Seidlitz L, et al. Age and suicidal ideation in older depressed inpatients. Am J Geriatr Psychiatry 1999;7(4):289–96.

[4] Gallo JJ, Anthony JC, Muthen BO. Age differences in the symptoms of depression: a latent trait analysis. J Gerontol 1994;49(6):251–64.

[5] Callahan CM, Nienaber NA, Hendrie HC, et al. Depression of elderly outpatients: primary care physicians' attitudes and practice patterns. J Gen Intern Med 1992;7(1): 26–31.

[6] Nutting PA, Rost K, Smith J, et al. Competing demands from physical problems: effect on initiating and completing depression care over 6 months. Arch Fam Med 2000;9(10): 1059–64.

[7] U.S. Preventive Services Task Force. Screening for depression: recommendations and rationale. Ann Intern Med 2002;136(10):760–4.

[8] Crosby AE, Cheltenham MP, Sacks JJ. Incidence of suicidal ideation and behavior in the United States, 1994. Suicide Life Threat Behav 1999;29(2):131–40.

[9] Fremouw WJ, dePerczel M, Ellis TE. Suicide risk: assessment and response guidelines. New York: Pergamon Press; 1990.

[10] McIntosh JL, Santos JF, Hubbard RW, et al. Elder suicide: research, theory, and treatment. Washington, DC: American Psychological Association; 1994.

[11] Conwell Y, Duberstein PR, Cox C, et al. Age differences in behaviors leading to completed suicide. Am J Geriatr Psychiatry 1998;6(2):122–6.

[12] Centers for Disease Control and Prevention. Web-based injury statistics query and reporting system. Available at: http://www.cdc.gov/ncipc/WISQARS/. Accessed October 15, 2007.

[13] World Health Organization - Mental Health. Suicide prevention (SUPRE). Available at: http://www.who.int/mental_health/prevention/suicide/suicideprevent/en/WorldHealth Organization. Accessed October 16, 2007.

[14] Gibbons RD, Hur K, Bhaumik DK, et al. The relationship between antidepressant medication use and rate of suicide. Arch Gen Psychiatry 2005;62(2):165–72.

[15] Erlangsen A, Canudas-Romo V, Conwell Y. Increased use of antidepressants and decreasing suicide rates: a population-based study using Danish register data. J Epi Commun Health, in press.

[16] Moscicki EK. Identification of suicide risk factors using epidemiologic studies. Psychiatr Clin North Am 1997;3:499–517.

[17] Beck AT, Brown GK, Steer RA, et al. Suicide ideation at its worst point: a predictor of eventual suicide in psychiatric outpatients. Suicide Life Threat Behav 1999;29(1):1–9.

[18] Beautrais AL. Suicides and serious suicide attempts: two populations or one? Psychol Med 2001;31(5):837–45.

[19] Conwell Y, Lyness JM, Duberstein P, et al. Completed suicide among older patients in primary care practices: a controlled study. J Am Geriatr Soc 2000;48(1):23–9.

[20] Conwell Y, Rotenberg M, Caine ED. Completed suicide at age 50 and over. J Am Geriatr Soc 1990;38(6):640–4.

[21] Hawton K, Appleby L, Platt S, et al. The psychological autopsy approach to studying suicide: a review of methodological issues. J Affect Disord 1998;50(2–3):269–76.

[22] Barraclough BM. Suicide in the elderly: recent developments in psychogeriatrics. British Journal of Psychiatry 1971;Spec. Suppl.#6:87–97.

[23] Carney SS, Rich CL, Burke PA, et al. Suicide over 60: the San Diego study. J Am Geriatr Soc 1994;42(2):174–80.

[24] Clark DC. Suicide among the elderly. Final report to the AARP Andrus Foundation 1991.

[25] Conwell Y, Duberstein PR, Cox C, et al. Relationships of age and axis I diagnoses in victims of completed suicide: a psychological autopsy study. Am J Psychiatry 1996;153(8):1001–8.

[26] Henriksson MM, Marttunen MJ, Isometsa ET, et al. Mental disorders in elderly suicide. Int Psychogeriatr 1995;7(2):275–86.

[27] Chiu HF, Yip PS, Chi I, et al. Elderly suicide in Hong Kong—a case-controlled psychological autopsy study. Acta Psychiatr Scand 2004;109(4):299–305.

[28] Waern M, Runeson B, Allebeck P, et al. Mental disorder in elderly suicides. Am J Psychiatry 2002;159(3):450–5.

[29] Duberstein PR, Conwell Y, Conner KR, et al. Suicide at 50 years of age and older: perceived physical illness, family discord and financial strain. Psychol Med 2004;34(1):137–46.

[30] Duberstein PR, Conwell Y, Conner KR, et al. Poor social integration and suicide: fact or artifact? A case-control study. Psychol Med 2004;34(7):1331–7.

[31] Beautrais AL. A case control study of suicide and attempted suicide in older adults. Suicide Life Threat Behav 2002;32(1):1–9.

[32] Harwood D, Hawton K, Hope T, et al. Psychiatric disorder and personality factors associated with suicide in older people: a descriptive and case-control study. Int J Geriatr Psychiatry 2001;16(2):155–65.

[33] Rubenowitz E, Waern M, Wilhelmsson K, et al. Life events and psychosocial factors in elderly suicides—a case control study. Psychol Med 2001;31:1193–202.

[34] First MB, Spitzer RL, Gibbon M, et al. Structured clinical interview for DSM-IV-TR axis I disorders - patient edition. New York: Biometrics Research Department, New York State Psychiatric Institute; 2001.

[35] Batchelor IRC, Napier MB. Attempted suicide in old age. Br Med J 1953;2:1186–90.

[36] Clark DC. Narcissistic crises of aging and suicidal despair. Suicide Life Threat Behav 1993;23(1):21–6.

[37] Duberstein PR. Openness to experience and completed suicide across the second half of life. Int Psychogeriatr 1995;7(2):183–98.

[38] Costa PT, McCrae RR. Revised NEO personality inventory and NEO five factor inventory: professional manual. Odessa (FL): PAR; 1992.

[39] Duberstein PR. Are closed-minded people more open to the idea of killing themselves? Suicide Life Threat Behav 2001;31(1):9–14.

[40] Beck AT, Steer RA, Beck JS, et al. Hopelessness, depression, suicidal ideation, and clinical diagnosis of depression. Suicide Life Threat Behav 1993;23(2):139–45.

[41] Beck AT, Steer RA, Kovacs M, et al. Hopelessness and eventual suicide: a 10-year prospective study of patients hospitalized with suicidal ideation. Am J Psychiatry 1985;142(5):559–63.

[42] Hill RD, Gallagher D, Thompson LW, et al. Hopelessness as a measure of suicide intent in the depressed elderly. Psychol Aging 1988;3:230–2.

[43] Ross RK, Bernstein L, Trent L, et al. A prospective study of risk factors for traumatic death in the retirement community. Prev Med 1990;19:323–34.

[44] Szanto K, Reynolds CF III, Conwell Y, et al. High levels of hopelessness persist in geriatric patients with remitted depression and a history of attempted suicide. J Am Geriatr Soc 1998;46(11):1401–6.

[45] Harris EC, Barraclough B. Suicide as an outcome for mental disorders. A meta-analysis. Br J Psychiatry 1997;170:205–28.

[46] Juurlink DN, Herrmann N, Szalai JP, et al. Medical illness and the risk of suicide in the elderly. Arch Intern Med 2004;164(11):1179–84.

[47] Quan H, Arboleda-Florez J, Fick GH, et al. Association between physical illness and suicide among the elderly. Soc Psychiatry Psychiatr Epidemiol 2002;37(4):190–7.

[48] Turvey CL, Conwell Y, Jones MP, et al. Risk factors for late-life suicide: a prospective, community-based study. Am J Geriatr Psychiatry 2002;10(4):398–406.

[49] Miller M. Geriatric suicide: the Arizona study. Gerontologist 1978;18:488–95.

[50] Tsoh J, Chiu HF, Duberstein PR, et al. Attempted suicide in elderly Chinese persons: a multi-group, controlled study. Am J Geriatr Psychiatry 2005;13(7):562–71.

[51] Conwell Y, Duberstein PR, Connor K, et al. Access to firearms and risk for suicide in middle-aged and older adults. Am J Geriatr Psychiatry 2002;10(4):407–16.

[52] Mann JJ, Waternaux C, Haas GL, et al. Toward a clinical model of suicidal behavior in psychiatric patients. Am J Psychiatry 1999;156(2):181–9.

[53] Mann JJ. Neurobiology of suicidal behaviour. Nat Rev Neurosci 2003;4(10):819–28.

[54] Alexopoulos GS, Meyers BS, Young RC, et al. 'Vascular depression' hypothesis. Arch Gen Psychiatry 1997;54(10):915–22.

[55] Alexopoulos GS, Kiosses DN, Klimstra S, et al. Clinical presentation of the "depression-executive dysfunction syndrome" of late life. Am J Geriatr Psychiatry 2002;10(1):98–106.

[56] Keilp JG, Sackeim HA, Brodsky BS, et al. Neuropsychological dysfunction in depressed suicide attempters. Am J Psychiatry 2001;158(5):735–41.

[57] King DA, Conwell Y, Cox C, et al. A neuropsychological comparison of depressed suicide attempters and nonattempters. J Neuropsychiatry Clin Neurosci 2000;12(1):64–70.

[58] Ahearn EP, Jamison KR, Steffens DC, et al. MRI correlates of suicide attempt history in unipolar depression. Biol Psychiatry 2001;50:266–70.

[59] Luoma JB, Martin CE, Pearson JL. Contact with mental health and primary care providers before suicide: a review of the evidence. Am J Psychiatry 2002;159(6):909–16.

[60] Bruce ML, McAvay GJ, Raue PJ, et al. Major depression in elderly home health care patients. Am J Psychiatry 2002;159(8):1367–74.

[61] Osgood NJ, Brant BA. Suicidal behavior in long-term care facilities. Suicide Life Threat Behav 1990;20(2):113–22.

[62] Abrams RC, Young RC, Holt JH, et al. Suicide in New York City nursing homes: 1980–1986. Am J Psychiatry 1988;145(11):1487–8.

[63] Florio ER, Rockwood TH, Hendryx MS, et al. A model gatekeeper program to find the at-risk elderly. J Case Manag 1996;5:106–14.

[64] Institute of Medicine. Reducing risks for mental disorders: frontiers for preventive intervention research. Washington, DC: National Academy Press; 1994.

[65] Bruce ML, Ten Have T, Reynolds CF III, et al. Reducing suicidal ideation and depressive symptoms in depressed older primary care patients: a randomized controlled trial. JAMA 2004;291(9):1081–91.

[66] Unützer J, Katon W, Callahan CM, et al. IMPACT Investigators. Improving Mood-Promoting Access to Collaborative Treatment. Collaborative care management of late-life depression in the primary care setting: a randomized controlled trial. JAMA 2002;288(22):2836–45.

[67] Unützer J, Tang L, Oishi S, et al, for the IMPACT Investigators. Reducing suicidal ideation in depressed older primary care patients. J Am Geriatr Soc 2006;54(10):1550–6.

[68] DeLeo D, Dello BM, Dwyer J. Suicide among the elderly: the long-term impact of a telephone support and assessment intervention in northern Italy. Br J Psychiatry 2002;181:226–9.

[69] Hawton K, Townsend E, Deeks J, et al. Effects of legislation restricting pack sizes of paracetamol and salicylate on self poisoning in the United Kingdom: before and after study. BMJ 2001;322(7296):1203–7.

[70] Ludwig J, Cook PJ. Homicide and suicide rates associated with implementation of the Brady Handgun Violence Prevention Act. JAMA 2000;284(5):585–91.

[71] Oyama H, Koida J, Sakashita T, et al. Community-based prevention for suicide in elderly by depression screening and follow-up. Community Ment Health J 2004;40(3):249–63.

[72] Oyama H, Ono Y, Watanabe N, et al. Local community intervention through depression screening and group activity for elderly suicide prevention. Psychiatry Clin Neurosci 2006;60(1):110–4.

[73] Oyama H, Watanabe N, Ono Y, et al. Community-based suicide prevention through group activity for the elderly successfully reduced the high suicide rate for females. Psychiatry Clin Neurosci 2005;59(3):337–44.

[74] Oyama H, Fujita M, Goto M, et al. Outcomes of community-based screening for depression and suicide prevention among Japanese elders. Gerontologist 2006;46(6):821–6.

[75] Oyama H, Goto M, Fujita M, et al. Preventing elderly suicide through primary care by community-based screening for depression in rural Japan. Crisis 2006;27(2):58–65.

[76] U.S. Preventive Services Task Force. Screening for suicide risk: recommendation and rationale. Ann Intern Med 2004;140(10):820–1.

[77] Yesavage JA. Geriatric depression scale. Psychopharmacol Bull 1988;24(4):709–11.

[78] Kroenke K, Spitzer RL, Williams JB. The PHQ-9: validity of a brief depression severity measure. J Gen Intern Med 2001;16(9):606–13.

Psychiatr Clin N Am 31 (2008) 357–362

PSYCHIATRIC CLINICS
OF NORTH AMERICA

ELSEVIER
SAUNDERS

INDEX

0193-953X/08/$ – see front matter
doi:10.1016/S0193-953X(08)00049-X